Cancer Treatment and Research

Volume 186

Series Editor

Steven T. Rosen, Duarte, CA, USA

This book series provides detailed updates on the state of the art in the treatment of different forms of cancer and also covers a wide spectrum of topics of current research interest. Clinicians will benefit from expert analysis of both standard treatment options and the latest therapeutic innovations and from provision of clear guidance on the management of clinical challenges in daily practice. The research-oriented volumes focus on aspects ranging from advances in basic science through to new treatment tools and evaluation of treatment safety and efficacy. Each volume is edited and authored by leading authorities in the topic under consideration. In providing cutting-edge information on cancer treatment and research, the series will appeal to a wide and interdisciplinary readership. The series is listed in PubMed/Index Medicus.

Timothy A. Yap · Geoffrey I. Shapiro
Editors

Targeting the DNA Damage Response for Cancer Therapy

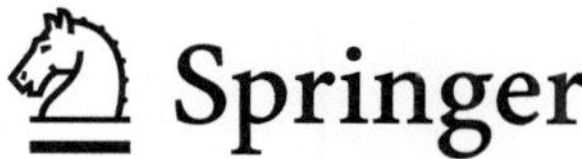 Springer

Editors
Timothy A. Yap
The University of Texas MD Anderson
Cancer Center
Houston, TX, USA

Geoffrey I. Shapiro
Dana-Farber Cancer Institute
Boston, MA, USA

ISSN 0927-3042 ISSN 2509-8497 (electronic)
Cancer Treatment and Research
ISBN 978-3-031-30067-7 ISBN 978-3-031-30065-3 (eBook)
https://doi.org/10.1007/978-3-031-30065-3

This Springer imprint is published by the registered company Springer Nature Switzerland AG
The registered company address is: Gewerbestrasse 11, 6330 Cham, Switzerland

Preface

Malignant transformation is associated with genomic instability in part related to underlying defects in DNA repair. While such defects may promote the evolution of oncogenesis, they may also be exploited for therapeutic benefit through the identification of targetable synthetic lethal interactions. The clinical benefit afforded by inhibitors of poly(ADP-ribose) polymerase (PARP) enzymes in *BRCA1/2* and other homologous recombination repair (HRR)-defective tumor cells has served as proof-of-principle for the concept of synthetic lethality. Seminal preclinical findings were first described in 2005, leading to an established role for PARP inhibitors in the armamentarium for HRR-deficient ovarian, breast, prostate, and pancreatic cancers. Additionally, while foundational science has led to important clinical progress, the availability of PARP inhibitor pharmacological agents has enabled an improved basic understanding of HRR and of other DNA repair and DNA damage response pathways. These advances have been made through the study of the mechanisms by which PARP inhibitors induce cytotoxicity, as well as by elucidation of mechanisms of intrinsic and acquired resistance. This work has also facilitated the identification of combinatorial strategies that may ultimately enhance response or overcome resistance.

In this volume, we have assembled chapters authored by leaders in the field that review accomplishments achieved over the past two decades of basic discovery and clinical work, and that point to new strategies poised to translate to benefit for patients with cancers harboring DNA repair deficiencies. These chapters focus on multiple pressing issues for the field beginning with the evolution of PARP inhibitor drug development, the biology of synthetic lethality, our current understanding of mechanisms of PARP inhibitor resistance, and the development of predictive biomarkers for response to these agents (Chaps. 1–4). Thereafter, individual chapters review up-to-date evidence supporting the use of PARP inhibitors in appropriate subsets of patients with ovarian, breast, prostate, and pancreatic cancers (Chaps. 5–8). Subsequently, the complex state of the field of combinatorial strategy development is addressed, including combinations of PARP inhibitors with chemotherapy, HRR targeting agents, other agents targeting the DNA damage response, as well as with immunotherapy. These sections, Chaps. 9–12, cover mechanisms of synergism, supporting preclinical data, as well as available clinical results, including both efficacy and toxicity considerations. Finally, reviews are presented in Chaps. 13–17 that cover other targets beyond PARP enzymes for which preclinical and clinical data are now accumulating, including the oxidative DNA repair protein human MutT homolog 1 (MTH1), ataxia telangiectasia and Rad3-related (ATR), polymerase theta (POLθ), DNA-PK, and the Werner syndrome ATP-dependent helicase (WRN).

The field of DNA repair and DNA damage response pathway targeting with pharmacological agents is rapidly moving forward. Additionally, there is growing recognition of larger numbers of patients who may ultimately benefit from these agents. These include individuals with pathogenic germline variants in DNA repair genes whose tumors may harbor functional DNA repair deficiencies based on inherited predisposition, who may be identified as germline testing becomes more widespread. Similarly, many somatic alterations that could also lead to functional DNA repair deficiency have yet to be characterized. Consequently, we present in this volume an authoritative state-of-the-art review of the field, with the goal of providing a foundation for a wide audience, as basic, translational, and clinical science continue to evolve.

Houston, USA   Timothy A. Yap
Boston, USA   Geoffrey I. Shapiro

Contents

About the Editors

Dr. Timothy A. Yap is a Medical Oncology Physician-Scientist and tenured Professor based at the University of Texas MD Anderson Cancer Center. He is a Professor in the Department for Investigational Cancer Therapeutics (Phase I Program), and the Department of Thoracic/Head and Neck Medical Oncology.

Dr. Yap is Vice President and Head of Clinical Development in the Therapeutics Discovery Division, a drug discovery biopharmaceutical division where drug discovery and clinical translation are seamlessly integrated.

He is also the Associate Director of Translational Research in the Institute for Personalized Cancer Therapy, which is an integrated research and clinical trials program aimed at implementing personalized cancer therapy and improving patient outcomes.

Dr. Yap's main research focuses on the first-in-human and combinatorial development of molecularly targeted agents and immunotherapies, and their acceleration through clinical studies using novel predictive and pharmacodynamic biomarkers. His main interests include the targeting of the DNA damage response (DDR) with novel therapeutics through clinical trials and translational studies. These including targets such as ATR, PARP1, WEE1, POLQ, USP1, PARG, CHK1, ATM and DNA-PK inhibitors, next generation CDK4 and CDK2-selective inhibitors, WRN inhibitors, SMARCA2 inhibitors, YAP/TEAD inhibitors, as well as the development of novel immunotherapeutics.

Prior to his current position, Dr. Yap was a Consultant Medical Oncologist at The Royal Marsden Hospital in London, UK and National Institute for Health Research BRC Clinician Scientist at The Institute of Cancer Research, London, UK.

Dr. Geoffrey I. Shapiro currently serves as Senior Vice President, Developmental Therapeutics, at the Dana-Farber Cancer Institute (DFCI). In this role, he co-leads the Developmental Therapeutics Program for the Dana-Farber/Harvard Cancer Center (DF/HCC) as well as the Cancer Center's activities in the NCI-Cancer Therapy Evaluation Program (NCI-CTEP) Experimental Therapeutics Clinical Trials Network (ETCTN). He additionally serves as the Clinical Director for the DFCI Center for DNA Damage and Repair, where he has developed multiple predictive and pharmacodynamic biomarkers for DNA repair inhibitor agents, including those targeting PARP, the ATR-CHK1-WEE1 axis, and polymerase theta. Dr. Shapiro practices within the DFCI Center for Cancer Therapeutic Innovation, where he develops and leads multiple early phase trials focused primarily on cell cycle and DNA repair inhibitor therapeutics and provides mentorship to early career investigators. He has made proof-of-mechanism studies a mission of his program and has worked closely with basic and translational scientists at his institution and elsewhere to establish robust preclinical rationale for many trials. He also leads a complimentary laboratory effort where he studies resistance to these agents and their interaction with the immune microenvironment to inform the development of rational combinations.

Evolution of the Development of PARP Inhibitors

Ruth Plummer

1.1 Introduction

The poly (ADP-ribose)polymerases (PARPs), a family of highly conserved enzymes found in plants and animals, were first described nearly 60 years ago [1]. This family of enzymes has multiple roles within the cell, being involved in the maintenance of genomic stability, regulation of DNA repair, telomer replication and cellular transport [2, 3], and longevity [4]. However, it is now known that there are at least 22 ADP-ribosylating enzymes with a variety of cellular functions, with some now known to be mono-ribosylating, hence the family now being known generically as ADPRTs ((ADP-ribosyl)-transferases) rather than PARPs [5]. The NAD^+ catalytic binding site is the most highly conserved region of the family of enzymes.

The common action of the poly-ribosylators is to form polymers of ADP-ribose from NAD^+ on acceptor molecules, which include glutamate residues on the PARP enzyme itself—automodification. The common mechanism of action of all PARP enzymes is shown in Fig. 1.1, NAD^+ binds in the catalytic site and is cleaved to release nicotinamide and ADP-ribose. This monomer subunit is then attached to other subunits to form long branched or linear polymers.

PARP-1 is the most abundant form of the enzyme and is highly conserved between species. It is located in the nucleus, acting as a "molecular nick sensor" to signal DNA single strand breaks and assist in their repair [6]. A second nuclear PARP (PARP-2) was discovered in the late 1990s [7].

R. Plummer (✉)
Translational and Clinical Research Institute, Newcastle University, Newcastle Upon Tyne, UK
e-mail: Ruth.plummer@ncl.ac.uk

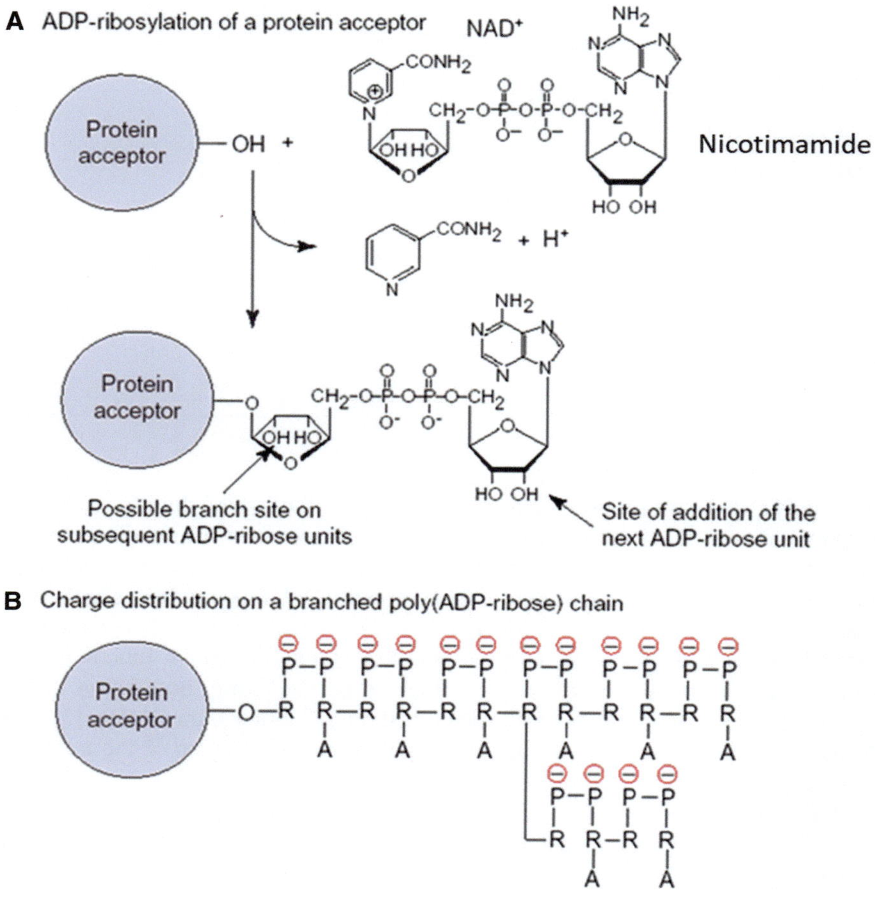

Fig. 1.1 Catalytic mechanism of PARP enzymes. **A)** PARP cleaves NAD+ releasing nicotinamide and covalently attaches linear and branched polymers of ADP-ribose, which may >100 units long, to acceptor proteins. **B)** charge distribution on polymer

It is now known that both PARP-1 and PARP-2, the two nuclear forms of the enzyme, function as part of the DNA Damage Response signalling pathway, protecting the genome. PARP-1 and 2 double knockout is embryologically lethal [8], showing the essential nature of these enzymes. Single knockout animals are viable but have increased sensitivity to DNA-damaging agents with cell lines developed from the animals showing increased genomic instability [9–11].

Although much of the early research into the function of PARP was focussed on the role of activation in inflammation and acute injury it was evidence that loss of PARP, or its inhibition, increased sensitivity to DNA damaging agents which led to the development of PARP inhibitors as potential anti-cancer agents. The first description of inhibition of this reaction, using the nicotinamide analogue and weak PARP inhibitor, 3-amino-benzamide, enhancing the cytotoxicity of a DNA damaging agent was by Durkacz et al. in 1980 [12], and this seminal paper had the visionary conclusion that inhibition of PARP might be a way to overcome resistance to chemotherapy and improve cancer treatment outcomes. In the concluding paragraph of this paper the authors suggested that this "potentiation of cell killing by alkylating agents and PARP inhibitors may be of use in the treatment of human leukaemia". This concept of chemo- or indeed radio-potentiation led to the active development of potential clinical compounds.

Chicken PARP-1 protein was purified in 1996 [13] with human PARP-1 being cloned in 2001 [14]. This enabled crystal structures to be developed and rational drug design of the next generation of more potent inhibitors. Hence over the 1990s and early 2000s a number of academic groups and pharma developed series of potent inhibitors, with the majority of the first series of molecules being competitive inhibitors of NAD^+ at the highly conserved substrate binding site, (reviewed in [15, 16]. For this reason, the first generation of PARP inhibitors to be granted drug registration inhibit multiple PARP enzymes [17].

PARP inhibitors therefore first entered the clinic in 2003 in combination with DNA damaging cytotoxic agents, based on the early preclinical data showing both chemo- and radio-potentiation with this class of compounds. At the time there was also considerable ongoing preclinical research and interest in potential clinical indications outside cancer medicine based on the observations of the protective effects of PARP inhibition or the PARP knockout mutation in cerebral ischaemia, endotoxic shock, inflammatory disorders and reperfusion injury (reviewed in [18, 19]. The activation of PARP-1 and its putative role in necrotic cell death has led to the suggestion that PARP inhibitors might prevent such activation and decrease resultant cell death. It has been suggested that such agents could be used as a neuroprotective agent after ischaemic stroke and traumatic brain injury, could be cardioprotective after myocardial infarction, and could be used in the treatment of Alzheimer's disease and endotoxic shock (reviewed in [19]) although these clinical indications have not been actively explored to date. The two modes for cell kill where PARPs play a critical role and hence the potential clinical applications are summarised in Fig. 1.2.

Further research, happening in parallel to the first early cancer medicine clinical trials, identified the potential single agent activity in the context of synthetic lethality which is where the clinical development of the class of compounds has subsequently been most successful and emerging data on a potential role of PARP in signalling through immune activation has led to a third area of clinical interest—combination with immunotherapy.

These first chemo-potentiation studies and the evolution of preclinical science widening the field of potential clinical applications are summarised below, with reference to the other relevant chapters in this manuscript where current clinical applications for this class of agents is covered in more detail.

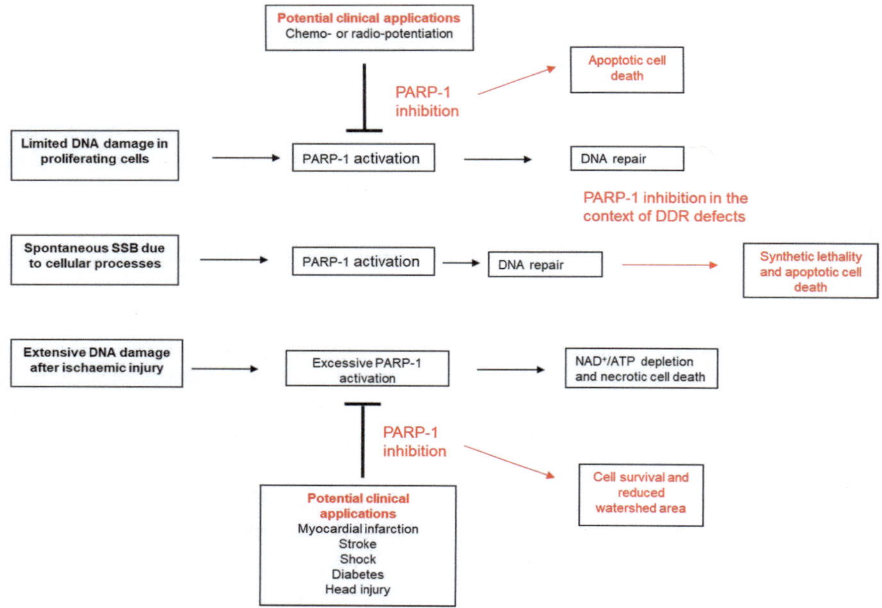

Fig. 1.2 PARP activation in response to DNA damage and potential clinical scenarios when PARP inhibition may be of benefit

1.2 FIH/FIC Trials and PARP Inhibition Biomarker Development—Chemo Potentiation

It was in an attempt to demonstrate the potentiation of the antitumour effect of the monofunctional alkylating agent, temozolomide, that PARP inhibitors first entered clinical trials in cancer patients. At this time, given there was no data to support single agent PARP inhibitor activity and the concept of synthetic lethality between PARP and BRCA defects had not emerged, it was considered ethical to perform a first-in-human combination study. In addition, the investigators were able to demonstrate a clear mechanistic rationale for the potentiation proposed when discussing with regulatory authorities.

Temozolomide methylates DNA at the O^6- and N^7-position of guanine and the N^3-position of adenine. The most cytotoxic of these lesions is O^6-methylguanine, because, unless it is repaired by MGMT prior to replication, it will miss-pair triggering the mismatch repair (MMR) proteins to initiate futile repair cycles, resulting in apoptosis [20]. It is now recognised that MGMT methylation is a predictive biomarker of temozolomide resistance [21]. The N-methylpurines, (~80% of the methylation species), are targets for BER and usually rapidly repaired by PARP-1 and 2 playing no role in cytotoxicity with single agent use of temoxolomide. The hypothesis that blocking the repair of these methylation species with a

PARP inhibitor would lead to chemopotentiation was backed by a range of pre-clinical studies. PD128763 and NU1025 increased temozolomide-induced DNA strand breakage and caused a four to seven-fold potentiation of cytotoxicity [22]. CEP-6800 and GPI 15427 increased temozolomide-induced DNA damage and cytotoxicity or growth inhibition in human glioblastoma cells and enhanced the antitumour activity of temozolomide in mice bearing gliomas, including intracranially implanted tumours [23, 24]. It was this background, together with the lack of evidence at the time of any single agent activity in preclinical models, led to rucaparib entering the clinic in 2003 in a pharmacodynamically driven dose finding study in combination with temozolomide [25].

This potent tricyclic indole PARP inhibitor, (AG014699, PF-01367338), was developed in collaboration between Newcastle University, Cancer Research UK and Agouron Pharmacueticals (part of Pfizer GRD) and subsequently by Clovis Oncology, and was the first-in-class PARP inhibitor to enter clinical development in 2003. The trial was designed to explore combination dosing—however it had a novel phase 0/I design and included a single agent test dose was given in cycle one to allow safety, pharmacokinetic (PK) and pharmacodynamic (PD) evaluation [25]. This study was also one of the first to be driven by a pharmacodynamic end-point, establishing a PARP inhibitory dose of the novel agent, before attempting to evaluate the maximum tolerated dose (MTD) of the combination. PARP inhibition in surrogate normal tissues, peripheral blood lymphocytes (PBLs), was a primary endpoint of the study with a >50% inhibition for 24 hours being the target based on the preclinical efficacy studies. Inhibition of the target enzyme was demonstrated in peripheral blood cells and tumour biopsies and the combination taken into a phase II study in metastatic melanoma. However, this second trial demonstrated enhanced temozolomide-induced myelosuppression when full dose temozolomide was combined with a PARP inhibitory does of AG014699 to a wider population of patients. Following a 25% dose reduction of the temozolomide dose the regi-men was well tolerated and this small phase II study reported an increase in the response rate and median time to progression compared to temozolomide alone [26]. These data have not been further progressed in the clinic following the shift in focus of PARP inhibitor development towards single agent activity and away from chemo-combinations.

This enhanced normal tissue toxicity recapitulated experience with previous DNA damage response modulators, O^6-benzyl guanine and lomaguatrib [27–30] and has been a common theme with all DDR inhibitors when clinical development has tried to safely combine with a DNA damaging agents. Enhanced normal tissue toxicity, especially myelosuppression, is a predictable but common dose-limiting problem.

In an NCI-sponsored combination study of olaparib with cisplatin and gemc-itabine, dose-limiting toxicity of myelosuppression was reported at the first dose level explored. The investigators de-escalated the dose to establish a MTD [31]. Similarly, veliparib in combination with topotecan, was also investigated by the NCI, and dose-limiting myelosuppression was observed at the first dose level and the MTD established with the PARP inhibitory dose was a significantly reduced dose of topotecan at 0.6 mg/m^2 days 1–5 [32].

Enhanced normal tissue toxicity has also been reported with olaparib in combination with dacarbazine [33] cyclophosphamide [34] and paclitaxel [35]. In the case of the latter agent, it may be that inhibition of telomerase (PARP-4) is responsible for this enhanced toxicity as inhibition of SSB repair would not be expected to increase the myelosuppression caused by an antimitotic agent. As discussed above the majority of PARP inhibitors in the clinic target the highly conserved substrate binding site in the enzyme family and will therefore inhibit to differing degrees various enzymes in the ADP-ribosylating family.

First reports of the agent iniparib (BSI-201 (BiPar, Sanofi Aventis) in combination with carboplatin and gemcitabine did not present this toxicity challenge [36, 37]. Clinical trials with this agent explored an intermittent twice weekly schedule and reported no increase in normal tissue toxicity [37, 38]. A randomised phase II study of a total 120 triple negative breast cancer patients where treatment with BSI-201 on the biweekly schedule (days 1, 4, 8, 11) combined with carboplatin (AUC2) and gemcitabine 1000 mg/m^2 days 1 and 8 was compared to treatment with carboplatin and gemcitabine alone showed an increased objective response rate (48 v 16%, p = 0.002), median progression free survival (6.9 v 3.3 months, p < 0.0001) and overall survival (9.6 v 7.5 months, p = 0.0005). However, this striking result was not recapitulated in the phase III confirmatory study [39] and recent studies investigating its mechanism of action suggest that iniparib should not be considered a PARP inhibitor [40, 41].

All these early studies with proven PARP inhibitors demonstrated the same clinical challenge—inhibiting the repair of DNA strand breaks also enhances normal tissue toxicity especially myelosuppression, which is dose limiting with many cytotoxic agents. In addition, the complexities of the iniparib development story may further have reduced enthusiasm for investigators and drug developers pursuing this potential mode of action for the clinical utility of PARP inhibitors and this avenue of clinical utility was largely abandoned for a number of years and the focus of clinical development moved to single agent use. The subsequent progress more recently in chemo-combinations is discussed in more detail in Chap. 9.

1.3 Emergence of Concept of Synthetic Lethality and Change in Development Path

The publication in 2005 of paired papers in Nature from the academic research groups in Sheffield/Newcastle and ICR, London/Cambridge revolutionised the clinical development of PARP inhibitors [42, 43]. These preclinical cell line and xenograft experiments demonstrated that cells which have lost the homologous recombination DSB repair pathway due to BRCA 1 or 2 mutations are hypersensitive to blockade of single strand break repair with a PARP inhibitor. The proposed mechanism of cytotoxicity is that blocking the repair of spontaneously occurring SSB leads to the formation of double strand breaks at the replication fork in dividing cells. In normal or heterozygote cells the DSB repair mechanisms can resolve the lesion and DNA replication and cell division continues. However, in cells where DSB repair is not functional, such as those with a homozygous mutation in BRCA1 or BRCA2, the loss of two DNA repair pathways causes synthetic lethality and cell death [42, 43].

This observation was first tested clinically with Olaparib (KU59436, AZD2281; KuDos/AstraZeneca). This agent was the second drug in the class to enter the clinic in 2005 and the investigators based their phase I trial design on the preclinical results described above. Therefore they did a single agent, continuous dosing phase I escalation study with an expanded cohort of patients with known germ line mutations in BRCA1 or BRCA2 genes. These patients have presumed loss of the second allele by mutation or methylation as a tumour-forming event [44]. This study used an oral formulation of an inhibitor and explored dosing from 10 mg daily for two out of three weeks, increasing to 600 mg twice daily on a continuous dosing schedule to achieve optimal PK and PD parameters. Dose limiting toxicities were myelosuppression and central nervous system side effects. The recommended phase II dose is 400 mg twice daily as continuous dosing, using the original capsule formulation of Olaparib. 9/23 patients developed confirmed partial responses on this phase I study, all of these had confirmed BRCA mutations, and this represented a 39% response rate in this population. Toxicities were similar in the germline BRCA-mutated and normal population. The investigators also demonstrated an increase in γH2AX foci in plucked eyebrow hair follicles 6 hours after olaparib treatment. These foci indicate the accumulation of DNA double strand breaks, indicating a proof of mechanism of the process of *synthetic lethality* where preservation of SSB by PARP inhibition leads to the formation of DNA DSB. It must be noted that this mechanistic proof was demonstrated in normal tissue not in the tumour. These data do raise a concern over the potential dangers of continuous dosing over a long period if there is accumulation of DNA damage within normal tissue, with a theoretical risk of secondary malignancies.

This early sign of single agent activity in genomically selected populations was confirmed by 2 small phase II studies of olaparib in BRCA1 or BRCA2 mutant carriers in breast and ovarian cancer respectively. These studies were also the first to indicate that dose and therefore degree and duration of PARP inhibition may be important when used in the context of synthetic lethality. Both these studies explored response and toxicity in two sequential cohorts of patients treated with 400 mg twice daily and 100 mg twice daily. The activity as a single agent was confirmed in the 400 mg cohorts but there was less activity in the lower dose cohorts suggesting that the degree of PARP inhibition is important for response. In the breast cancer study 27 patients with metastatic disease were treated at each of the doses. The response rate in the 400 mg cohort was 41%, falling to 22% with the lower dose [45]. Toxicities were less on the lower dose cohort but mild overall, with fatigue, nausea and vomiting the commonest toxicities with this generally well tolerated agent. This dose response was confirmed in the ovarian study where 33 patients were treated at 400 mg bd and 24 at 100 mg bd with a 33% confirmed partial response rate at the higher dose and 13% at the lower dose [46]. Further confirmation of this strategy to induce synthetic lethality was also demonstrated in a phase II study with rucaparib [47], although initially in this trial rucaparib was in use as an intravenous preparation limiting the ability to give prolonged coverage, which has been shown to be important in this context both clinically and preclinically [48].

The early demonstration of efficacy, with good tolerability, utilising the concept of synthetic lethality has certainly driven the development of subsequent PARP inhibitors to enter the clinic and also the first registrations of this new class of anti-cancer agents. The clinical development path and current indications are described in more detail in Chaps. 2, 5, 6, 7 and 8.

1.4 Interaction with the Immune System—Widening the Field

The most recent "evolution" in the clinical development of the PARP inhibitors has arisen from the hypothesis that PARP inhibition can cause activation of interferon pathways—causing immune activation similar to that seen after a viral infection. This "signature" was first reported by the group in Belfast exploring signatures observed in breast cancer samples following DNA damage [49] and was proposed by them as a potential clinical scenario to explore. The activation of the cGAS STING pathway using PARP inhibitors has subsequently been confirms by multiple groups [50, 51], and, in addition, it has been shown that PARP inhibition can also increase PDL-1 expression in tumour models [52, 53]. These observations have led to multiple clinical trials combining PARP inhibitors with immune checkpoint inhibitors [54]—and this field is reviewed in detail in Chap. 12.

1.5 Conclusion

PARP inhibitors have been in clinical development in cancer medicine for nearly 20 years, with now four approved agents, olaparib, rucaparib, niraparib, talazoparib, and multiple others in clinical development. The history of their clinical development illustrates the importance of translational research and the bench to bedside approach of cancer drug development. Whilst the class of agents entered the clinic in the early 2000s as chemo-potentiating agents based on the available preclinical data and clinical development paths rapidly adapted to parallel preclinical research. As is illustrated in the following chapters we now have a powerful class of drugs available to patients in our armamentarium to treat cancer and ongoing clinical development is increasing the groups of patients who may benefit from treatment with a PARP inhibitor.

References

1. Chambon P, Weil J, Mandel P (1963) Nicotinamide mononucleotide activation of a new DNA-dependent polyadenylic acid sythesizing nuclear enzyme. Biochem Biophy Res Commun 11:39
2. Burkle A (2001) Physiology and pathophysiology of poly(ADP-ribosyl)ation. BioEssays 29:795–806
3. Chiarugi A (2002) Poly(ADP-ribose) polymerase: killer or conspirator? The "suicide hypothesis" revisited. Trends Pharmacol. Sci 23(3):122–9
4. Burkle A (2000) Poly(ADP-ribosyl)ation: a posttranslational protein modification linked with genome protection and mammalian longevity. Biogerontology 1:41–46
5. Liu C, Yu X (2015) ADP-ribosyltransferases and poly ADP-ribosylation. Curr Protein Pept Sci 16(6):491–501
6. de Murcia G, Menissier de Murcia J (1994) Poly(ADP-ribose) polymerase: a molecular nicksensor. Trends Biochem Sci 9(4):172–6
7. Ame JC, Rolli V, Schreiber V, Niedergang C, Apiou F, Decker P et al (1999) PARP-2, A novel mammalian DNA damage-dependent poly(ADP-ribose) polymerase. J Biol Chem 274(25):17860–17868
8. Menissier de Murcia J, Ricoul M, Tartier L, Niedergang C, Huber A, Dantzer F et al (2003) Functional interaction between PARP-1 and PARP-2 in chromosome stability and embryonic development in mouse. Embo J 22(9):2255–63
9. Wang Z-Q, Auer B, Stingl L, Berghammer H, Haidacher D, Schweiger M et al (1995) Mice lacking ADPRT and poly(ADP-ribosyl)ation develop normally but are susceptible to skin disease. Genes Dev 9:509–520
10. Simbulan-Rosenthal CM, Haddad BR, Rosenthal DS, Weaver Z, Coleman A, Luo R et al (1999) Chromosomal aberrations in PARP(-/-) mice: genome stabilization in immortalized cells by reintroduction of poly(ADP-ribose) polymerase cDNA. Proc Natl Acad Sci U S A 96(23):13191–13196
11. Schreiber V, Ame JC, Dolle P, Schultz I, Rinaldi B, Fraulob V et al (2002) Poly(ADP-ribose) polymerase-2 (PARP-2) is required for efficient base excision DNA repair in association with PARP-1 and XRCC1. J Biol Chem 277(25):23028–23036
12. Durkacz B, Omidiji O, Gray D, Shall S (1980) (ADP-ribose)$_n$ participates in DNA excision repair. Nature 283:593–596
13. Ruf A, de Murcia G, Schulz GE (1998) Inhibitor and NAD+ binding to poly(ADP-ribose) polymerase as derived from crystal structures and homology modeling. Biochemistry 37(11):3893–3900
14. Knight MI, Chambers PJ (2001) Production, extraction, and purification of human poly(ADP-ribose) polymerase-1 (PARP-1) with high specific activity. Protein Expr Purif 23(3):453–458
15. Griffin RJ, Pemberton LC, Rhodes D, Bleasdale C, Bowman K, Calvert AH et al (1995) Novel potent inhibitors of the DNA repair enzyme poly(ADP-ribose)polymerase (PARP). Anticancer Drug Des 10(6):507–514
16. Li JH, Zhang J (2001) PARP inhibitors. IDrugs 4(7):804–812
17. Thorsell AG, Ekblad T, Karlberg T, Low M, Pinto AF, Tresaugues L et al (2017) Structural basis for potency and promiscuity in poly(ADP-ribose) polymerase (PARP) and tankyrase inhibitors. J Med Chem 60(4):1262–1271
18. Virag L, Szabo C (2002) The therapeutic potential of poly(ADP-ribose) polymerase inhibitors. Pharmacol Rev 54:375–429
19. Tentori L, Portarena I, Graziani G (2002) Potential clinical applications of poly(ADP-ribose) polymerase (PARP) inhibitors. Pharmacol Res 45(2):73–85
20. Bignami M, O'Driscoll M, Aquilina G, Karran P (2000) Unmasking a killer: DNA O(6)-methylguanine and the cytotoxicity of methylating agents. Mutat Res 462(2–3):71–82

21. Hegi ME, Diserens AC, Godard S, Dietrich PY, Regli L, Ostermann S et al (2004) Clinical trial substantiates the predictive value of O-6-methylguanine-DNA methyltransferase promoter methylation in glioblastoma patients treated with temozolomide. Clin Cancer Res 10(6):1871–1874
22. Boulton S, Pemberton LC, Porteous JK, Curtin NJ, Griffin RJ, Golding BT et al (1995) Potentiation of temozolomide-induced cytotoxicity: a comparative study of the biological effects of poly(ADP-ribose) polymerase inhibitors. Br J Cancer 72(4):849–856
23. Miknyoczki SJ, Jones-Bolin S, Pritchard S, Hunter K, Zhao H, Wan W et al (2003) Chemopotentiation of temozolomide, irinotecan, and cisplatin activity by CEP-6800, a poly(ADP-ribose) polymerase inhibitor. Mol Cancer Ther 2(4):371–382
24. Tentori L, Portarena I, Barbarino M, Balduzzi A, Levati L, Vergati M et al (2003) Inhibition of telomerase increases resistance of melanoma cells to temozolomide, but not to temozolomide combined with poly (adp-ribose) polymerase inhibitor. Mol Pharmacol 63(1):192–202
25. Plummer R, Jones C, Middleton M, Wilson R, Evans J, Olsen A et al (2008) Phase I study of the poly(ADP-Ribose) polymerase inhibitor, AG014699, in combination with temozolomide in patients with advanced solid tumors. Clin Cancer Res 14(23):7917–7923
26. Plummer R, Lorigan P, Evans J, Steven N, Middleton M, Wilson R et al (2006) First and final report of a phase II study of the poly(ADP-ribose) polymerase (PARP) inhibitor, AG014699, in combination with temozolomide (TMZ) in patients with metastatic malignant melanoma (MM). J Clin Oncol 24(18s):8013
27. Quinn JA, Pluda J, Dolan ME, Delaney S, Kaplan R, Rich JN et al (2002) Phase II trial of carmustine plus O(6)-benzylguanine for patients with nitrosourea-resistant recurrent or progressive malignant glioma. J Clin Oncol 20(9):2277–2283
28. Quinn JA, Desjardins A, Weingart J, Brem H, Dolan ME, Delaney SM et al (2005) Phase I trial of temozolomide plus O6-benzylguanine for patients with recurrent or progressive malignant glioma. J Clin Oncol 23(28):7178–7187
29. Schilsky RL, Dolan ME, Bertucci D, Ewesuedo RB, Vogelzang NJ, Mani S et al (2000) Phase I clinical and pharmacological study of O6-benzylguanine followed by carmustine in patients with advanced cancer. Clin Cancer Res 6(8):3025–3031
30. Ranson M, Middleton MR, Bridgewater J, Lee SM, Dawson M, Jowle D et al (2006) Lomeguatrib, a potent inhibitor of O6-alkylguanine-DNA-alkyltransferase: phase I safety, pharmacodynamic, and pharmacokinetic trial and evaluation in combination with temozolomide in patients with advanced solid tumors. Clin Cancer Res 12(5):1577–1584
31. Rajan A, Carter CA, Kelly RJ, Gutierrez M, Kummar S, Szabo E et al (2012) A phase I combination study of olaparib with cisplatin and gemcitabine in adults with solid tumors. Clin Cancer Res 18(8):2344–2351
32. Kummar S, Chen A, Ji J, Zhang Y, Reid JM, Ames M et al (2011) Phase I study of PARP inhibitor ABT-888 in combination with topotecan in adults with refractory solid tumors and lymphomas. Cancer Res 71(17):5626–5634
33. Khan OA, Gore M, Lorigan P, Stone J, Greystoke A, Burke W, et al. A phase I study of the safety and tolerability of olaparib (AZD2281, KU0059436) and dacarbazine in patients with advanced solid tumours. Br J Cancer 104(5):750–5
34. Kummar S, Ji J, Morgan R, Lenz HJ, Puhalla SL, Belani CP et al (2012) A phase I study of veliparib in combination with metronomic cyclophosphamide in adults with refractory solid tumors and lymphomas. Clin Cancer Res 18(6):1726–1734
35. Dent RA, Lindeman GJ, Clemons M, Wildiers H, Chan A, McCarthy NJ, et al (2010) Safety and efficacy of the oral PARP inhibitor olaparib (AZD2281) in combination with paclitaxel for the first- or second-line treatment of patients with metastatic triple-negative breast cancer: results from the safety cohort of a phase I/II multicenter trial. J Clin Oncol 28(Suppl):Abstract 1018
36. O'Shaughnessy J, Osborne C, Pippen J, Yoffe M, Patt D, Monaghan G et al (2010) Final efficacy and safety results of a randomized phase II study of the PARP inhibitor iniparib (BSI-201) in combination with gemcitabine/carboplatin (G/C) in metastatic triple negative breast cancer (TNBC). ESMO, Milan, Italy, p Abstract LBA11

37. Kopetz S, Mita M, Mok I, Sankhala K, Moseley J, Sherman B et al (2008) First in human phase I study of BSI-201, a small molecule inhibitor of poly ADP-ribose polymerase (PARP) in subjects with advanced solid tumors. J Clin Oncol 26(May 20 Suppl):3577

38. Mahany J, Lewis N, Heath E, LoRusso P, Mita M, Rodon J et al (2008) A phase IB study evaluating BSI-201 in combination with chemotherapy in subjects with advanced solid tumors. J Clin Oncol 26(May 20 Suppl):3579

39. O'Shaughnessy J, Schwartzberg L, Danso MA, Miller KD, Rugo HS, Neubauer M et al (2014) Phase III study of iniparib plus gemcitabine and carboplatin versus gemcitabine and carboplatin in patients with metastatic triple-negative breast cancer. J Clin Oncol 32(34):3840–3847

40. Liu X, Shi Y, Maag DX, Palma JP, Patterson MJ, Ellis PA et al (2012) Iniparib nonselectively modifies cysteine-containing proteins in tumor cells and is not a bona fide PARP inhibitor. Clin Cancer Res 18(2):510–523

41. Patel AG, De Lorenzo SB, Flatten KS, Poirier GG, Kaufmann SH (2012) Failure of iniparib to inhibit poly(ADP-Ribose) polymerase in vitro. Clin Cancer Res 18(6):1655–1662

42. Bryant HE, Schultz N, Thomas HD, Parker KM, Flower D, Lopez E et al (2005) Specific killing of BRCA2-deficient tumours with inhibitors of poly(ADP-ribose) polymerase. Nature 434(7035):913–917

43. Farmer H, McCabe N, Lord CJ, Tutt AN, Johnson DA, Richardson TB et al (2005) Targeting the DNA repair defect in BRCA mutant cells as a therapeutic strategy. Nature 434(7035):917–921

44. Fong P, Boss D, Yap T, Tutt A, Wu P, Mergui-Roelvink M et al (2009) Inhibition of poly(ADP-Ribose) polymerase in tumors from BRCA mutation carriers. N Engl J Med 361(2):123–134

45. Tutt A, Robson M, Garber J, Domchek S, Audeh M, Weitzel J et al (2009) Phase II trial of the oral PARP inhibitor olaparib in BRCA-deficient advanced breast cancer. J Clin Oncol 27(18s):CRA501

46. Audeh M, Penson R, Friedlander M, Powell B, B-M KM, Scott C, Weitzel J, C J et al (2009) Phase II trial of the oral PARP inhibitor olaparib (AZD2281) in BRCA-deficient advanced ovarian cancer J Clin Oncol 27(15s):5500

47. Drew Y, Ledermann J, Hall G, Rea D, Glasspool R, Highley M et al (2016) Phase 2 multicentre trial investigating intermittent and continuous dosing schedules of the poly(ADP-ribose) polymerase inhibitor rucaparib in germline BRCA mutation carriers with advanced ovarian and breast cancer. Br J Cancer 114(12):e21

48. Murray J, Thomas H, Berry P, Kyle S, Patterson M, Jones C et al (2014) Tumour cell retention of rucaparib, sustained PARP inhibition and efficacy of weekly as well as daily schedules. Br J Cancer

49. Parkes EE, Walker SM, Taggart LE, McCabe N, Knight LA, Wilkinson R et al (2017) Activation of STING-dependent innate immune signaling by S-Phase-specific DNA damage in breast cancer. J Natl Cancer Inst 109(1)

50. Chabanon RM, Muirhead G, Krastev DB, Adam J, Morel D, Garrido M et al (2019) PARP inhibition enhances tumor cell-intrinsic immunity in ERCC1-deficient non-small cell lung cancer. J Clin Invest 129(3):1211–1228

51. Pantelidou C, Sonzogni O, De Oliveria TM, Mehta AK, Kothari A, Wang D et al (2019) PARP inhibitor efficacy depends on CD8(+) T-cell recruitment via intratumoral STING pathway activation in BRCA-deficient models of triple-negative breast cancer. Cancer Discov 9(6):722–737

52. Jiao S, Xia W, Yamaguchi H, Wei Y, Chen MK, Hsu JM et al (2017) PARP inhibitor upregulates PD-L1 expression and enhances cancer-associated immunosuppression. Clin Cancer Res 23(14):3711–3720

53. Ding L, Kim HJ, Wang Q, Kearns M, Jiang T, Ohlson CE et al (2018) PARP inhibition elicits STING-dependent antitumor immunity in Brca1-deficient ovarian cancer. Cell Rep 25(11):2972–80 e5

54. Brown JS, Sundar R, Lopez J (2018) Combining DNA damaging therapeutics with immunotherapy: more haste, less speed. Br J Cancer 118(3):312–324

Exploiting Cancer Synthetic Lethality in Cancer—Lessons Learnt from PARP Inhibitors

Stephen J. Pettitt, Colm J. Ryan, and Christopher J. Lord

2.1 Introduction

One of the more pervasive hallmarks of many cancers are defects in the complex network of proteins and processes comprising the DNA damage response (DDR) network that normally maintain the integrity of the genome. Defects in the DDR likely foster tumourigenesis by enabling mutations to occur that give cells new, oncogenic, properties and historically were identified by noting that many cancers have highly disordered genomes and are sensitive to agents that cause DNA damage (e.g. radiotherapy or DNA-damaging chemotherapies) [1]. More recently though, the molecular basis of cancer-specific defects in DNA repair has been established by the identification of multiple cancer driver genes whose dysfunction either causes defects in the DDR (e.g. tumour suppressors such as the "caretakers", *BRCA1*, *BRCA2*, *PALB2*, *RAD51C*, *RAD51D*, the Fanconi's Anaemia (FANC) family of genes and *ATM*), those whose dysfunction contributes to the formation of cancer by disturbing the normal progression, repair and restart of replication forks e.g. *CCNE1* (a phenotype known as replication fork stress [2]) and those genes whose dysfunction allows the result of these DDR defects (i.e. mutations

S. J. Pettitt · C. J. Lord (✉)
The CRUK Gene Function Laboratory and Breast Cancer Now Toby Robins Research Centre, The Institute of Cancer Research, London SW3 6JB, UK
e-mail: Chris.Lord@icr.ac.uk

S. J. Pettitt
e-mail: Stephen.Pettitt@icr.ac.uk

C. J. Ryan
School of Computer Science and Systems Biology Ireland, University College Dublin, Dublin, Ireland
e-mail: Colm.Ryan@ucd.ie

© The Author(s), under exclusive license to Springer Nature Switzerland AG 2023
T. A. Yap and G. I. Shapiro (eds.), *Targeting the DNA Damage Response for Cancer Therapy*, Cancer Treatment and Research 186,
https://doi.org/10.1007/978-3-031-30065-3_2

and gross chromosomal rearrangements) to be passed onto daughter cells ('gate-keepers" such as *p53*). Rather ironically, many of the vulnerabilities that arise in cancer cells because of a dysregulated DDR, include the targeting of components of the DDR itself [3]. Aside from the use of radiotherapy and classical chemotherapies (which target DDR defects by overwhelming tumour cells with DNA damage they are unable to effectively repair) perhaps the most well-understood example of a cancer-specific DDR defect being therapeutically targeted via inhibition of a DDR component is that of PARP inhibitors (PARPi) that inhibit the function of the DNA repair protein PARP1 [4]. As discussed throughout this book, PARPi are particularly effective in killing tumour cells [5, 6] and treating cancers [7] that have defects in the genes that control DNA repair by homologous recombination (HR e.g. *BRCA1, BRCA2, PALB2, RAD51C, RAD51D* etc.). Moreover, the sensitivity of HR defective tumours to PARPi provides perhaps the best example of the application of the synthetic lethal principle, the biological concept that describes how a particular combination (or "synthesis") of defects in a cell causes cell death (e.g. defect in *BRCA1/2* plus inhibition of PARP1, the target of PARPi), whereas the same defects, when occurring in isolation, do not [8–11].

The details of how the BRCA/PARPi synthetic lethality was identified and how this effect has been exploited therapeutically are discussed in detail throughout this book. Here we discuss what lessons have been learnt from studying this particular synthetic lethality and how these lessons and principles could inform how inhibitors of other DNA repair proteins could be used.

2.2 Lesson 1: Synthetic Lethal Penetrance Is Important

For a synthetic lethal interaction to be of practical use in biomarker-driven cancer treatment, loss of one partner should be highly predictive of profound vulnerability to loss or inhibition of the other, regardless of other molecular differences that may exist in different tumours and patients In genetic terms, this is referred to as highly penetrant or robust [12]. For example, one of the features of the *BRCA1/BRCA2* plus PARPi synthetic lethality is that the effect achieved is profound in a number of contexts including cell lines from multiple cancer types (e.g. breast, ovarian, pancreatic), cell lines from different species and in both *in vitro* and *in vivo* model systems [5, 6, 13]. One of the lessons learnt from large-scale shRNA, CRISPR-Cas9 and drug sensitivity screens is that such highly penetrant cancer-associated synthetic lethality effects are the rarity rather than the norm. This issue of penetrance has been one of the challenges that has limited the identification of actionable synthetic lethal interactions associated with commonly occurring oncogenes such as *KRAS*, where a number of real and profound synthetic lethal effects have been identified, but these tend to be private to individual model systems [14]. It is therefore important to discriminate experimentally identified synthetic lethal interactions that are private to a very particular context (e.g. seen in one isogenic system) from those that apply more generally. These latter, highly penetrant, interactions can be identified empirically by validating interactions across large panels of cell lines, tumour organoids, tumour xenografts etc. or by using genetic perturbation technologies to assess how robust a synthetic lethal effect is in the face of mutation (Fig. 2.1).

Based on these principles and observations from large-scale genetic perturbation screens, heuristics for the identification of such highly penetrant effects have been proposed, including: (i) the molecular pathway targetted being broadly essential or having an essential role in tumours, (ii) the synthetic lethal partners having a close functional relationship such as membership of a common pathway; (iii) lack of cell type specificity in expression of the synthetic lethal genes and (iv) conservation of synthetic lethal effects across species barriers [12]. While these heuristics seem like intuitive approaches to identify more penetrant effects, to date only the use of a close functional relationship (as suggested by a protein–protein interaction) has been empirically demonstrated to have utility in identifying robust synthetic lethals [15]. The routine assessment of penetrance when describing a synthetic lethality is likely to be important in ensuring that only robust effects are progressed to

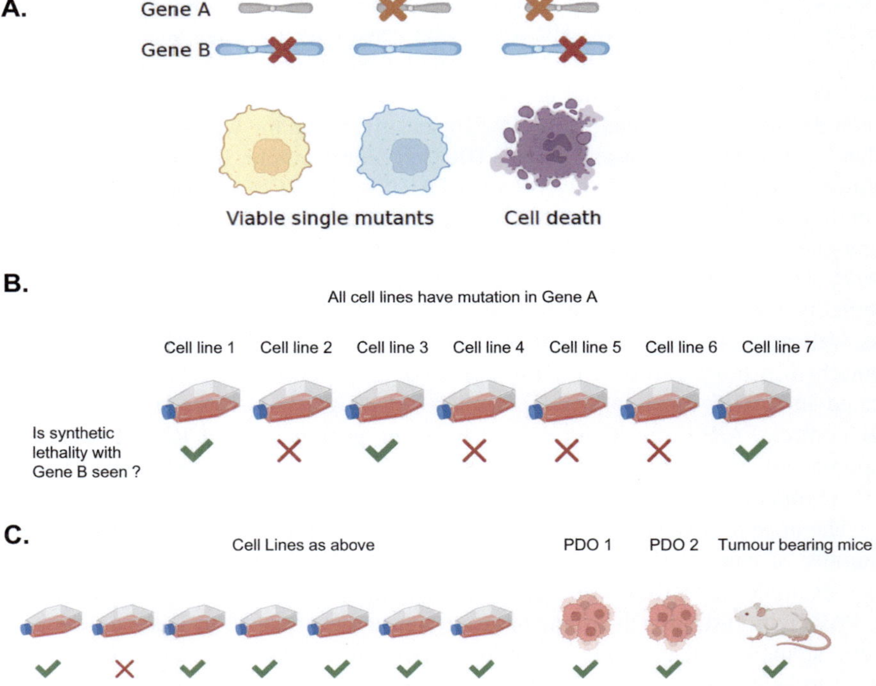

Fig. 2.1 Synthetic lethal penetrance. A. Illustration of the principle of genetic synthetic lethality. Deletion of either gene A or gene B is viable, but deletion of both in the same cell results in loss of viability. **B.** A low penetrance synthetic lethal effect operates in a limited range of cell line models, likely due to further dependency on genetic background or cell type. **C.** Ideally, a therapeutically useful synthetic lethality is applicable across a wide range of cell line backgrounds, tumour and *in vivo* models

biomarker-driven trials. For example, a number of newer DNA repair inhibitors are now either in pre-clinical or clinical development as synthetic lethal treatments for cancer, including inhibitors of ATM, ATR, DNAPK or Polθ (see other chapters in this book). Based on the understanding that the penetrance of a synthetic lethal interaction might determine its eventual clinical effectiveness, determining how penetrant the synthetic lethal interactions are with these inhibitors might be seen as a key objective.

2.3 Lesson 2: Synthetic Lethal Phenocopy Effects Provide Additional Indications for DDR Inhibitors

Prior to the discovery of the BRCA/PARPi synthetic lethality [5, 6], the concept of BRCAness was defined, i.e. the existence of tumours that do not have germ-line mutations in either *BRCA1* or *BRCA2* (*gBRCAm*) but which exhibit many of the phenotypes of *gBRCAm* cancers [16]. These phenotypes include histological features, transcriptomic profiles that resemble *gBRCAm* cancers, a defect in homologous recombination, distinct mutational patterns or scars in the genome that are a consequence of defective HR, or indeed sensitivity to drugs such as platinum salts that target defective HR [16, 17]. The introduction of PARPi into clinical use and large-scale tumour genomic DNA sequencing has extended this definition to include those cancers that exhibit PARPi sensitivity and the wider group of cancers that have mutations that also impair HR [17]. For example, shortly after the identification of synthetic lethality between PARPi and BRCA1 or BRCA2 defects, a small-scale short-hairpin (sh)RNA interference screen demonstrated that defects in any one of a series of genes involved in HR (*RAD51, RAD54, DSS1, RPA1, NBS1, ATR, ATM, CHK1, CHK2, FANCD2, FANCA,* or *FANCC*) cause PARPi synthetic lethality [18], observations confirmed by hypothesis-driven experiments [19–22] as well as a whole genome shRNA screen, where 74 DDR genes, significantly enriched in those involved in HR (e.g. *CDK12, RAD51C, RAD51D*) were implicated in PARPi sensitivity [23]. Similar sets of genes have been demonstrated to control PARPi sensitivity in more recent genome-wide CRISPR screening approaches, which has further revealed the role of genes outside the well-known HR regulators, such as the *RNASEH2* family [24].

The appeal of phenocopies from a therapeutic point of view is to exapand the number of patients that could potentially benefit from a synthetic lethal therapy. For example, a "BRCAness" gene panel is now approved to direct the use of a PARPi in castration resistant prostate cancer, whereas in gynaecological cancers, signatures of genomic instability derived from tumour sequencing data are used to select patients for PARPi treatment, even in the absence of a germ-line or somatic BRCA1/2 mutation [4]. This observation that multiple members of a specific pathway may display similar synthetic lethal effects is consistent with systematic studies in model organisms [25, 26], suggesting that it is unlikely to be specific to PARPi. The same phenocopy paradigm might therefore be used to direct the use of some of the newer DDR inhibitors in development. For example,

ATR inhibitor synthetic lethality is seen in models of gynaecological cancer that have a mutation in the SWI/SNF tumour suppressor gene *ARID1A* [27]. The SWI/SNF complex is involved in chromatin remodeling and includes proteins encoded by other tumour suppressors such as *SMARCA4* and *PBRM1*. Defects in these genes cause ATRi sensitivity [28–30] as do defects in other SWI/SNF complex proteins present in synovial sarcomas [31]. As such, some consideration could be given to whether ATRi synthetic lethality is a common feature of "SWI/SNFness" in the same way that BRCAness is characterised by PARPi sensitivity.

2.4 Lesson 3: Resistance Can Emerge via Modulation of Either Synthetic Lethal Partner

The first clinical approval for a PARPi was in 2014 [32] and so at the time of writing (2021) PARPi have only been in widespread clinical use for a relatively short time. Because of this, the ability to study and understand how drug resistance to a synthetic lethal DDR therapy has been limited, when compared to, for example, standard-of-care targeted therapies such as endocrine agents that have been in use for decades. Nevertheless, there is some understanding of how PARPi resistance occurs, most of which has been delineated by pre-clinical investigation. Although this is discussed in other chapters of this book, in brief, PARPi resistance can occur via: (i) modulation of the drug target, PARP1 itself, for example via mutations in *PARP1* or via changes in PARP1 PARylation caused by loss of PARG [33]; (ii) modulation of the synthetic lethal partner, for example, via loss of *BRCA1* promoter hypermethylation or reversion mutation that restores the open reading frame and function of a BRCAness gene; (iii) compensatory changes in other DNA repair genes, such as *TP53BP1, MAD2L2, SHLD1/2/3*, that restore HR in BRCA1 mutant tumour cells [34]; (iv) pharmacokinetic changes that reduce the cellular concentration of PARPi, such as upregulation of P-glycoprotein pumps [35] (Fig. 2.2). In totality, the discovery of these different mechanisms suggests that for synthetic lethal treatments, drug resistance might not simply emerge via modulation of the drug target or the drug itself, as is common for many other targeted therapies, but also via modulation of the synthetic lethal partner (e.g. reversion mutation), a phenomenon termed synthetic lethal resistance [36]. It will be interesting to see whether resistance to other synthetic lethal effects in cancer also emerges via synthetic lethal resistance or whether modulation of drug and/or drug target is a more dominant mechanism; of course, whether this occurs might be very dependent upon the precise synthetic lethal pairing under consideration as it is possible that: (i) some drug targets do not tolerate mutations that restore function and/or prevent inhibition; (ii) some cancer driver genes involved in synthetic lethal interactions are not able to revert, as their continued dysfunction is critical to the fitness of the tumour cell. Nevertheless, the study of how drug resistance develops in the BRCA/PARP inhibitor synthetic lethality has certainly indicated that a focus on just the drug target might not be wise when one is looking for mechanisms of drug resistance.

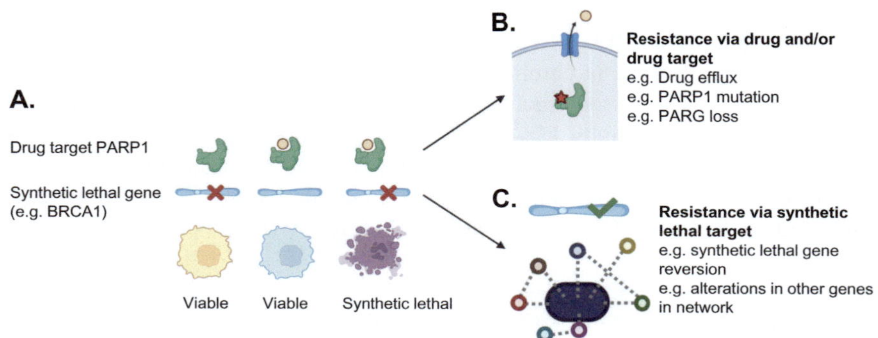

Fig. 2.2 Resistance to synthetic lethal therapies can occur via modulation of either partner. **A**. An example synthetic lethal interaction exploited via a drug inhibiting one of the partners (e.g. PARP1-BRCA1). **B**. Resistance occurring via effects proximal to the drug target, e.g. resistance-causing PARP1 mutation or upregulation of drug efflux. **C**. Resistance may also occur by bypassing the genetic mutation, e.g. via reversion mutation or pathway bypass of the synthetic lethal partner

2.5 Lesson 4: Synthetic Lethal Interactions that Appear to Be Digenic Are Probably Polygenic and Complex

Knowingly or not, when synthetic lethal interactions in cancer are discussed there is often an implicit assumption that a phenotype controlled by only two genes (a *digenic* effect) is being considered. Of course, for a fully penetrant effect (e.g. defect in gene A + defect in gene B *always* causes cell death with no exceptions) the synthetic lethality is indeed digenic. However, it is likely that many of the synthetic lethal effects currently being developed as cancer therapies are actually *polygenic*, i.e. like many cellular phenotypes these are controlled by multiple genes. Furthermore, they may also be complex, i.e. influenced by both genetic and environmental factors and potentially interactions between the two. Strictly speaking, the fact that a synthetic lethal effect is not fully penetrant (there are some contexts where dysfunction in A and B do not cause cell death), implies other modifiers, either genetic or environmental, are involved. Indeed, we already know this to be the case for PARPi synthetic lethality. For example, the synthetic lethal interaction between *BRCA1* and PARPi in model systems is not simply a digenic interaction between BRCA1 and PARP1 but is a polygenic phenotype controlled by additional genes such as *53BP1, REV7, SHLD1/2/3* etc. Likewise, the ultimate therapeutic effect of PARPi in *in vivo* models of *gBRCAm* cancer is modified by the presence or absence of an adaptive immune response [37], suggesting an even more complex interaction between *BRCA* genes, PARP1 and the genes and environmental factors that control the immune response. Whether this is the case for many other synthetic lethal effects in cancer remains to be empirically established, but given that none identified thus far appear fully penetrant, the suggestion is that most are indeed polygenic and/or complex. What does this mean for the continued study of and application of synthetic lethal effects in cancer? Two obvious things:

(i) the likely polygenicity and complexity of cancer synthetic lethals suggests that trying to identify modifiers of an apparently digenic synthetic lethal effect might be very worthwhile, especially if the aim is to develop predictive biomarkers that effectively stratify patients for treatment; and (ii) an acceptance that the most accurate biomarkers of a favourable response to a synthetic lethal treatment are likely to be polygenic biomarkers that take into account not just the status of the drug target and its synthetic lethal cancer driver gene, but also the known polygenic modifiers of the synthetic lethality.

2.6   Lesson 5: Drug Resistance Could Be Targeted via Evolutionary Double Binds

The observation of synthetic lethality in cancer suggests that although a cancer driver gene alteration might provide a tumour cell with a fitness advantage, it also imparts a synthetic lethal vulnerability. The same logic could also be applied to thinking about how to target therapy resistance. For example, the study of drug resistance to PARPi has shown that although loss of *53BP1, REV7, SHLD1/2/3* etc. cause PARPi resistance in BRCA1m cells, these alterations also impart ATR inhibitor [38], Polθ inhibitor [39, 40] or radiosensitivity [41] onto tumour cells. In evolutionary terms, this could be viewed as a double bind [42]; the selective pressure of an initial treatment (PARPi) forces the evolution of a tumour cell population down a particular molecular route (e.g. loss of *53BP1*), which whilst initially providing a fitness advantage to the cell, also imposes a phenotypic fitness cost, which in this case is (for example) Polθ inhibitor sensitivity [39, 40]. This example also neatly illustrates why the study of therapy resistance to synthetic lethal effects is necessary—not just so that biomarkers can be identified that could monitor the early emerge of therapy resistant tumour clones, but also so that new vulnerabilities put in place by the resistance mechanism can be therapeutically exploited. Is this something peculiar to PARPi? Almost certainly not; much of what is known about double binds when applied to cancer treatment has come from the study of targeted treatments that exploit effects such as oncogene addiction [42]. Nevertheless, the concept of double binds might be very relevant to optimising not just PARPi synthetic lethality but also other DDR inhibitor related synthetic lethals. For example, early studies examining ATR inhibitor resistance identified loss of CDC25 as a driver [43]. Whilst loss of CDC25 allows cells to stall the cell cycle to repair DNA damage prior to mitosis (something that is less likely when an ATR inhibitor is present), it does now impose a dependency upon the WEE1 cell cycle checkpoint kinase, which can be exploited using WEE1 inhibitors [43].

2.7 Horizon Scanning—What's Next ?

There remain several highly mutated tumour suppressor genes for which a synthetic lethal target has yet to be identified and/or developed. Chief among these is p53—although it is likely that many active cancer treatments target p53 deficiency to some extent, there are no agents for which a p53 defect is a sensitive and specific biomarker of efficacy. As synthetic lethal effects are typically identified by comparing models with an alteration of a driver gene to models without that alteration, the near ubiquitous deregulation of the p53 pathway can make this approach problematic. Loss of p53, or some phenocopy thereof, is likely so critical to the cancer phenotype (or even immortalisation of normal cells in culture) that currently used models and methods of synthetic lethal identification in cell lines may be ill equipped to identify these effects. This has also presented difficulties with other common tumour suppressor genes such as *RB1* as most cancer cell lines harbour a genetic alteration of at least one member of the RB pathway. Nonetheless several recent studies have identified promising synthetic lethal effects associating mutation of RB1 with increased sensitivity to *Aurora A/B, TSC2* or *SKP2* inhibition [44–48]. As with tumour suppressors, the identification of highly-penetrant synthetic lethal interactions for a number of common oncogenes (KRAS, MYC) also remains challenging.

While synthetic lethality serves well as a principle for identifying genetic vulnerabilities in cancer, there are several ways in which the concept could be developed to better suit the genetic diversity encountered in tumours and the tools available for therapy. The synthetic lethal experimental approach is often predicated on cells having exactly one null mutation in a query gene and being effectively assessed against a large number of null mutations in other genes to discover synthetic lethal partners. However, cancers develop from a diverse range of cell types, acquire multiple driver mutations, are associated with stromal cells and may have mutations that do not lead to complete loss of function. These characteristics can be taken into account to some extent in the analysis and prioritisation of synthetic lethal interactions.

One possibility to tackle the problem of multiple driver events in cells is to combine synthetic lethal treatments. This strategy could either exploit synthetic lethal interactions with two driver mutations in distinct pathways or consider a particular common combination of alterations as a single "query" for synthetic lethal discovery. For example, although *KRAS* mutations are uncommon in *BRCA*-associated breast and ovarian cancers, they occur frequently in pancreatic cancers with *BRCA*-gene mutations. This may represent an opportunity, which would not be present in breast or ovarian cancer, for combination of PARP inhibitors with agents targeting *KRAS* mutations such as MEK inhibitors.

In the example above, two interventions would be combined that target separate mutations that occur within the same tumour (MEK inhibitors targeting RAS mutations; PARP inhibitors targeting BRCA1/2 mutations). Such an approach relies primarily on the identification of pairwise synthetic lethal relationships. However, it is also possible, and indeed likely, that individual driver gene alterations may sensitise cells to specific combinations of therapies. For example, KRAS mutation has been shown in preclinical models to be associated with increased sensitivity to a combination of CHEK1 and MK2 inhibitors [49]. Such higher-order synthetic lethal effects could potentially be exploited therapeutically, but the major challenge is in identifying them. The space of possible combinations of drugs to test is enormous, and therefore approaches to prioritise those most likely to be synergistic in specific contexts are required.

Acknowledgements C. J. L. and S. J. P. thank the following for funding work in our laboratories: Breast Cancer Now as part of Programme Funding to the Breast Cancer Now Toby Robins Research Centre and Cancer Research UK, as part of Programme funding. C. J. R. thanks Science Foundation for funding under grant number 20/FFP-P/8641. This work represents independent research supported by the National Institute for Health Research (NIHR) Biomedical Research Centre at The Royal Marsden NHS Foundation Trust and the Institute of Cancer Research, London. The views expressed are those of the author(s) and not necessarily those of the NIHR or the Department of Health and Social Care. Figures were created with BioRender.com.

Disclosures C. J. L. makes the following disclosures: receives and/or has received research funding from: AstraZeneca, Merck KGaA, Artios. Received consultancy, SAB membership or honoraria payments from: Syncona, Sun Pharma, Gerson Lehrman Group, Merck KGaA, Vertex, AstraZeneca, Tango, 3rd Rock, Ono Pharma, Artios, Abingworth, Tesselate, Dark Blue Therapeutics, Pontifax, Astex, Neophore, Glaxo Smith Kline. Has stock in: Tango, Ovibio, Hysplex, Tesselate. C. J. L. is also a named inventor on patents describing the use of DNA repair inhibitors and stands to gain from their development and use as part of the ICR "Rewards to Inventors" scheme and also reports benefits from this scheme associated with patents for PARP inhibitors paid into CJL's personal account and research accounts at the Institute of Cancer Research. S. J. P. makes the following disclosure: named inventor on patents describing the use of DNA repair inhibitors and stands to gain from their development and use as part of the ICR "Rewards to Inventors" scheme.

References

1. Jeggo PA, Pearl LH, Carr AM (2016) DNA repair, genome stability and cancer: a historical perspective. Nat Rev Cancer 16(1):35–42
2. Zeman MK, Cimprich KA (2014) Causes and consequences of replication stress. Nat Cell Biol 16(1):2–9
3. O'Connor MJ (2015) Targeting the DNA damage response in cancer. Mol Cell 60(4):547–560
4. Lord CJ, Ashworth A (2017) PARP inhibitors: synthetic lethality in the clinic. Science 355(6330):1152–1158
5. Farmer H, McCabe N, Lord CJ, Tutt AN, Johnson DA, Richardson TB et al (2005) Targeting the DNA repair defect in BRCA mutant cells as a therapeutic strategy. Nature 434(7035):917–921
6. Bryant HE, Schultz N, Thomas HD, Parker KM, Flower D, Lopez E et al (2005) Specific killing of BRCA2-deficient tumours with inhibitors of poly(ADP-ribose) polymerase. Nature 434(7035):913–917
7. Fong PC, Boss DS, Yap TA, Tutt A, Wu P, Mergui-Roelvink M et al (2009) Inhibition of poly(ADP-ribose) polymerase in tumors from BRCA mutation carriers. N Engl J Med 361(2):123–134
8. Bridges C (1922) The origin of variations in sexual and sex-limited characters. Am Nat 56:51–63
9. Brummelkamp TR, Bernards R (2003) New tools for functional mammalian cancer genetics. Nat Rev Cancer 3(10):781–789

10. Dobzhansky T (1946) Genetics of natural populations. Xiii. Recombination and variability in populations of drosophila pseudoobscura. Genetics 31(3):269–90

11. Kaelin WG Jr (2005) The concept of synthetic lethality in the context of anticancer therapy. Nat Rev Cancer 5(9):689–698

12. Ryan CJ, Bajrami I, Lord CJ (2018) Synthetic lethality and cancer—penetrance as the major barrier. Trends Cancer. 4(10):671–683

13. Rottenberg S, Jaspers JE, Kersbergen A, van der Burg E, Nygren AO, Zander SA et al (2008) High sensitivity of BRCA1-deficient mammary tumors to the PARP inhibitor AZD2281 alone and in combination with platinum drugs. Proc Natl Acad Sci U S A 105(44):17079–17084

14. Downward J (2015) RAS synthetic lethal screens revisited: still seeking the elusive prize? Clin Cancer Res 21(8):1802–1809

15. Lord CJ, Quinn N, Ryan CJ (2020) Integrative analysis of large-scale loss-of-function screens identifies robust cancer-associated genetic interactions. eLife 9

16. Turner N, Tutt A, Ashworth A (2004) Hallmarks of 'BRCAness' in sporadic cancers. Nat Rev Cancer 4(10):814–819

17. Lord CJ, Ashworth A (2016) BRCAness revisited. Nat Rev Cancer 16(2):110–120

18. McCabe N, Turner NC, Lord CJ, Kluzek K, Bialkowska A, Swift S et al (2006) Deficiency in the repair of DNA damage by homologous recombination and sensitivity to poly(ADP-ribose) polymerase inhibition. Cancer Res 66(16):8109–8115

19. Min A, Im SA, Yoon YK, Song SH, Nam HJ, Hur HS et al (2013) RAD51C-deficient cancer cells are highly sensitive to the PARP inhibitor olaparib. Mol Cancer Ther 12(6):865–877

20. Loveday C, Turnbull C, Ramsay E, Hughes D, Ruark E, Frankum JR et al (2011) Germline mutations in RAD51D confer susceptibility to ovarian cancer. Nat Genet 43(9):879–882

21. Lord CJ, McDonald S, Swift S, Turner NC, Ashworth A (2008) A high-throughput RNA interference screen for DNA repair determinants of PARP inhibitor sensitivity. DNA Repair (Amst). 7(12):2010–2019

22. Murai J, Yang K, Dejsuphong D, Hirota K, Takeda S, D'Andrea AD (2011) The USP1/UAF1 complex promotes double-strand break repair through homologous recombination. Mol Cell Biol 31(12):2462–2469

23. Bajrami I, Frankum JR, Konde A, Miller RE, Rehman FL, Brough R et al (2013) Genome-wide profiling of genetic synthetic lethality identifies CDK12 as a novel determinant of PARP1/2 inhibitor sensitivity. Can Res 74(1):287–297

24. Zimmermann M, Murina O, Reijns MAM, Agathanggelou A, Challis R, Tarnauskaite Z et al (2018) CRISPR screens identify genomic ribonucleotides as a source of PARP-trapping lesions. Nature 559(7713):285–289

25. Lee I, Lehner B, Vavouri T, Shin J, Fraser AG, Marcotte EM (2010) Predicting genetic modifier loci using functional gene networks. Genome Res 20(8):1143–1153

26. Kelley R, Ideker T (2005) Systematic interpretation of genetic interactions using protein networks. Nat Biotechnol 23(5):561–566

27. Williamson CT, Miller R, Pemberton HN, Jones SE, Campbell J, Konde A et al (2016) ATR inhibitors as a synthetic lethal therapy for tumours deficient in ARID1A. Nat Commun 7:13837

28. Gupta M, Concepcion CP, Fahey CG, Keshishian H, Bhutkar A, Brainson CF et al (2020) BRG1 loss predisposes lung cancers to replicative stress and ATR dependency. Cancer Res 80(18):3841–3854

29. Kurashima K, Kashiwagi H, Shimomura I, Suzuki A, Takeshita F, Mazevet M et al (2020) SMARCA4 deficiency-associated heterochromatin induces intrinsic DNA replication stress and susceptibility to ATR inhibition in lung adenocarcinoma. NAR Cancer 2(2):zcaa005

30. Chabanon RM, Morel D, Eychenne T, Colmet-Daage L, Bajrami I, Dorvault N et al (2021) PBRM1 deficiency confers synthetic lethality to DNA repair inhibitors in cancer. Cancer Res 81(11):2888–2902

31. Jones SE, Fleuren EDG, Frankum J, Konde A, Williamson CT, Krastev DB et al (2017) ATR is a therapeutic target in synovial sarcoma. Cancer Res

32. Deeks ED (2015) Olaparib: first global approval. Drugs 75(2):231–240

33. Gogola E, Duarte AA, de Ruiter JR, Wiegant WW, Schmid JA, de Bruijn R et al (2019) Selective loss of PARG restores PARylation and counteracts PARP inhibitor-mediated synthetic lethality. Cancer Cell 35(6):950–952

34. Liptay M, Barbosa JS, Rottenberg S (2020) Replication fork remodeling and therapy escape in DNA damage response-deficient cancers. Front Oncol 10:670

35. Henneman L, van Miltenburg MH, Michalak EM, Braumuller TM, Jaspers JE, Drenth AP et al (2015) Selective resistance to the PARP inhibitor olaparib in a mouse model for BRCA1-deficient metaplastic breast cancer. Proc Natl Acad Sci U S A 112(27):8409–8414

36. Lord CJ, Ashworth A (2013) Mechanisms of resistance to therapies targeting BRCA-mutant cancers. Nat Med 19(11):1381–1388

37. Pantelidou C, Sonzogni O, De Oliveria TM, Mehta AK, Kothari A, Wang D et al (2019) PARP inhibitor efficacy depends on CD8(+) T-cell recruitment via intratumoral STING pathway activation in BRCA-deficient models of triple-negative breast cancer. Cancer Discov 9(6):722–737

38. Yazinski SA, Comaills V, Buisson R, Genois MM, Nguyen HD, Ho CK et al (2017) ATR inhibition disrupts rewired homologous recombination and fork protection pathways in PARP inhibitor-resistant BRCA-deficient cancer cells. Genes Dev 31(3):318–332

39. Zatreanu D, Robinson HMR, Alkhatib O, Boursier M, Finch H, Geo L et al (2021) Pol-theta inhibitors elicit BRCA-gene synthetic lethality and target PARP inhibitor resistance. Nat Commun 12(1):3636

40. Zhou J, Gelot C, Pantelidou C, Li A, Yucel H, Davis RE et al (2021) A first-in-class polymerase theta inhibitor selectively targets homologous-recombination-deficient tumors. Nat Cancer. 2(6):598–610

41. Barazas M, Gasparini A, Huang Y, Kucukosmanoglu A, Annunziato S, Bouwman P et al (2019) Radiosensitivity is an acquired vulnerability of PARPi-resistant BRCA1-deficient tumors. Cancer Res 79(3):452–460

42. Gatenby RA, Brown J, Vincent T (2009) Lessons from applied ecology: cancer control using an evolutionary double bind. Cancer Res 69(19):7499–7502

43. Ruiz S, Mayor-Ruiz C, Lafarga V, Murga M, Vega-Sendino M, Ortega S et al (2016) A genome-wide CRISPR screen identifies CDC25A as a determinant of sensitivity to ATR inhibitors. Mol Cell 62(2):307–313

44. Brough R, Gulati A, Haider S, Kumar R, Campbell J, Knudsen E et al (2018) Identification of highly penetrant Rb-related synthetic lethal interactions in triple negative breast cancer. Oncogene 37(43):5701–5718

45. Oser MG, Fonseca R, Chakraborty AA, Brough R, Spektor A, Jennings RB et al (2018) Cells lacking the RB1 tumor suppressor gene are hyperdependent on aurora B kinase for survival. Cancer Discov 9(2):230–247

46. Li B, Gordon GM, Du CH, Xu J, Du W (2010) Specific killing of Rb mutant cancer cells by inactivating TSC2. Cancer Cell 17(5):469–480

47. Nittner D, Lambertz I, Clermont F, Mestdagh P, Köhler C, Nielsen SJ et al (2012) Synthetic lethality between Rb, p53 and Dicer or miR-17–92 in retinal progenitors suppresses retinoblastoma formation. Nat Cell Biol 14(9):958–965

48. Gong X, Du J, Parsons SH, Merzoug FF, Webster Y, Iversen PW et al (2019) Aurora A kinase inhibition is synthetic lethal with loss of the RB1 tumor suppressor gene. Cancer Discov 9(2):248–263

49. Dietlein F, Kalb B, Jokic M, Noll EM, Strong A, Tharun L et al (2015) A synergistic interaction between Chk1- and MK2 inhibitors in KRAS-mutant cancer. Cell 162(1):146–159

Mechanisms of PARP Inhibitor Resistance

3

Mark J. O'Connor and Josep V. Forment

3.1 Introduction

Poly(ADP-ribose) polymerase (PARP) inhibitors (PARPi) represent the first cancer medicines based on the targeting of the DNA Damage Response (DDR) and have transformed the therapeutic landscape for advanced ovarian cancer as well as expanding treatment options for other tumor types, including breast, pancreatic and prostate cancer. In spite of the success of PARPi, not all patients can gain clinical benefit from them, either because of primary resistance, or because of acquired resistance during treatment.

The mechanism of action of PARPi as single agents was originally described as a synthetic lethality (SL) relationship between mutations in the breast cancer susceptibility and tumour suppressor genes *BRCA1* and *BRCA2* (*BRCA* genes) when combined with the inhibition of PARP enzymes [1, 2]. Later, this SL relationship was extended to other genes that played a role in the homologous recombination repair (HRR) of DNA double-strand breaks (DSBs) [3]. Cancers that do not contain defined HRR deficiencies (HRD) are unlikely to respond well to single-agent PARPi in preclinical models [4] or as monotherapy in the clinic [5–8]. Thus, HRR proficiency (HRP), represents a primary mechanism of resistance to PARPi. While there have been a number of additional PARPi resistance mechanisms described over the last 15 years, it has emerged that the majority of those observed in clinical material, either samples analysed directly from patients or from patient-derived

M. J. O'Connor (✉) · J. V. Forment
Oncology R&D, AstraZeneca, Discovery Centre, Cambridge Biomedical Campus, 1 Francis Crick Avenue, Cambridge CB2 0AA, UK
e-mail: mark.j.oconnor@astrazeneca.com

J. V. Forment
e-mail: josep.forment@astrazeneca.com

  25
T. A. Yap and G. I. Shapiro (eds.), *Targeting the DNA Damage Response for Cancer Therapy*, Cancer Treatment and Research 186,
https://doi.org/10.1007/978-3-031-30065-3_3

tumour models, involve reactivation of HRR to some degree or other, leading to effective DNA DSB repair following PARPi treatment and consequently PARPi resistance.

3.2 Overview of PARP Inhibitor Mechanisms of Resistance

The first PARPi to be tested as monotherapy in *BRCA*-deficient cancer patients was olaparib [8] with the Phase 1 clinical trial initiated in 2005. The first mechanism of PARPi resistance published was in 2008 and this described the emergence of secondary mutations within the *BRCA* genes that led to a regain of function [9–11]. Since then, there have been a number of PARPi resistance mechanisms described (Fig. 3.1). These can be divided into those where the BRCA functionality (or HRR proficiency) status of the tumor cells is key in determining PARPi response, or those operating independently of HRR status. Not all of these proposed mechanisms of resistance have had the same level of validation, some being observed only in cancer cell lines *in vitro*, others also in patient-derived *in vivo* models, and only a small number identified in patient's tumour samples directly from the clinic. Here, we will focus primarily on mechanisms of resistance that modulate tumor BRCA/HRR status and are consistently observed clinically or in patient-derived xenograft (PDX) models in relevant disease settings.

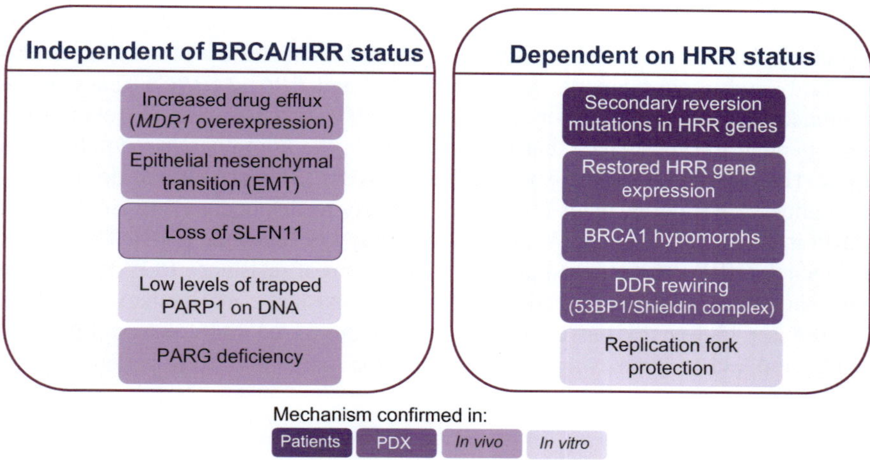

Fig. 3.1 Mechanisms of PARP inhibitor resistance can be divided into those that are independent of HRR status and those that are not. MDR (multi-drug resistance); HRR (homologous recombination repair); DDR (DNA damage response); PDX (Patient Derived eXplant *in vivo* models)

3.3 BRCA/HRR-Independent Mechanisms of PARPi Resistance

3.3.1 Increased P-glycoprotein Expression and Drug Efflux

Olaparib resistance was first observed in BRCA1 and BRCA2 knockout (KO) genetically engineered mouse models (GEMMs) after long-term treatment duration. Olaparib is a P-glycoprotein (P-gp) substrate and the mouse ATP-binding cassette (ABC) drug efflux transporter P-glycoprotein ABCB1, also known as MDR1 in humans, can be upregulated in response to drug treatment. Overexpression of P-gp was one of the earlier mechanisms of PARPi resistance to be described [12, 13]. Indeed, the propensity for this to drive olaparib resistance in these syngeneic mouse models effectively masked the ability to identify other mechanisms of PARPi resistance. The generation of AZD2461, an olaparib-related PARP1/ 2 inhibitor, that was not a substrate for P-gp [14], has facilitated the discovery of several additional potential routes by which PARPi resistance in BRCA1 and BRCA2 KO GEMMs can be generated, as described in the sections below.

Many drugs, including some PARPi, are ABC drug efflux substrates. Upregulation of MDR1 has been found in small numbers of chemotherapy-resistant and/ or PARPi-resistant high-grade serous ovarian cancer patient tumours [15, 16]. In the case of PARPi-resistant tumours, MDR1 overexpression was accompanied by other alterations linked to resistance [15] and as such, it is still not clear how clinically relevant this mechanism of PARPi resistance may be.

3.3.2 Epithelial-Mesenchymal Transition

Epithelial-mesenchymal transition (EMT), where epithelial cells lose their cell polarity and gain migratory and invasive properties, is essential for numerous developmental processes [17] but it is also associated with cancer metastasis and drug resistance [18]. Two independent studies using BRCA2 KO GEMMs identified EMT as being associated with PARPi resistance [19, 20]. In the first, a subset of mammary tumors generated in the *K14cre; Brca2; Tp53* KO mice were characterized as EMT-like sarcomatoid and were associated with multi-drug resistance, including to the PARPi olaparib. However, in this case, poor response was associated with high P-gp expression and could be overcome using a P-gp inhibitor in combination with olaparib [19]. In the second study, the use of the non-P-gp substrate PARPi AZD2461 in a *BlgCre Brca2/Tp53*-mutant mouse mammary model resulted in an increase in the proportion of metaplastic spindle cell carcinoma cells that was also associated with an increase in P-gp expression. However, the increase in P-gp was not the cause of resistance to PARPi, since there was no impact on tumour PARPi levels or the level of PARP1 PARylation inhibition in the resistant tumours. Moreover, in this study, there was also no observable downregulation of PARP1 levels or the re-establishment of DNA DSB repair by HRR associated with tumour outgrowth, suggesting PARPi resistance was likely a product of an as-yet unidentified mechanism associated with a rapid transition to the mesenchymal phenotype [20].

In addition to these two studies in GEMMs, a study in small-cell lung cancer PDX models and cell lines has also identified a link between EMT and PARPi resistance [21]. In the same study, high SLFN11 expression levels were associated with PARPi response and resistance with low levels of SLFN11.

3.3.3 Loss of SLFN11 Expression

A member of the schlaffen (SLFN) family of proteins, found only in mammals, SLFN11 is a putative nuclear DNA/RNA helicase, the expression level of which has one of the strongest genomic correlations with sensitivity to anti-replicative agents such as topotecan, etoposide, cisplatin and PARPi [22]. As indicated by its name (schlaffen is German for 'sleep'), SLFN11 enforces irreversible cell cycle arrest in S-phase upon the induction of DNA damage that can induce replication stress [22]. Under these circumstances SLFN11, recruited to chromatin by phospho-RPA, binds the extended single strand DNA that results following replication fork stalling, and arrests replication by blocking the replicative helicase complex. Loss of SLFN11 has been proposed to induce resistance to a variety of DNA damaging agents (but not radiation) as well as PARPi [23, 24], presumably by removing this important protective mechanism against genome instability [22]. The relevance of SLFN11 as a mechanism of resistance, both in PDX models and in the clinic, is still to be determined, since there was no obvious correlation with PARPi resistance in a large cohort of breast PDX models [24] and only a trend for the correlation of high SLFN11 expression with better progression-free survival (PFS) in an ovarian cancer maintenance trial where olaparib treatment was compared to placebo [25]. Further analyses of both the SLFN11 mechanism and importance as a biomarker of PARPi response are needed.

3.3.4 Low Levels of Trapped PARP1 on DNA

PARPi that demonstrate monotherapy activity in the clinic in HRD cancers, not only inhibit PARP enzymatic activity (inhibition of poly(ADP-ribose) (PAR) formation) but also physically trap PARP onto DNA [26]. The importance of PARP trapping as an integral component of PARPi activity has previously been described [27–29]. The implication is that the potential for PARPi-associated DNA replication fork stalling and DSB induction will be influenced by the number of PARP trapping events, which in turn could be determined by the cellular levels of PARP protein, the number of genomic DNA single-strand breaks (SSBs) and the ability of PARP protein to bind to them. This is supported by evidence that low levels of basal total or activated PARP1 (determined by either total PARP1 protein and/or PARP1 auto-PARylation) is associated with poor PARP inhibitor response

[30, 31]. Genetic backgrounds that can act as modifiers of PARPi response in HRD cancer cell backgrounds have been identified, a recent example being the loss of 2'-Deoxynucleoside 5'-Phosphate N-Hydrolase 1 (DNPH1), a hydrolase that removes a specific modified nucleotide, 5-hydroxymethyl-deoxyuridine monophosphate (hmdU), which when removed by the SMUG1 glycosylase results in increased DNA SSBs, PARP trapping and HRD cancer cell death [32]. It is therefore likely that the reverse is also true, and the loss of glycosylases that generate DNA SSBs, such as MUTYH, have been linked to a decrease in DNA SSB formation and PARP activation [33]. More recently, *in vitro* studies have shown that PARP1 mutant proteins that have lost their ability to bind DNA also confer resistance to PARPi [34, 35]. How frequently a reduction in PARP trapping is associated with PARPi response is difficult to gauge currently, since there is little in the way of clinical evidence for it.

3.3.5 PARG Deficiency

Poly(ADP-ribose) glycohydrolase (PARG) essentially catalyses the opposite reaction of PARPs (1 and 2) by degrading PAR chains [36]. PARG loss associated with PARPi resistance has been described in a BRCA2 KO GEMM model treated with AZD2461 [37]. Mechanistically, it has been shown that loss of PARG expression allows for some PARylation to occur even in the presence of PARPi, including PARP1 auto-PARylation, important to allow PARP1 dissociation from DNA facilitating DNA repair. Consequently, PARG deficiency led to reduced PARP1 trapping and DNA damage accumulation [37]. To date, there is little evidence that this mechanism represents an important one in the clinic.

3.4 BRCA/HRR-Dependent Mechanisms of PARPi Resistance

3.4.1 The Importance of Dynamic Markers of HRR Status

As described earlier, the primary driver of PARPi single agent sensitivity in a tumor is HRD and for innate resistance it is HRP. As we shall see from the examples below, current literature suggests that in most cases, acquired resistance will likely result from the reactivation of HRR and that there are multiple mechanisms by which this can occur. Moreover, reactivation of HRR can occur in the presence of the original *BRCA1*, *BRCA2* or non-*BRCA* HRR gene mutations or genomic 'scars' associated with HRD, making it difficult to predict the current HRR status in the tumour and therefore likely response to PARPi.

In order to overcome these limitations, there are current efforts to develop dynamic functional biomarkers of HRR status for use in the clinic. One such promising approach that has already been extremely useful in preclinical studies of PARPi resistance, is the quantification of the RAD51 protein in discrete, sub-nuclear structures termed "foci" by immunofluorescence (IF) microscopy [38,

39]. RAD51 is a key mediator of HRR and its recruitment to DNA damage sites by the complex of BRCA1-PALB2-BRCA2 proteins, is essential for effective repair of DNA DSBs by HRR (Fig. 3.2). This recruitment can be measured by IF using RAD51-specific antibodies on FFPE sections at baseline without the need to apply exogenous DNA damage to the samples, providing an indicator of HRR status—low RAD51 counts predicting HRD and better PARPi sensitivity than those with high RAD51 foci counts [38, 39] (Fig. 3.2). This greatly simplifies its application in clinical material and early comparisons with existing, less dynamic approaches for correlative potential with PARPi response are encouraging [40]. Although there is still some way to go before RAD51 IF assays can become straight forward in determining the HRR status of cancers to make treatment decisions, it has been demonstrated to be extremely effective in PDX models, where an impressive correlation with PARPi responses could be observed [4]. Although most of these analyses have been carried out in tumours of breast cancer origin, emerging data suggest that the same could be applied to tumours of prostate [41] or ovarian origin [42]. Restoration of RAD51 foci formation, and HRP as a key mechanism of acquired PARPi resistance in the clinic, has still to be fully addressed (primarily due to the challenges of accessing post-PARPi treated tumour biopsies). There have been reports of restoration of RAD51 foci in breast cancer tumours collected on PARPi and platinum agent progression [43]. In this section, the use of RAD51 foci analysis has facilitated our understanding of how different mechanisms can lead to HRR reactivation and PARPi resistance.

3.4.2 Secondary Reversion Mutations in HRR Genes

Sensitivity to PARPi due to mutations in HRR genes can be reversed if secondary mutations occur within the mutated gene in a manner that restores function (the so-called reversion mutations, see Fig. 3.3) and were one of the earliest mechanisms of PARPi and/or platinum resistance described [9–11]. Most of the information on reversion mutations come from the study of germline *BRCA* gene mutations, which are mostly missense or nonsense mutations or small insertions-deletions that lead to frameshifts and premature STOP codons. This likely explains the prevalence of reversion mutations as a mechanism of resistance since they can either delete or reverse the original mutation to either partially, or fully, restore BRCA function. Consistent with this, reversion mutations have been shown to restore RAD51 foci formation [43].

Since those first descriptions of revertant mutations, BRCA reversions have been identified in many tumours from patients progressing on PARPi treatment in all of the disease settings where PARPi are approved, making this the only clinically validated mechanism of resistance to PARPi described to date [44, 45]. Given that ovarian cancer is where PARPi have been approved the longest, it is not surprising that the majority of reversions have been identified in this disease setting, where they account for approximately 25% of the cases of progression after platinum or PARPi treatment [45]. Interestingly, a study of long-term patient

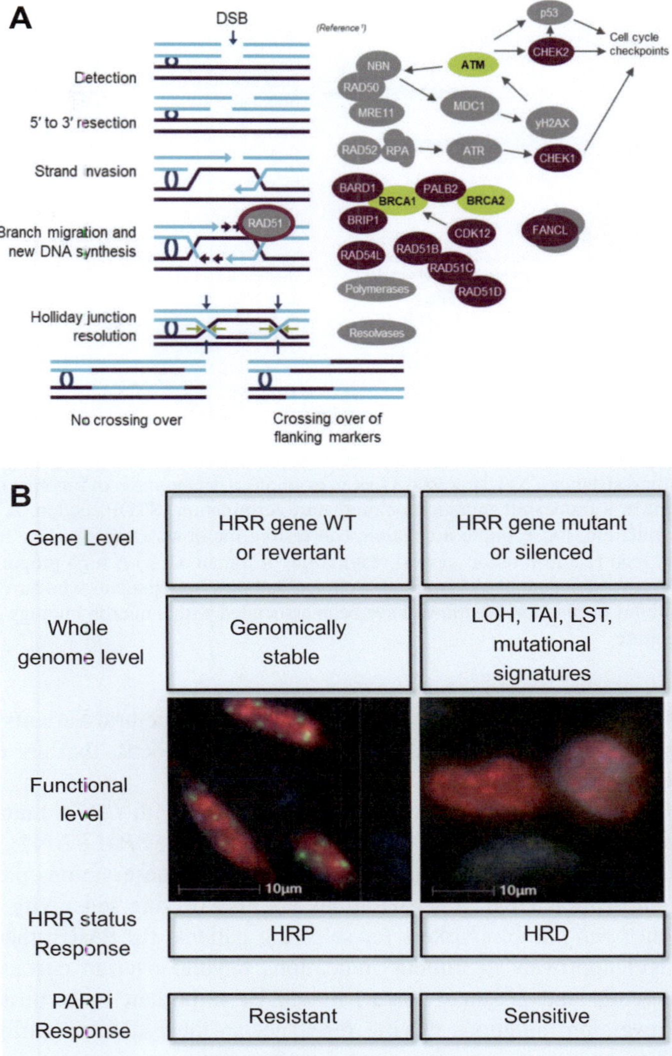

Fig. 3.2 RAD51 is a key mediator of HRR, and detection of foci is an indicator of functionality and PARP inhibitor response (A) Schematic of the different stages of homologous recombination repair (HRR) and the proteins involved in this mechanism of DNA double strand break (DSB) repair. (B) HRR pathway status can be assessed at multiple levels from gene sequencing to measuring genomic rearrangements but quantification of nuclear RAD51 foci in S/G2 phase cells is a representation of HRR functionality and likely response to PARP inhibitors

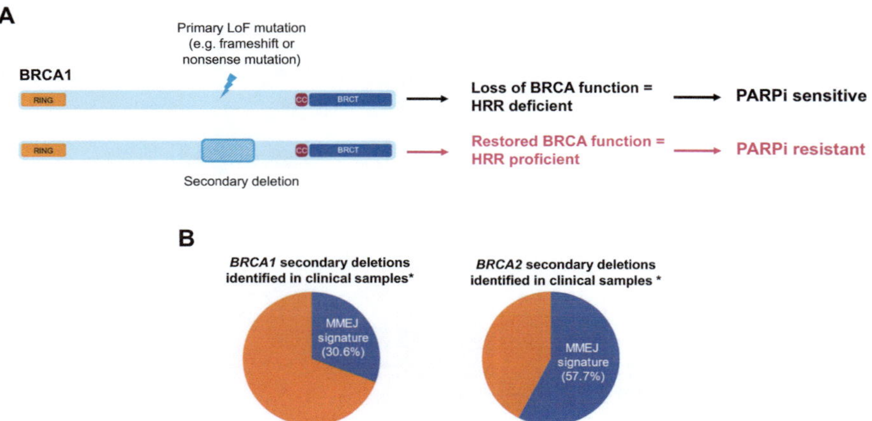

Fig. 3.3 Secondary reversion mutations of BRCA genes restore BRCA functionality and lead to PARP inhibitor resistance. (A) Using *BRCA1* as an example, a primary loss of function (LoF) mutation can result in a frameshift mutation or premature termination (STOP) codon. A subsequent (secondary) mutation, for example a deletion, can restore the downstream reading frame of the gene and may lead to a restoration, or part restoration, of function. (B) A high proportion of secondary BRCA reversion mutations identified in clinical samples from patients who have progressed on PARP inhibitor or platinum treatment have been associated with a microhomology end-joining (MMEJ) signature

responders to PARPi has identified the enrichment of structural variants of *BRCA* mutations, such as homozygous deletions of the entire locus, that are inherently incapable of undergoing reversion [46].

Reversions have not only been detected in tumours with *BRCA* mutations but also in tumours with mutations in other HRR genes such as *PALB2* [47], *RAD51C* and *RAD51D* [48] (Fig. 3.2). It can be argued that these observations provide evidence that non-*BRCA* HRR gene mutations are also driving sensitivity to PARPi and represent *bona fide* biomarkers for selecting patients for PARPi therapy. Following PARPi approvals in tumour indications beyond ovarian cancer, namely, breast, pancreatic and prostate cancer, it will be important to confirm the frequency of reversion mutations driving resistance in these disease settings. Since these reversion mutations are often found at low allelic frequencies in all disease settings, understanding the true prevalence of HRR gene reversions is likely to be dependent on the use of advances in DNA sequencing quality and depth, using non-invasive methods to follow cancer progression, such as liquid biopsies [49].

Recently, an important insight into the mechanism by which HRR gene reversions may arise has been described [44, 45]. The detailed analyses of a large number of clinical tumor sample reversion events, highlighted that most amino acid sequences encoded by exon 11 in *BRCA1* and *BRCA2* are dispensable to generate resistance to platinum or PARPi, whereas other regions were more refractory to sizeable amino acid losses. Importantly, these findings highlighted the role of mutagenic micro-homology end-joining (MMEJ) repair in generating reversions, especially in those in the *BRCA2* gene, where just under 60% of the reversion mutations were associated with microhomologies with around 30% being observed in the *BRCA1* gene [45] (see Fig. 3.3).

3.4.3 Restoration of HRR Gene Expression

HRR gene silencing resulting from promoter hypermethylation has previously been described for *BRCA1* and *RAD51C* in ovarian and breast tumours [50] and is associated with HRD [51] and PARPi sensitivity [52, 53]. In addition, a recently published study has highlighted XRCC3 deficiency as a driver of PARPi sensitivity and that in prostate cancer there is evidence for a high incidence of gene silencing due to promoter methylation [54].

A potential mechanism of resistance to PARPi in these tumours would be the reactivation of gene expression through loss of promoter hypermethylation. Indeed, analyses of paired biopsies pre- and post-platinum progression of ovarian cancer have shown that loss of silencing of BRCA1 is linked to platinum resistance [16]. No such correlation has yet been established in post-PARPi clinical progressions, but there have been several cases of acquired PARPi resistance in PDX models of breast [38, 55] and ovarian [56] cancer where this has been observed, with restored BRCA1 expression correlating with regained ability of the tumour to form RAD51 foci [38]. In addition to the demethylation of the previously silenced *BRCA1* gene promoter as a cause of re-expression, it has also been observed that gene fusions placing *BRCA1* under the transcriptional control of a heterologous promoter can restore expression and the acquisition of PARPi resistance [56].

3.4.4 Expression of BRCA1 Hypomorphs

A hypomorph is a gene or protein variant with partial activity compared with the corresponding wild-type version. In the case of BRCA1, there is evidence that BRCA1 hypomorphic proteins may increase cancer risk following loss of the wild type allele and these have been characterized and shown to have one or more entire domains missing [57–61] (see Fig. 3.4). BRCA1 has a complex and multi-faceted role within HRR and has several well-defined functions that contribute towards overall proficiency [62], although the coiled-coil domain that facilitates the interaction between BRCA1 and PALB2, and therefore RAD51 loading onto DNA, appears to be the most critical for HRR-dependent DNA DSB repair. In contrast, loss of the BRCA1 RING domain and exon 11 are defective for the fork protection role of BRCA1 but retain the ability to provide residual HRR and can play a role in PARPi resistance. Some BRCA1 missense mutations have been shown to produce full-length proteins but with hypomorphic activity, such as the BRCA1^{C61G} mutant that lacks a functional RING domain. This hypomorph is associated with an increased risk of breast and ovarian cancer and normally confers PARPi sensitivity. However, over-expression of this hypomorph results

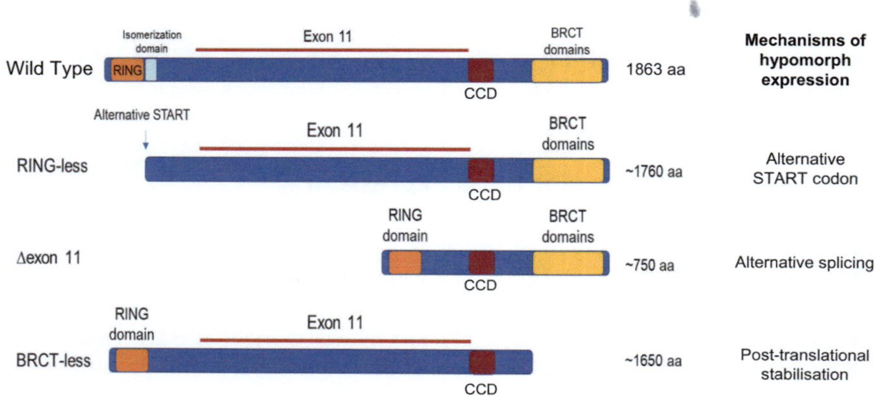

Fig. 3.4 BRCA hypomorph expression can provide resistance to PARP inhibitors. Both the BRCA1 (shown here) and BRCA2 proteins contain multiple domains involved in various aspects of DNA double strand break (DSB) repair and replication fork biology. BRCA hypomorphs either consist of protein truncations or domain function mutations that lead to sub-optimal functionality compared to wild type protein. Hypomorphs are associated with increased cancer risk but can retain sufficient DSB repair function to confer PARP inhibitor resistance. The different domains highlighted are the RING (E3-ubiquitin ligase interaction), CCD (coiled-coil for PALB2/RAD51 binding) and BRCT (for phospho-peptide, DNA and PAR binding)

in PARPi resistance [63]. In situations where the BRCA1 hypomorphic mutant protein is not expressed at high enough levels to confer HRR activity, secondary mutations that restore the reading frame and expression of the full-length protein could promote PARPi resistance [64]. There are fewer reports on the existence of BRCA2 hypomorphs and the limited number of studies linking them to resistance are only from *in vitro* settings [65].

Although initially BRCA1 hypomorphs were only described *in vitro*, there are now several reports of their identification in PARPi-resistant PDX models, where they occur at high frequency and are linked to the restoration of RAD51 foci [38, 39]. There is a need to develop capabilities to detect the various BRCA1 hypomorphs in patient samples as well as testing in preclinical models the levels of PARPi resistance that can be achieved *in vivo* by expressing these hypomorphs. Emerging data suggest in fact that the ectopic overexpression of truncated BRCA1 proteins only provides partial or low levels of HRR and PARPi resistance. Thus, BRCA1 hypomorphs may promote more robust PARPi resistance when in combination with additional events. Consistent with this is the observation that reductions in 53BP1 protein levels have been seen in conjunction with BRCA1 hypomorph expression [61, 62].

3.4.5 DDR Re-wiring to Promote End-Resection and HRR

In the previous sections, we have described the mechanisms of PARPi resistance that led to reactivation of HRR and the presence of basal RAD51 foci by altering the *BRCA* genes and/or the levels of expression of BRCA proteins. These paths to PARPi resistance represent the majority of observed cases, at least in PDX models. However, alternative ways to regaining HRR proficiency, specifically in *BRCA1* mutated cancer cells, have been described that do not affect the original *BRCA1* mutant status of the cell. The best studied mechanism involves the loss of the TP53BP1 (53BP1) protein and the 53BP1-RIF1-shieldin complex. While BRCA1 promotes processing of DNA DSBs, the 53BP1-RIF1-shieldin complex inhibits it (Fig. 3.5, reviewed in [66]). Loss of 53BP1 as a mechanism of PARPi resistance was first described in a *Brca1* mutant mouse knockout model [67], but since then there have been a plethora of examples where loss of the 53BP1-RIF1-shieldin complex components results in restoration of RAD51 foci formation and reactivation of HRR in the absence of fully functional BRCA1 protein [68–70]. To date, only 53BP1 loss has been identified in a clinical sample [43] and, since all of these examples have been identified in breast cancer, it will be important to understand their prevalence in other disease settings and the clinical relevance of the other components of the 53BP1-RIF1-shieldin complex, other than 53BP1 itself and in backgrounds beyond *BRCA1* mutated tumors [70].

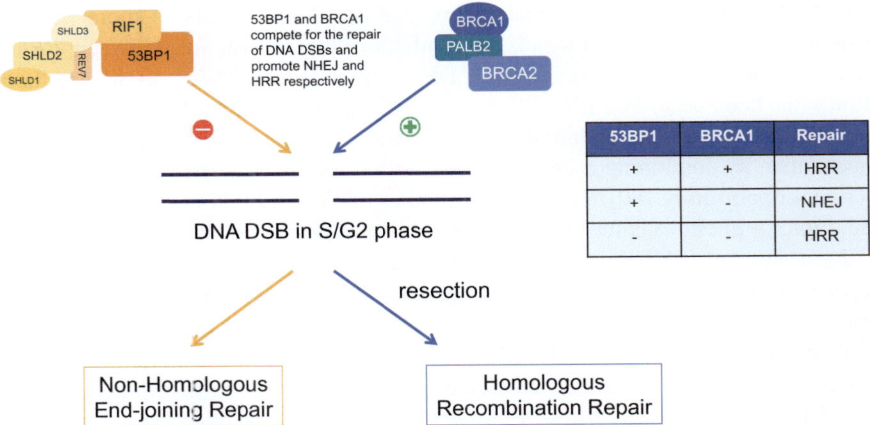

53BP1	BRCA1	Repair
+	+	HRR
+	-	NHEJ
-	-	HRR

Fig. 3.5 The BRCA1/PALB2/BRCA2 and 53BP1/RIF1/SHLD complexes compete to decide which DNA DSB repair pathway is utilized. BRCA1 and 53BP! Compete for the repair of DNA double strand breaks (DSBs). In the presence of both complexes BRCA1 will drive the resection of the DNA DSB end to facilitate RAD51 binding and homologous recombination repair (HRR). In the absence of BRCA1, 53BP1 will initiate Non-homologous end-joining (NHEJ). Even in the presence of BRCA1 deficiency, the loss of any of the 53BP1 RIF1 SHLD complex can result in HRR, thus providing a mechanism of PARP inhibitor resistance

3.4.6 Restoration of Replication Fork Protection

BRCA proteins play a role in DNA replication fork protection (RFP) that prevents stalled and regressed replication forks from being degraded by the action of DNA nucleases [71]. This activity is independent of their canonical roles in HRR as shown by the existence of separation of function mutants [71–73]. As such, deficiency in the recruitment of these nucleases to stalled replication forks, or defective remodelling of the forks that is required for their processing, have been shown to cause a moderate level of PARPi resistance in BRCA mutant cell lines [74]. However, the relevance of restoration of RFP acting as a driver of PARPi resistance is potentially in question based on two observations. Firstly, separation of function mutations in BRCA1 [75] or BRCA2 [71] that affect their RFP function, still leave their HRR role intact and do not confer sensitivity to PARPi. Secondly, the loss of 53BP1, that causes PARPi resistance in *BRCA1* mutant settings, restores RAD51 foci formation and HRR but not RFP [74]. Since this putative mechanism of resistance has only been described *in vitro*, we will have to wait for further evidence from *in vivo* data to be able to assess its likely importance in clinical settings.

3.5 Strategies to Overcome PARP Inhibitor Resistance

PARPi, particularly in earlier lines of therapy, are providing significant benefit to patients [26]. Although many tumours eventually develop PARPi resistance, current data support the idea that earlier use of PARPi results in more durable responses [76, 77]. More recently, a synthetic lethal interaction between *BRCA* mutations and loss of the key MMEJ DNA repair factor DNA polymerase theta (Polθ) has been described [78, 79]. Given the importance of MMEJ in the generation of *BRCA* reversion mutations, the potential to delay or prevent this resistance mechanism by combining a Polθ inhibitor with a PARPi in earlier lines of therapy is a real opportunity [80]. There are a number of Polθ inhibitors either already in the clinic or about to enter the clinic, so this concept can be tested.

In a number of the scenarios involving mechanisms of PARPi resistance described in this chapter, the underlying mutations in *BRCA* or other HRR genes remain. Even in those situations where in *BRCA* mutated cancers, there has been sufficient HRR reactivated with the associated detection of RAD51, there remains a deficiency in RFP and a dependency on replication stress proteins such as ATR and WEE1 [81]. There are now a number of preclinical studies where combining either ATR or WEE1 inhibitors with PARPi results in the re-sensitization of PARPi resistant tumors [82–84]. Moreover, emerging data from clinical trials suggests there is a real opportunity for these combinations in clinical settings [85, 86].

In addition, combinations with targeted therapies that can enhance the number of DNA SSBs and provide tumor selective increases in cell kill offer opportunities to enhance both activity and the therapeutic window of PARPi. One such exciting example of this is the inhibition of DNPH1, a nucleotide sanitizer that normally prevents incorporation of hmdU during replication and the inhibition of which leads to glycosylase-mediated generation of DNA SSBs. DNPH1 was identified in a synthetic lethal screen with olaparib and its inhibition shown to potentiate PARPi activity specifically in HRD cancer cell backgrounds. Moreover, inhibition of DNPH1 and increased hmdU when combined with olaparib resulted in the ability to overcome 53BP1 loss, associated with PARPi resistance in a *BRCA1* mutated cell line model [32].

3.6 Conclusions

PARPi represent a new approach to the treatment of cancers harboring HRD. Inevitably, we are now seeing emerging resistance to this targeted therapy. However, our increased understanding of the mechanisms of PARPi resistance in the clinic means there are now a growing number of approaches in which this resistance can be addressed. The wide range of PARPi resistance mechanisms described in pre-clinical models is not matched by our understanding of how relevant many of these models are in the clinic, since actual clinical data are relatively scarce. To date, most clinical data confirm the prevalence of reversion mutations as a primary driver of PARPi failure. The lack of clinical data highlight the need to evaluate PARPi resistance in post-PARPi tumour biopsies. One way to do this would be to increase the number of clinical trials in the post-PARPi patient population with mandatory biopsies on enrolment, as it will be key to have a dynamic measure of the tumour HRD status at the time of treatment to provide the best therapeutic options going forward. In addition, this will have the benefit of revealing the true diversity of resistance mechanisms in patients. Access to such samples, together with improvements on sensitivity of new technologies such as DNA sequencing in both solid and liquid biopsies and non-genetic methods of detection of resistance, such as protein biomarkers or promoter methylation status, will help direct the focus of pre-clinical and drug development efforts on the most clinically relevant PARPi resistance mechanisms.

References

1. Farmer H, McCabe N, Lord CJ, Tutt ANJ, Johnson DA, Richardson TB et al (2005) Targeting the DNA repair defect in BRCA mutant cells as a therapeutic strategy. Nature 434:917. https://doi.org/10.1038/nature03445 https://www.nature.com/articles/nature03445#supplementary-information
2. Bryant HE, Schultz N, Thomas HD, Parker KM, Flower D, Lopez E et al (2005) Specific killing of BRCA2-deficient tumours with inhibitors of poly(ADP-ribose) polymerase. Nature 434:913. https://doi.org/10.1038/nature03443 https://www.nature.com/articles/nature03443#supplementary-information
3. McCabe N, Turner NC, Lord CJ, Kluzek K, Białkowska A, Swift S et al (2006) Deficiency in the repair of DNA damage by homologous recombination and sensitivity to poly(ADP-Ribose) polymerase inhibition. Can Res 66(16):8109–8115. https://doi.org/10.1158/0008-5472.Can-06-0140

4. Pellegrino B, Herencia-Ropero A, Llop-Guevara A, Pedretti F, Moles-Fernández A, Viaplana C et al (2022) Preclinical in vivo validation of the RAD51 test for identification of homologous recombination-deficient tumors and patient stratification. Can Res 82(8):1646–1657. https://doi.org/10.1158/0008-5472.CAN-21-2409

5. Pujade-Lauraine E, Ledermann JA, Selle F, Gebski V, Penson RT, Oza AM et al (2017) Olaparib tablets as maintenance therapy in patients with platinum-sensitive, relapsed ovarian cancer and a BRCA1/2 mutation (SOLO2/ENGOT-Ov21): a double-blind, randomised, placebo-controlled, phase 3 trial. Lancet Oncol 18(9):1274–1284. https://doi.org/10.1016/S1470-204 5(17)30469-2

6. Coleman RL, Oza AM, Lorusso D, Aghajanian C, Oaknin A, Dean A et al (2017) Rucaparib maintenance treatment for recurrent ovarian carcinoma after response to platinum therapy (ARIEL3): a randomised, double-blind, placebo-controlled, phase 3 trial. Lancet 390(10106):1949–1961. https://doi.org/10.1016/S0140-6736(17)32440-6

7. Mirza MR, Monk BJ, Herrstedt J, Oza AM, Mahner S, Redondo A et al (2016) Niraparib maintenance therapy in platinum-sensitive, recurrent ovarian cancer. N Engl J Med 375(22):2154–2164. https://doi.org/10.1056/NEJMoa1611310

8. Fong PC, Boss DS, Yap TA, Tutt A, Wu P, Mergui-Roelvink M et al (2009) Inhibition of poly(ADP-Ribose) polymerase in tumors from BRCA mutation carriers. N Engl J Med 361(2):123–134. https://doi.org/10.1056/NEJMoa0900212

9. Edwards SL, Brough R, Lord CJ, Natrajan R, Vatcheva R, Levine DA et al (2008) Resistance to therapy caused by intragenic deletion in BRCA2. Nature 451:1111. https://doi.org/10.1038/nature06548 https://www.nature.com/articles/nature06548#supplementary-information

10. Swisher EM, Sakai W, Karlan BY, Wurz K, Urban N, Taniguchi T (2008) Secondary BRCA1 mutations in BRCA1-mutated ovarian carcinomas with platinum resistance. Cancer Res 68(8):2581–2586. https://doi.org/10.1158/0008-5472.CAN-08-0088

11. Sakai W, Swisher EM, Karlan BY, Agarwal MK, Higgins J, Friedman C et al (2008) Secondary mutations as a mechanism of cisplatin resistance in BRCA2-mutated cancers. Nature 451:1116. https://doi.org/10.1038/nature06633 https://www.nature.com/articles/nature06633#supplementary-information

12. Rottenberg S, Jaspers JE, Kersbergen A, van der Burg E, Nygren AOH, Zander SAL et al (2008) High sensitivity of BRCA1-deficient mammary tumors to the PARP inhibitor AZD2281 alone and in combination with platinum drugs. Proc Natl Acad Sci 105(44):17079–17084. https://doi.org/10.1073/pnas.0806092105

13. Hay T, Matthews JR, Pietzka L, Lau A, Cranston A, Nygren AOH et al (2009) Poly(ADP-Ribose) polymerase-1 inhibitor treatment regresses autochthonous Brca2/p53-mutant mammary tumors in vivo and delays tumor relapse in combination with carboplatin. Can Res 69(9):3850–3855. https://doi.org/10.1158/0008-5472.CAN-08-2388

14. Oplustil O'Connor L, Rulten SL, Cranston AN, Odedra R, Brown H, Jaspers JE et al (2016) The PARP inhibitor AZD2461 provides insights into the role of PARP3 inhibition for both synthetic lethality and tolerability with chemotherapy in preclinical models. Cancer Res 76(20):6084–6094. https://doi.org/10.1158/0008-5472.CAN-15-3240

15. Lheureux S, Oaknin A, Garg S, Bruce JP, Madariaga A, Dhani NC et al (2020) EVOLVE: a multicenter open-label single-arm clinical and translational Phase II trial of cediranib plus olaparib for ovarian cancer after PARP inhibition progression. Clin Cancer Res 26(16):4206–4215. https://doi.org/10.1158/1078-0432.CCR-19-4121%JClinicalCancerResearch

16. Patch A-M, Christie EL, Etemadmoghadam D, Garsed DW, George J, Fereday S et al (2015) Whole–genome characterization of chemoresistant ovarian cancer. Nature 521:489. https://doi.org/10.1038/nature14410 https://www.nature.com/articles/nature14410#supplementary-information

17. Lamouille S, Xu J, Derynck R (2014) Molecular mechanisms of epithelial–mesenchymal transition. Nat Rev Mol Cell Biol 15(3):178–196. https://doi.org/10.1038/nrm3758

18. Singh A, Settleman J (2010) EMT, cancer stem cells and drug resistance: an emerging axis of evil in the war on cancer. Oncogene 29(34):4741–4751. https://doi.org/10.1038/onc.2010.215

19. Jaspers JE, Sol W, Kersbergen A, Schlicker A, Guyader C, Xu G et al (2015) BRCA2-deficient Sarcomatoid mammary tumors exhibit multidrug resistance. Cancer Res 75(4):732–741. https://doi.org/10.1158/0008-5472.CAN-14-0839%JCancerResearch

20. Ordonez LD, Hay T, McEwen R, Polanska UM, Hughes A, Delpuech O et al (2019) Rapid activation of epithelial-mesenchymal transition drives PARP inhibitor resistance in Brca2 -mutant mammary tumours. Oncotarget 10(27)

21. Allison Stewart C, Tong P, Cardnell RJ, Sen T, Li L, Gay CM et al (2017) Dynamic variations in epithelial-to-mesenchymal transition (EMT), ATM, and SLFN11 govern response to PARP inhibitors and cisplatin in small cell lung cancer. Oncotarget 8(17):28575–28587. https://doi.org/10.18632/oncotarget.15338

22. Zoppoli G, Regairaz M, Leo E, Reinhold WC, Varma S, Ballestrero A et al (2012) Putative DNA/RNA helicase Schlafen-11 (SLFN11) sensitizes cancer cells to DNA-damaging agents. Proc Natl Acad Sci U S A. 201205943. https://doi.org/10.1073/pnas.1205943109

23. Murai J, Tang S-W, Leo E, Baechler SA, Redon CE, Zhang H et al (2018) SLFN11 blocks stressed replication forks independently of ATR. Mol Cell 69(3):371–84.e6. https://doi.org/10.1016/j.molcel.2018.01.012

24. Winkler C, Armenia J, Jones GN, Tobalina L, Sale MJ, Petreus T et al (2021) SLFN11 informs on standard of care and novel treatments in a wide range of cancer models. Br J Cancer 124(5):951–962. https://doi.org/10.1038/s41416-020-01199-4

25. Willis SE, Winkler C, Roudier MP, Baird T, Marco-Casanova P, Jones EV et al (2021) Retrospective analysis of Schlafen11 (SLFN11) to predict the outcomes to therapies affecting the DNA damage response. Br J Cancer 125(12):1666–1676. https://doi.org/10.1038/s41416-021-01560-1

26. Pilié PG, Tang C, Mills GB, Yap TA (2019) State-of-the-art strategies for targeting the DNA damage response in cancer. Nat Rev Clin Oncol 16(2):81–104. https://doi.org/10.1038/s41571-018-0114-z

27. Murai J, Huang S-yN, Das BB, Renaud A, Zhang Y, Doroshow JH et al (2012) Trapping of PARP1 and PARP2 by clinical PARP inhibitors. Cancer Res 72(21):5588–99. https://doi.org/10.1158/0008-5472.CAN-12-2753

28. Maede Y, Shimizu H, Fukushima T, Kogame T, Nakamura T, Miki T et al (2014) Differential and common DNA repair pathways for topoisomerase I- and II-targeted drugs in a genetic DT40 repair cell screen panel. Mol Cancer Ther 13(1):214–220. https://doi.org/10.1158/1535-7163.Mct-13-0551

29. Pommier Y, O'Connor MJ, de Bono J (2016) Laying a trap to kill cancer cells: PARP inhibitors and their mechanisms of action. Sci Transl Med 8(362):362ps17. https://doi.org/10.1126/scitranslmed.aaf9246

30. Oplustilova L, Wolanin K, Mistrik M, Korinkova G, Simkova D, Bouchal J et al (2012) Evaluation of candidate biomarkers to predict cancer cell sensitivity or resistance to PARP-1 inhibitor treatment. Cell Cycle 11(20):3837–3850. https://doi.org/10.4161/cc.22026

31. Pettitt SJ, Rehman FL, Bajrami I, Brough R, Wallberg F, Kozarewa I et al (2013) A genetic screen using the PiggyBac transposon in haploid cells identifies PARP1 as a mediator of olaparib toxicity. PLoS ONE 8(4):e61520. https://doi.org/10.1371/journal.pone.0061520

32. Fugger K, Bajrami I, Silva Dos Santos M, Young SJ, Kunzelmann S, Kelly G et al (2021) Targeting the nucleotide salvage factor DNPH1 sensitizes BRCA-deficient cells to PARP inhibitors. Science 372(6538):156–65. https://doi.org/10.1126/science.abb4542

33. Oka S, Ohno M, Tsuchimoto D, Sakumi K, Furuichi M, Nakabeppu Y (2008) Two distinct pathways of cell death triggered by oxidative damage to nuclear and mitochondrial DNAs. EMBO J 27(2):421–432. https://doi.org/10.1038/sj.emboj.7601975

34. Pettitt SJ, Krastev DB, Brandsma I, Dréan A, Song F, Aleksandrov R et al (2018) Genome-wide and high-density CRISPR-Cas9 screens identify point mutations in PARP1 causing PARP inhibitor resistance. Nat Commun 9(1):1849. https://doi.org/10.1038/s41467-018-03917-2

35. Herzog M, Puddu F, Coates J, Geisler N, Forment JV, Jackson SP (2018) Detection of functional protein domains by unbiased genome-wide forward genetic screening. Sci Rep 8(1):6161. https://doi.org/10.1038/s41598-018-24400-4

36. Pascal JM, Ellenberger T (2015) The rise and fall of poly(ADP-ribose): an enzymatic perspective. DNA Repair 32:10–16. https://doi.org/10.1016/j.dnarep.2015.04.008
37. Gogola E, Duarte AA, de Ruiter JR, Wiegant WW, Schmid JA, de Bruijn R et al (2018) Selective loss of PARG restores parylation and counteracts PARP inhibitor-mediated synthetic lethality. Cancer Cell 33(6):1078–93 e12. https://doi.org/10.1016/j.ccell.2018.05.008
38. Castroviejo-Bermejo M, Cruz C, Llop-Guevara A, Gutiérrez-Enríquez S, Ducy M, Ibrahim YH et al (2018) A RAD51 assay feasible in routine tumor samples calls PARP inhibitor response beyond BRCA mutation. EMBO Mol Med. https://doi.org/10.15252/emmm.201809172
39. Cruz C, Castroviejo-Bermejo M, Gutiérrez-Enríquez S, Llop-Guevara A, Ibrahim YH, Gris-Oliver A et al (2018) RAD51 foci as a functional biomarker of homologous recombination repair and PARP inhibitor resistance in germline BRCA-mutated breast cancer. Ann Oncol mdy099-mdy. https://doi.org/10.1093/annonc/mdy099
40. Eikesdal HP, Yndestad S, Elzawahry A, Llop-Guevara A, Gilje B, Blix ES et al (2021) Olaparib monotherapy as primary treatment in unselected triple negative breast cancer. Ann Oncol 32(2):240–249. https://doi.org/10.1016/j.annonc.2020.11.009
41. Carreira S, Porta N, Arce-Gallego S, Seed G, Llop-Guevara A, Bianchini D et al (2021) Biomarkers associating with PARP inhibitor benefit in prostate cancer in the TOPARP-B Trial. Cancer Discov. https://doi.org/10.1158/2159-8290.CD-21-0007
42. Guffanti F, Alvisi MF, Anastasia A, Ricci F, Chiappa M, Llop-Guevara A et al (2021) Basal expression of RAD51 foci predicts olaparib response in patient-derived ovarian cancer xenografts. Br J Cancer. https://doi.org/10.1038/s41416-021-01609-1
43. Waks AG, Cohen O, Kochupurakkal B, Kim D, Dunn CE, Buendia Buendia J et al (2020) Reversion and non-reversion mechanisms of resistance to PARP inhibitor or platinum chemotherapy in BRCA1/2-mutant metastatic breast cancer. Ann Oncol. https://doi.org/10.1016/j.annonc.2020.02.008
44. Pettitt SJ, Frankum JR, Punta M, Lise S, Alexander J, Chen Y et al (2020) Clinical BRCA1/2 reversion analysis identifies hotspot mutations and predicted neoantigens associated with therapy resistance. Cancer Discov. https://doi.org/10.1158/2159-8290.CD-19-1485
45. Tobalina L, Armenia J, Irving E, O'Connor MJ, Forment JV (2021) A meta-analysis of reversion mutations in BRCA genes identifies signatures of DNA end-joining repair mechanisms driving therapy resistance. Ann Oncol 32(1):103–112. https://doi.org/10.1016/j.annonc.2020.10.470
46. Swisher EM, Kristeleit RS, Oza AM, Tinker AV, Ray-Coquard I, Oaknin A et al (2021) Characterization of patients with long-term responses to rucaparib treatment in recurrent ovarian cancer. Gynecol Oncol. https://doi.org/10.1016/j.ygyno.2021.08.030
47. Goodall J, Mateo J, Yuan W, Mossop H, Porta N, Miranda S et al (2017) Circulating cell-free DNA to guide prostate cancer treatment with PARP inhibition. Cancer Discov 7(9):1006–1017. https://doi.org/10.1158/2159-8290.cd-17-0261
48. Kondrashova O, Nguyen M, Shield-Artin K, Tinker AV, Teng NNH, Harrell MI et al (2017) Secondary somatic mutations restoring RAD51C and RAD51D associated with acquired resistance to the PARP inhibitor rucaparib in high-grade ovarian carcinoma. Cancer Discov 7(9):984–998. https://doi.org/10.1158/2159-8290.cd-17-0419
49. Siravegna G, Mussolin B, Venesio T, Marsoni S, Seoane J, Dive C et al (2019) How liquid biopsies can change clinical practice in oncology. Ann Oncol 30(10):1580–1590. https://doi.org/10.1093/annonc/mdz227
50. Knijnenburg TA, Wang L, Zimmermann MT, Chambwe N, Gao GF, Cherniack AD et al (2018) Genomic and molecular landscape of DNA damage repair deficiency across the cancer genome atlas. Cell Rep 23(1):239–54.e6. https://doi.org/10.1016/j.celrep.2018.03.076
51. Min A, Kim K, Jeong K, Choi S, Kim S, Suh KJ et al (2020) Homologous repair deficiency score for identifying breast cancers with defective DNA damage response. Sci Rep 10(1):12506. https://doi.org/10.1038/s41598-020-68176-y
52. Min A, Im S-A, Yoon Y-K, Song S-H, Nam H-J, Hur H-S et al (2013) RAD51C-deficient cancer cells are highly sensitive to the PARP inhibitor olaparib. Mol Cancer Ther 12(6):865–877. https://doi.org/10.1158/1535-7163.MCT-12-0950

53. Kondrashova O, Topp M, Nesic K, Lieschke E, Ho G-Y, Harrell MI et al (2018) Methylation of all BRCA1 copies predicts response to the PARP inhibitor rucaparib in ovarian carcinoma. Nat Commun 9(1):3970. https://doi.org/10.1038/s41467-018-05564-z

54. Jamal K, Galbiati A, Armenia J, Illuzzi G, Hall J, Bentouati S et al (2022) Drug–gene interaction screens coupled to tumor data analyses identify the most clinically relevant cancer vulnerabilities driving sensitivity to PARP inhibition. Cancer Res Commun 2(10):1244–1254. https://doi.org/10.1158/2767-9764.CRC-22-0119

55. ter Brugge P, Kristel P, van der Burg E, Boon U, de Maaker M, Lips E et al (2016) Mechanisms of therapy resistance in patient-derived xenograft models of BRCA1-deficient breast cancer. JNCI: J Natl Cancer Inst 108(11). https://doi.org/10.1093/jnci/djw148

56. Hurley RM, McGehee CD, Nesic K, Correia C, Weiskittel Taylor M, Kelly Rebecca L et al (2021) Characterization of a RAD51C-silenced high-grade serous ovarian cancer model during development of PARP inhibitor resistance. NAR Cancer 3(3). https://doi.org/10.1093/narcan/zcab028

57. Wang Y, Krais JJ, Bernhardy AJ, Nicolas E, Cai KQ, Harrell MI et al (2016) RING domain–deficient BRCA1 promotes PARP inhibitor and platinum resistance. J Clin Investig 126(8):3145–3157. https://doi.org/10.1172/JCI87033

58. Wang Y, Bernhardy AJ, Nacson J, Krais JJ, Tan Y-F, Nicolas E et al (2019) BRCA1 intronic Alu elements drive gene rearrangements and PARP inhibitor resistance. Nat Commun 10(1):5661. https://doi.org/10.1038/s41467-019-13530-6

59. Wang Y, Bernhardy AJ, Cruz C, Krais JJ, Nacson J, Nicolas E et al (2016) The BRCA1-Delta11q alternative splice isoform bypasses germline mutations and promotes therapeutic resistance to PARP inhibition and cisplatin. Cancer Res 76(9):2778–2790. https://doi.org/10.1158/0008-5472.CAN-16-0186

60. Drost R, Dhillon KK, van der Gulden H, van der Heijden I, Brandsma I, Cruz C et al (2016) BRCA1185delAG tumors may acquire therapy resistance through expression of RING-less BRCA1. J Clin Invest 126(8):2903–2918. https://doi.org/10.1172/JCI70196

61. Johnson N, Johnson SF, Yao W, Li Y-C, Choi Y-E, Bernhardy AJ et al (2013) Stabilization of mutant BRCA1 protein confers PARP inhibitor and platinum resistance. Proc Natl Acad Sci 110(42):17041–17046. https://doi.org/10.1073/pnas.1305170110

62. Krais JJ, Johnson N (2020) BRCA1 mutations in cancer: coordinating deficiencies in homologous recombination with tumorigenesis. Can Res 80(21):4601–4609. https://doi.org/10.1158/0008-5472.CAN-20-1830

63. Drost R, Bouwman P, Rottenberg S, Boon U, Schut E, Klarenbeek S et al (2011) BRCA1 RING function is essential for tumor suppression but dispensable for therapy resistance. Cancer Cell 20(6):797–809. https://doi.org/10.1016/j.ccr.2011.11.014

64. Lord CJ, Ashworth A (2013) Mechanisms of resistance to therapies targeting BRCA-mutant cancers. Nat Med 19(11):1381–1388. https://doi.org/10.1038/nm.3369

65. Park PH, Yamamoto TM, Li H, Alcivar AL, Xia B, Wang Y et al (2020) Amplification of the mutation-carrying BRCA2 allele promotes RAD51 loading and PARP inhibitor resistance in the absence of reversion mutations. Mol Cancer Ther 19(2):602–613. https://doi.org/10.1158/1535-7163.MCT-17-0256%JMolecularCancerTherapeutics

66. Mirman Z, de Lange T (2020) 53BP1: a DSB escort. Genes Dev 34(1–2):7–23. https://doi.org/10.1101/gad.333237.119

67. Jaspers JE, Kersbergen A, Boon U, Sol W, van Deemter L, Zander SA et al (2013) Loss of 53BP1 causes PARP inhibitor resistance in <em>Brca1</em>-mutated mouse mammary tumors. Cancer Discov 3(1):68–81. https://doi.org/10.1158/2159-8290.Cd-12-0049

68. Callen E, Zong D, Wu W, Wong N, Stanlie A, Ishikawa M et al (2020) 53BP1 enforces distinct pre- and post-resection blocks on homologous recombination. Mol Cell 77(1):26-38.e7. https://doi.org/10.1016/j.molcel.2019.09.024

69. Zong D, Adam S, Wang Y, Sasanuma H, Callén E, Murga M et al (2019) BRCA1 haploinsufficiency is masked by RNF168-mediated chromatin ubiquitylation. Mol Cell. https://doi.org/10.1016/j.molcel.2018.12.010

70. Belotserkovskaya R, Raga Gil E, Lawrence N, Butler R, Clifford G, Wilson MD et al (2020) PALB2 chromatin recruitment restores homologous recombination in BRCA1-deficient cells depleted of 53BP1. Nat Commun 11(1):819. https://doi.org/10.1038/s41467-020-14563-y

71. Schlacher K, Wu H, Jasin M (2012) A distinct replication fork protection pathway connects Fanconi anemia tumor suppressors to RAD51-BRCA1/2. Cancer Cell 22(1):106–116. https://doi.org/10.1016/j.ccr.2012.05.015

72. Tye S, Ronson GE, Morris JR (2021) A fork in the road: Where homologous recombination and stalled replication fork protection part ways. Semin Cell Dev Biol 113:14–26. https://doi.org/10.1016/j.semcdb.2020.07.004

73. Berti M, Cortez D, Lopes M (2020) The plasticity of DNA replication forks in response to clinically relevant genotoxic stress. Nat Rev Mol Cell Biol 21(10):633–651. https://doi.org/10.1038/s41580-020-0257-5

74. Ray Chaudhuri A, Callen E, Ding X, Gogola E, Duarte AA, Lee JE et al (2016) Replication fork stability confers chemoresistance in BRCA-deficient cells. Nature 535(7612):382–387. https://doi.org/10.1038/nature18325

75. Daza-Martin M, Starowicz K, Jamshad M, Tye S, Ronson GE, MacKay HL et al (2019) Isomerization of BRCA1–BARD1 promotes replication fork protection. Nature 571(7766):521–527. https://doi.org/10.1038/s41586-019-1363-4

76. Moore K, Colombo N, Scambia G, Kim BG, Oaknin A, Friedlander M et al (2018) Maintenance olaparib in patients with newly diagnosed advanced ovarian cancer. N Engl J Med 379(26):2495–2505. https://doi.org/10.1056/NEJMoa1810858

77. DiSilvestro P, Banerjee S, Colombo N, Scambia G, Kim B-G, Oaknin A et al (2022) Overall survival with maintenance olaparib at a 7-year follow-up in patients with newly diagnosed advanced ovarian cancer and a BRCA mutation: the SOLO1/GOG 3004 Trial. J Clin Oncol 0(0):JCO.22.01549. https://doi.org/10.1200/jco.22.01549

78. Ceccaldi R, Liu JC, Amunugama R, Hajdu I, Primack B, Petalcorin MI et al (2015) Homologous-recombination-deficient tumours are dependent on Poltheta-mediated repair. Nature 518(7538):258–262. https://doi.org/10.1038/nature14184

79. Mateos-Gomez PA, Gong F, Nair N, Miller KM, Lazzerini-Denchi E, Sfeir A (2015) Mammalian polymerase theta promotes alternative NHEJ and suppresses recombination. Nature 518(7538):254–257. https://doi.org/10.1038/nature14157

80. Higgins GS, Boulton SJ (2018) Beyond PARP—POLθ as an anticancer target. Science 359(6381):1217–1218. https://doi.org/10.1126/science.aar5149

81. Forment JV, O'Connor MJ (2018) Targeting the replication stress response in cancer. Pharmacol Ther 188:155–167. https://doi.org/10.1016/j.pharmthera.2018.03.005

82. Kim H, Xu H, George E, Hallberg D, Kumar S, Jagannathan V et al (2020) Combining PARP with ATR inhibition overcomes PARP inhibitor and platinum resistance in ovarian cancer models. Nat Commun 11(1):3726. https://doi.org/10.1038/s41467-020-17127-2

83. Fang Y, McGrail DJ, Sun C, Labrie M, Chen X, Zhang D et al (2019) Sequential therapy with PARP and WEE1 inhibitors minimizes toxicity while maintaining efficacy. Cancer Cell 35(6):851–67.e7. https://doi.org/10.1016/j.ccell.2019.05.001

84. Serra V, Wang AT, Castroviejo-Bermejo M, Polanska UM, Palafox M, Herencia-Ropero A et al (2022) Identification of a molecularly-defined subset of breast and ovarian cancer models that respond to WEE1 or ATR inhibition, overcoming PARP inhibitor resistance. Clin Cancer Res 28(20):4536–4550. https://doi.org/10.1158/1078-0432.CCR-22-0568

85. Shah PD, Wethington SL, Pagan C, Latif N, Tanyi J, Martin LP et al (2021) Combination ATR and PARP inhibitor (CAPRI): a phase 2 study of ceralasertib plus olaparib in patients with recurrent, platinum-resistant epithelial ovarian cancer. Gynecol Oncol 163(2):246–253. https://doi.org/10.1016/j.ygyno.2021.08.024

86. Westin SN, Coleman RL, Fellman BM, Yuan Y, Sood AK, Soliman PT et al (2021) EFFORT: efficacy of adavosertib in PARP resistance: a randomized two-arm non-comparative phase II study of adavosertib with or without olaparib in women with PARP-resistant ovarian cancer. J Clin Oncol 39(15_suppl):5505. https://doi.org/10.1200/JCO.2021.39.15_suppl.5505

Development of Homologous Recombination Functional Assays for Targeting the DDR

Ailsa J. Oswald and Charlie Gourley

4.1 Introduction

Accurate identification of homologous recombination deficiency (HRD) has become of increasing clinical importance since the discovery and development of PARP inhibitors (PARPi) [1]. Somatic and germline mutations of *BRCA1* and *BRCA2* are the archetypal defect of HRD [2]. However, it is clear that the HRD phenotype extends beyond those with *BRCA1/2* mutations in multiple cancer types [1, 3, 4]. This has been starkly demonstrated in high grade serous ovarian cancer (HGSOC), where around 50% of patients have genetic or epigenetic defects in homologous recombination (HR) repair genes, with somatic or germline *BRCA1/2* mutations only accounting for around 20% of patients [2, 5, 6]. This concept has been reinforced by outcomes in multiple clinical trials, where patients with HGSOC and no *BRCA1/2* mutation still benefitted from a PARPi [7, 8]. An accurate method of identifying an HRD phenotype, beyond *BRCA1/2* mutations, is paramount to accurately stratify which patient cohorts are most likely to benefit from PARPis [4].

Homologous recombination repair capability can change over a disease course, particularly in relation to previous therapies. Therefore, a real-time readout of current HR status is vital [9]. This is one of the major factors that has led to functional

A. J. Oswald (✉) · C. Gourley
Cancer Research UK Scotland Centre, University of Edinburgh, Edinburgh, UK
e-mail: ailsa.oswald@ed.ac.uk

C. Gourley
e-mail: Charlie.gourley@ed.ac.uk

© The Author(s), under exclusive license to Springer Nature Switzerland AG 2023
T. A. Yap and G. I. Shapiro (eds.), *Targeting the DNA Damage Response for Cancer Therapy*, Cancer Treatment and Research 186,
https://doi.org/10.1007/978-3-031-30065-3_4

HR assays being an appealing strategy to identify HRD, in comparison to alternative methods that may represent historic HR status, such as genomic signatures [4, 9].

In this chapter, we briefly outline different methods for measuring HRD and the rationale for functional assays. We describe major pre-clinical advances in the development of the main functional assay, the RAD51 foci assay. We discuss the clinical applicability of assays and outline the challenges in the development of a functional HR test ready for clinical practice.

4.2 Methods for Testing for Homologous Recombination Deficiency

Clinical selection, by identifying those with platinum sensitive disease, has been used historically as a method to assess likelihood of HRD. Specific methods for HRD testing can be classified into mutational/methylation sequencing, genomic scars/signatures or functional RAD51 assays.

4.2.1 Clinical Selection

Sensitivity to platinum confers a high likelihood of PARPi response, particularly in HGSOC and this was the basis for patient selection in early PARPi clinical trials [4]. Mechanistically, platinum agents create DNA crosslinks which can be repaired by homologous recombination or by non-homologous end joining (NHEJ) [10]. Therefore, HRD tumours are often platinum sensitive [11]. However, the overlap of sensitivity between platinum and PARPis is incomplete [12]. Clinically, some patients who become resistant to PARPis still respond to platinum and vice versa [13].

A further challenge with utilising platinum sensitivity as a clinical selection biomarker relates to assessability of response. For example, in the situation where a patient has had all visible tumour resected and is receiving adjuvant platinum therapy, assessment of platinum sensitivity is not possible. Also, if PARPi therapy is to be started soon after the end of adjuvant chemotherapy then the duration of platinum response (historically a marker of platinum sensitivity) cannot inform the PARPi treatment decision.

4.2.2 Sequencing

Panel-based sequencing for deleterious mutations in key HRD genes (certainly *BRCA1* and *BRCA2* but often also including *RAD51C, RAD51D, BRIP1* and *PALB2*) is routinely performed in many countries around the world. While loss of function events in *BRCA1* and *BRCA2* clearly result in HRD, the extent to which loss of other genes encoding known pathway members functionally impact HRD is less clear. Preclinical data suggests that the extent of impact on PARPi sensitivity from HRD gene knockout varies from gene to gene [14]. Also, in PARPi clinical trials, the impact of loss of non-BRCA HRD genes on sensitivity varies from disease to disease and from study to study [15–18]. In HGSOC, the extent of benefit in patients with non-BRCA HRD gene defects appears to be less than for *BRCA1/2* but is greater in the relapsed disease setting than it is in the first line setting [15, 17]. In addition, this testing modality does not identify all potentially PARPi sensitive patients. There are clearly patients without mutations in recognised HRD genes who still benefit from PARPi [17].

In HGSOC, there is evidence that *BRCA1* or *RAD51C* methylation result in an HRD phenotype [19]. However, utilising this as a biomarker for PARPi response has produced contradictory results, with concerns regarding technical factors with testing [19–22]. Therefore, the clinical validity of methylation of *BRCA1/RAD51C* predicting PARPi sensitivity is currently unclear [9].

Beyond BRCA-associated cancers (such as HGSOC, breast, pancreas, prostate), the role of mutational sequencing is less clear. In non BRCA-associated tumours, the frequency of *BRCA1/2* mutations is low (<5%) and mutational impact is less clear [23]. There is also evidence of loss of *BRCA1* and *BRCA2* by structural variation, which is not detectable by standard next generation sequencing (NGS), in a variety of human cancers. This is associated with loss of gene expression and may be another mechanism by which PARPi sensitivity can arise [24].

To summarise, in HGSOC, it is standard clinical practice to perform tumour sequencing of *BRCA1* and *BRCA2* (plus often additional genes) and this will identify a proportion of patients highly likely to have an HRD phenotype [9, 25]. However, testing for this alone will fail to identify a significant proportion of patients with HRD, in both HGSOC and other cancer types.

4.2.3 Genomic Scars/Signatures

Genomic scar assays and signatures identify HRD by measuring the underlying genomic features, irrespective of aetiology. This relies on the concept that HRD tumours are genomically unstable and DNA damage is likely to be repaired by error-prone repair pathways, such as NHEJ. This results in abnormal copy number profiles, small insertions or deletions, and large chromosomal rearrangements [5, 26].

A number of commercial genomic scar assays are available, such as the Myriad myChoice® assay and FoundationOne® LOH. The myChoice® assay is a NGS diagnostic test producing a genomic instability score (GIS), by algorithmic measurement of loss of heterozygosity (LOH), telomeric allelic imbalance and large scale transitions, from formalin-fixed paraffin embedded (FFPE) tumour samples [27, 28].

A major attraction of this method is the potential to identify HRD occurring from a wide range of molecular mechanisms without having to identify these individually. However, in HGSOC, there have been variable results from clinical trials using these companion diagnostic tests. Their main limitation in pre-planned exploratory subgroup analysis is a poor negative predictive value, with many trials being unable to identify a *BRCA*-wild-type subgroup who did not benefit from PARPis [7, 8, 29] However, the recent PAOLA-1 study, which tested the addition of olaparib (PARPi) to bevacizumab in the first line setting, included a subgroup analysis of HRD groups based on the myChoice® assay. This demonstrated an improvement in progression free survival (PFS) from the addition of olaparib in the HRD group, with no benefit in the homologous recombination proficient (HRP) subgroup [30]. This has led to FDA approval of olaparib and bevacizumab in the first line setting, in combination with the use of a HRD GIS assay [9, 30]. Recent European consensus guidelines have recommended HRD testing by GIS, to aid stratification of patients who may benefit from a PARPi [31].

In triple negative breast cancer (TNBC), the myChoice® assay was shown to predict response to neo-adjuvant chemotherapy [11]. However, this assay does not currently have licensed approval as a diagnostic companion in breast cancer.

Academically-developed signature based assays include HRDetect and classifier of homologous recombination deficiency (CHORD), which both utilise whole genome sequencing (WGS) data [3, 32]. HRDetect was developed using a breast cancer cohort, with scoring associated with platinum response in patients with advanced breast cancer [32, 33]. However, a major challenge with WGS technologies is they are largely reliant of fresh frozen tissue (as successful analysis using FFPE material has been variable) [34].

Overall, GIS HRD assays are beginning to be incorporated into specific clinical contexts as companion diagnostic tests to aid clinical decision-making [31]. However, use in different centres is variable and is limited to certain tumour types. WGS based tests are not currently routinely used in clinical practice [9].

4.2.4 The Rationale for Functional HRD Assays

One of the major drawbacks of the genomic sequencing or scarring assays is that they only demonstrate whether HRD was present at some time point, not necessarily the current HRD status (which may change, for example as a result of development of platinum or PARPi resistance mechanisms) [35]. Functional assays have the benefit of theoretically giving a real-time readout of the HR functionality, [4] therefore potentially identifying patients who are likely to benefit from the initiation of a PARPi at that current time point.

HR is a dynamic process that can evolve, particularly in relation to previous treatments. For example, secondary HRD gene mutations, loss of *BRCA1* or *RAD51C* methylation or mutations in Shieldin complex genes can restore HR function which will impact on sensitivity to therapeutics such as PARPi [4, 35–38]. Furthermore, different molecular events may have variable effects on the extent of HR function restoration [35]. Instead of attempting to identify and quantify the array of potential resistance mechanisms, it may be simpler to use functional assays to elucidate the nett effect of these mechanisms on HR status at any particular point in time.

4.3 Functional RAD51 Foci Assays: How Do They Work?

Homologous recombination (HR) is a high fidelity repair mechanism occurring in the S and G2 cell cycle phases, with RAD51 playing a key role. RAD51 searches for the homologous template and facilitates strand invasion into the sister chromatid to allow restoration of the original DNA sequence (Fig. 4.1). Vital proteins involved in this process are encoded by genes such as *BRCA1, BRCA2* and *PALB2,* which positively regulate RAD51 [39]. RAD51 also functions at stalled replication forks, by promoting replication fork reversal at times of fork-blocking lesions and reversing the direction to continue replication [40].

Given that HR is complex, measuring the effect of a single downstream event is the most appealing strategy to identify multiple potential alterations in upstream mechanisms. This rationale has led to nuclear RAD51 quantification being the most common functional biomarker test to determine functional HR status [41, 42, 43]. It allows assessment of the functional status of HR up to the stage of RAD51 loading [40].

RAD51 foci are the visible distinct protein cluster that can be visualised by immunofluorescence (IF) [41]. Visible foci indicate a tumour is likely to be HR proficient and likely PARPi resistant. If a tumour is HRD, the RAD51 foci will be absent because RAD51 will not be loaded on the areas of single stranded DNA breakage, as illustrated in Fig. 4.2 [43].

In practice, developing these assays has been technically challenging. In subsequent sections, we outline the development of RAD51 assays; firstly, the pre-clinical *in vitro* development and secondly, the clinical applicability and utility.

4.4 RAD51 Foci Assays: Pre-Clinical Data and Method Considerations

Over the last decade, various methods for RAD51 foci assays have been described (Table 4.1). We outline key method developments and considerations, along with supportive pre-clinical data.

4.4.1 Co-staining

At the times of DSB, histone H2AX is phosphorylated to γH2AX [45]. This sensitive indicator of DNA DSB can be visualised by IF as γH2AX foci and is often reported with RAD51 assays [41]. This allows confirmation that an absent RAD51

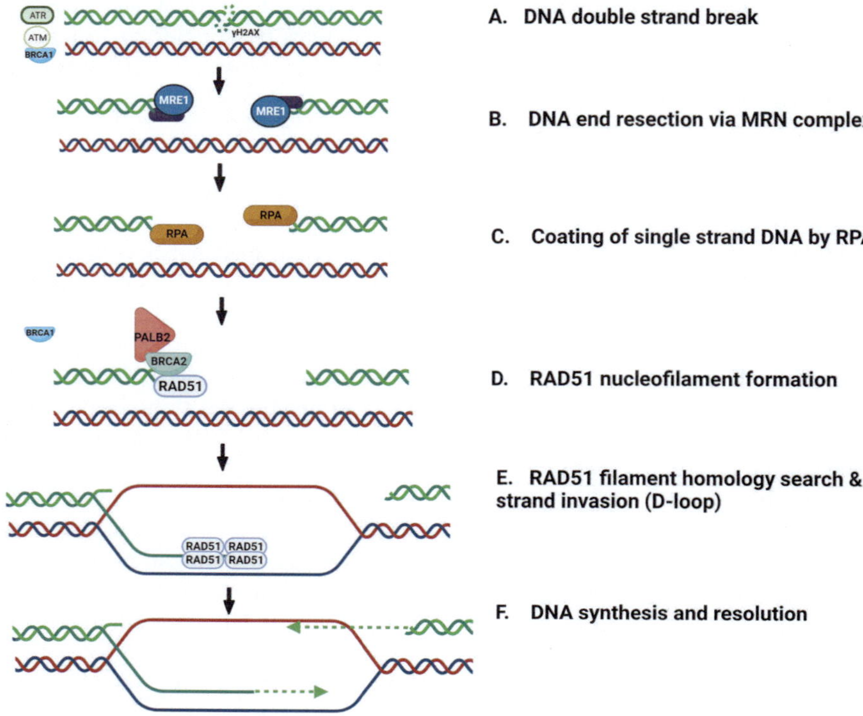

Fig. 4.1 Role of RAD51 in homologous recombination. A. Homologous recombination, a high fidelity process, is cell cycle phase dependent and only occurs in S/G2 phase. DNA double strand break occurs, from exogenous sources (e.g. irradiation or cytotoxic chemotherapy) or endogenous sources (e.g. replicative stress). DNA damage sensors are activated and recruitment of DNA repair proteins to the breakage area occurs. H2AX is phosphorylated to γH2AX by ATM and ATR [40]. BRCA1 is phosphorylated and activated by CHK2 and is involved in initiating the activation of the HR pathway [44]. An alternative process to DNA double strand breaks is non-homologous end joining (NHEJ), which is more error-prone (not visualised above). **B.** DNA ends are resected by MRN complex (MRE11-RAD50-NBS) to form 3' single strand DNA overhangs. **C.** These overhangs are coated by replication protein A (RPA) that consists of RFA1, RFA2, RFA3. This protects the single strand DNA from nucleases and prevents coiling. This forms a single strand DNA nucleofilament. **D.** BRCA2 (with PALB2) is recruited to the area of breakage by BRCA1. BRCA2 loads RAD51 onto the single strand DNA overhang, which displaces RPA. This forms a RAD51 nucleoprotein filament. **E.** RAD51 then invades the sister chromatid, to identify the matching homologous sequence. The strand invasion forms a displacement loop (D-loop). **F.** Once the homologous sequence is invaded, RAD51 is displaced to allow DNA polymerase to replicate the template. There will be crossover or non-crossover products, depending on whether the homologous chromosomes exchange parts with each other. *Image created with BioRender.com (2022)*

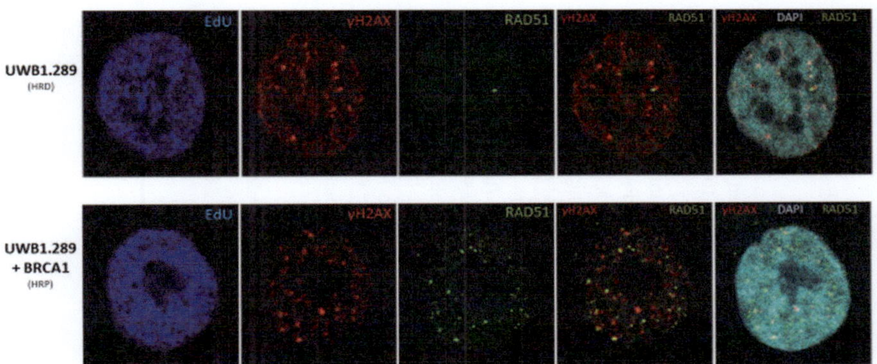

Fig. 4.2 **Immunofluorescence (IF) of two cancer cell lines demonstrating functional HR status**. UWB1.289 is a high grade serous ovarian cancer cell line, with a known germline *BRCA1* mutation (exon 11). It is homologous recombination deficient, as illustrated by a single RAD51 focus in response to DNA damage. UWB1.289 + BRCA1 is derived from UWB1.289, in which the wild type *BRCA1* has been restored. This behaves as HR proficient, with multiple RAD51 foci present in response to DNA damage. Above images were produced by authors and imaged using Olympus FV3000 confocal (×60). Coverslips were stained for DAPI, EdU (measurement of DNA synthesis), γH2AX and RAD51 after 4 hours of *in vitro* cisplatin exposure

focus is not simply due to a lack of DNA DSB occurring, which could erroneously appear suggestive of HRD [46]. Furthermore, γH2AX levels have been utilised to ensure variations in RAD51 foci are not simply related to pharmacokinetic variation of the DNA damage induction agent [47]. BRCA1 IF can also be performed, in order to elucidate aetiology of RAD51 response [46].

HR is cell cycle dependent, with RAD51 foci only forming in S and G2 phases. To control for variation in tumour proliferation, many studies co-stain for geminin (GMN), which is only expressed in S and G2 phases [48]. Cyclin A2 has been used as an alternative [49]. To adjust for proliferation rates, many studies use number of GMN expressing cells as the denominator, with number of RAD51 positive cells as the numerator [41].

The presence of stromal cells in sampling is a consideration, as their presence could cause a false negative result. Some studies have performed serial haematoxylin and eosin stained sections to determine tumour areas by morphology, or undergone cytokeratin 7 staining to identify epithelial cells [49, 50].

4.4.2 DNA Damage Induction

DDR pathways are dynamic and activated only at times of induced DNA damage. In early stages of RAD51 assay development, it was questioned whether basal levels of DNA damage would be sufficient to accurately identify HR status [42, 51]. This was observed in an early study by Graeser et al. who examined RAD51

Table 4.1 Pre-clinical data supporting the use of RAD51 foci assays

Author, Year	Tumour type (*source*)	Molecular group	N	Method (fixation time)	DNA damage agent	In *vitro* or *vivo* treatment	Main results
Mukhopadhyay [61]	Ovary (*Primary culture*)	Unselected	25	IF (24 hr)	Rucaparib	Rucaparib	• 16/25 had no increase in RAD51 foci (suggestive of HRD) • HRD status correlated with in-*vitro* PARPi response (93%–15/16 samples) by clonogenic assay or sulforhodamine B assay
Naipal [50]	Breast (*Fresh tumour PDX model*)	Unselected	54	IF + geminin (2 hr)	Ex vivo irradiation (5 Gy)	Olaparib	• Unable to analyse 9/54 samples (low GMN) • 11% (5/45) were HRD, with higher rates in TNBC samples • For the 5 HRD samples, all had *BRCA1/2* defects (mutations n = 3, *BRCA1* promoter hypermethylation n = 2) • PDX models showed in-*vitro* sensitivity to Olaparib

(continued)

Table 4.1 (continued)

Author, Year	Tumour type (*source*)	Molecular group	N	Method (fixation time)	DNA damage agent	In *vitro* or *vivo* treatment	Main results
Patterson [62]	Ovary, breast, lung (*Primary culture*)	Unselected	15	IF (24 hr)	Rucaparib	Rucaparib	• 4/15 samples HRD (lung, mesothelioma). No DDR mutations (by *NGS*), but probable loss of heterozygosity of FANCG, RPA1, PARP1
Cruz [52]*	Breast, ovary (*PDX model, FFPE*)	g*BRCA* mutations	PDX n = 12, FFPE n = 20	IF + geminin (NA)	None	Olaparib	• Association between low RAD51 score and response to PARPi in PDX models • Able to perform RAD51 foci testing in FFPE tissue without ex *vivo* irradiation
Castroviejo-Bermejo [46]*	Breast (*PDX model, FFPE*)	Varied in each cohort, but mainly BRCAwt	PDX n = 18,28 FFPE n = 23	IF + geminin (NA)	None	Olaparib	• RAD51 highly effective at predicting PARPi sensitivity in PDX models (*BRCA* wild-type, mixture of sensitive/resistant models). Included validation PDX cohort • FFPE samples identified 14/23 with HRD

(continued)

Table 4.1 (continued)

Author, Year	Tumour type (source)	Molecular group	N	Method (fixation time)	DNA damage agent	In vitro or vivo treatment	Main results
Meijer [53]*	Breast (Fresh tumour)	Unselected	170 (125 testable)	IF + geminin (2 hr)	Ex vivo irradiation (5 Gy)	NA	• Unable to analyse 26% due to lack of proliferating cancer cells • 19% HRD, 76% HRP, 5% intermediate • Unable to explain aetiology in 7/23 of HRD cases
Hill [58]	Ovary (Organoid)	Unselected	33	IHC + geminin (4 hr)	Ex vivo irradiation (10 Gy)	Olaparib	• Individual patient correlation of RAD51 and PARPi sensitivity. Unstable replication fork correlated with platinum sensitivity

(continued)

Table 4.1 (continued)

Author, Year	Tumour type (*source*)	Molecular group	N	Method (fixation time)	DNA damage agent	In *vitro* or *vivo* treatment	Main results
van Wijk [54]	Ovary (*Fresh—solid tumour, ascites*)	Unselected	49	IF + geminin (2 hr)	Ex vivo irradiation (5 Gy)	NA	• 20% HRD, 76% HRP and 4% intermediate • BRCA abnormalities in 89% (8/9) of HRD group • No DDR defects in HRP group
Van Wijk [56]*	Ovary, endometrium (*FFPE*)	Unselected	74	IF + geminin (NA)	None	NA	• Adapting their method using fresh tissue to FFPE material and optimising parameters. Quality control measures; tumour tissue $\geq 70\%$, γH2AX/GMN $+ \geq 25\%$ and minimum 40 GMN cells • RAD51-FFPE test detected BRCA mutant tumours with 90% sensitivity and HRD tumours (from fresh sample) with 87% sensitivity

Summary of main studies describing pre-clinical studies testing RAD51 foci, methods and main findings. Format adapted from: [41]
denotes key references (described in main text)

foci in patients with primary breast cancer, treated with neo-adjuvant chemotherapy. On baseline biopsies, they were unfortunately unable to visualise foci in most samples. They concluded the endogenous DNA damage level was below the sensitivity level for their assay. Therefore, they performed assays only on biopsies taken 24 hours after chemotherapy, as this would induce DNA damage [47].

Subsequent studies used *ex-vivo* radiation or *ex-vivo* systemic agents to induce DNA damage (Table 4.1). However, in 2018, Cruz et al. reported RAD51 foci testing in FFPE material without the requirement for DNA damage induction [46, 52]. They aimed to investigate *in vivo* mechanisms of PARPi resistance using g*BRCA1* mutated patient derived tumour xenografts (PDX). They unexpectedly identified evidence of endogenous DNA damage in untreated samples, which allowed RAD51 foci testing in PDX models. They also successfully tested ten untreated patient FFPE samples without DNA damage induction [52]. In this PDX cohort, RAD51 was highly effective at predicting PARPi response, with higher percentages of RAD51 positive cells present in PARPi resistant tumours [52].

This relationship was further validated in a PDX cohort of 28 TNBC models from a mixture of molecular backgrounds [46]. Using a RAD51 score $\leq$10%, they identified 25% of models as HRD and similarly this was highly predictive of PARPi response. They also scored RAD51 in clinical samples (n = 23) in patients beyond g*BRCA* mutations, such as those with g*PALB2* mutations and high clinical suspicion of hereditary breast cancer. Around 60% (14/23) had HRD, which included all 11 g*PALB2* mutant samples and a sample with *BRCA1* promoter hypermethylation. Ultimately, their work demonstrated RAD51 assays could successfully identify HRD effectively in patient FFPE samples (without exogenous DNA damage) and could be used to identify HRD tumours (including those beyond *BRCA1/2* mutations) [46].

4.4.3 Tissue Source

RAD51 testing on FFPE samples is much more feasible for implementation into clinical practice. However, many other studies relied on fresh tumour samples (Table 4.1*)*. This includes the functional REcombination CAPacity (RECAP) test, which has demonstrated use in multiple tumour types [50, 53, 54].

The RECAP test initially reported on fresh breast tumour samples, using ex-vivo irradiation and staining for RAD51/geminin [50]. In a feasibility study (n = 125), they successfully tested 74% of samples and the main reason for testing failure was lack of proliferating cells. They identified 19% as HRD, 76% HRP and 5% HR-intermediate. Though *BRCA1/2* mutations accounted for the majority of HRD, there were 7/23 HRD patients for whom they could not explain the HRD mechanism following extensive testing for *BRCA1/2* genetic or epigenetic defects. There was no matched clinical data to evaluate predictive value [53].

In ovarian cancer samples, the RECAP test included a protocol adaptation to improve suitability for solid tumour/ascites and similarly around 70% met quality control. Of the HGSOC subtype (n = 39), 26% were scored as HRD, with

8/9 having pathogenic *BRCA1/2* mutations. No pathogenic variants were found in HRP tumours. The HRD frequency reported in this study (26%) was significantly lower than expected HRD prevalence [6]. Therefore, it is possible the RECAP test underestimated HRD in this cohort [54]. The RECAP test has also been utilised in endometrial cancers (n = 25), with HRD being identified in 24%. All except one of the HRD cases had a pathogenic *BRCA1* mutation or alteration in HR related genes [55].

Following reports of successful RAD51 testing on FFPE samples without irradiation, those involved in developing the RECAP test aimed to adapt their methods from fresh tissue to FFPE without irradiation, to improve the clinical feasibility of testing [46, 52]. They reported the RAD51-FFPE test on 74 samples of ovarian and endometrial cancer [56]. They optimised co-IF staining protocols and confirmed optimal threshold for defining HRD. Ninety five percent of diagnostic FFPE tumour specimens passed quality control. Almost all (97%) of samples had satisfactory γH2AX scores, suggesting sufficient endogenous DNA damage for testing. Using matched RECAP data from fresh tissue, they recalibrated test parameters for RAD51 foci cut off and HRD threshold (15%). These thresholds resulted in high sensitivity for identifying *BRCA*-deficient (90%) and RECAP HRD (87%) cases. However, specificity for *BRCA*-wild-type and RECAP-HRP was lower (68%, 73%) and many RECAP HRP cases displayed low RAD51 FFPE scores. The reason for this was unclear. Authors considered whether the DNA damage (tested by γH2AX) in the low score RAD51-FFPE samples represented a sufficient substrate for HR. Overall, their work continued to support the consensus RAD51 testing is possible in FFPE tissue, without exogenous DNA damage and they demonstrate effective use in further tumour types (such as endometrium). The next steps for RAD51-FFPE testing will involve performance validation in large independent study cohorts, ideally with matched clinical and genomic data [56].

Primary culture from ascites or pleural fluid and RAD51 foci testing has demonstrated in-*vitro* sensitivity to PARP inhibitors in those identified as HRD [57]. However, utilising primary culture for RAD51 assays is not feasible in a routine clinical laboratory. Patient derived organoid HGSOC models have also been described to measure RAD51 expression and replication fork stability (Table 4.1) [58].

4.4.4 Other Method Considerations

4.4.4.1 Immunofluorescence Versus Immunohistochemistry

Immunofluorescence (IF) for RAD51 foci formation has been comprehensively evaluated in multiple tissue sources (Table 4.1). More recently, immunohistochemistry (IHC) has been successfully tested, as described below and in Table 4.2 [59, 60].

Table 4.2 Clinical correlation in observational studies

Author, Year	Tumour type (source)	Molecular group	N	Treatment background	RAD51 testing	DNA damage induction	Main findings
Graeser [47]	Breast (all subtypes) *FFPE*	Unselected No known *gBRCA1/2*	68	Treatment naïve	IF + geminin	Patient neoadjuvant treatment—*anthracycline chemotherapy*	• 26% had score in keeping with HRD (RAD51 score <10%) • Low RAD51 score associated with higher grade, high Ki67 score and TNBC subtype • Low RAD51 score was a predictive marker of pathCR
Mukhopadhyay [57]	Ovary (ascites) *Primary culture*	Unselected	50	Treatment naïve	IF	Ex vivo Rucaparib	• Identified 26/50 samples as HRD using RAD51 assay • Observational prospective comparison of HRD versus HRP group. HRD group had improved platinum sensitivity and longer PFS (11 m versus 8 m) and higher baseline CA125 • No routine *BRCA* sequencing, but there was a stronger family history of breast or ovarian cancer in the HRD group. One patient subsequently found to have *gBRCA2* mutation

(continued)

Table 4.2 (continued)

Author, Year	Tumour type (*source*)	Molecular group	N	Treatment background	RAD51 testing	DNA damage induction	Main findings
Tumiati [49]	Ovary (ascites and solid tumour) *Primary culture*	Not specified	23	Mixed—included platinum sensitive & resistant	IF + CK7/ CDA2	Ex vivo radiation 10 Gy	• Low HR score was associated with longer platinum free interval and improved OS • Independent tumour samples within a single patient demonstrated different HRD scores • When compared with sequencing and genomic signatures, there was suggestion functional assay may identify more HRD patients

(continued)

Table 4.2 (continued)

Author, Year	Tumour type *(source)*	Molecular group	N	Treatment background	RAD51 testing	DNA damage induction	Main findings
Van Wijk [54]	Ovary (ascites and solid tumour) *Fresh tumour*	Unselected	23 sub-group	Mixed	IF + geminin	Ex vivo radiation 5 Gy	• Similar rates to first line chemotherapy in both groups (87% HRD versus 81% HRP) • Clinically, trend towards superior OS and higher rates of complete response to subsequent chemotherapy in the HRD group
Waks [59]	Breast (TNBC, ER + ve) *FFPE*	g/s*BRCA* mutant	8	Previous PARPi or platinum, pre/post samples	IHC + geminin	Patient treatment—*PARPi or platinum*	• Absence or presence of RAD51 foci correlated well with response and resistance to platinum/ PARP inhibitors in pre/post samples • *BRCA1/2* reversion detected in 4/8 patients, with alternative resistance mechanism identified in 2/8 patients by whole exome sequencing

Summary of main studies describing RAD51 foci testing and observational clinical outcomes

4.4.4.2 Timing of Fixation

In the context of DNA damage induction agents, the time to fixation is an important consideration and summarised in Table 4.1. In *vitro* work suggests high levels of RAD51 are present between 2 and 8 hours following DNA damage agents, with a peak at around 4 hours [41].

4.5   Summary of Pre-clinical Development

Important technical factors in the development of RAD51 assays have included the confirmation of DNA DSB by measuring γH2AX and accounting for the number of proliferating cells by co-staining for geminin. The increasing evidence of satisfactory assay performance in FFPE material, without the requirement for DNA damage induction [46, 52, 56] has been a major step towards increasing feasibility of performing testing on patient samples.

4.6   Clinical Applicability

Following promising pre-clinical development of RAD51 foci assays, there are further considerations prior to use in clinical settings. These include correlation to clinical outcomes, practical issues and evaluating how RAD51 foci assays compare to and/or complement other testing modalities. The optimal clinical outcome to measure a HRD test against would be PARPi benefit, as this has the greatest clinical utility for accurate patient selection [9].

Until recently, correlation between RAD51 assays and clinical outcomes was mainly from small observational cohorts (Table 4.2). However, recent studies have performed testing on tumour samples from randomised controlled trials (RCT) with more robust matched clinical data. These aim to validate RAD51 as a predictive biomarker of treatment response.

4.6.1   Observational Data

4.6.1.1 Ovarian Cancer

An early study investigated HRD status by RAD51 IF in primary cultures from ascitic fluid in chemotherapy naïve molecularly unselected patients (n = 50). In their HRD group (51%), they noted higher platinum sensitivity rates and longer median PFS from prospective observational data. At this time, PARPi were not routinely use, but they demonstrated good correlation between *in vitro* platinum and PARPi sensitivity [57].

In the RECAP ovarian study, they reported observational clinical outcomes from a subgroup with newly diagnosed HGSOC who had undergone cytoreductive surgery and platinum chemotherapy (n = 24). There were similar responses to first line chemotherapy (81% HRP, 87% HRD group) but a trend towards higher rates of complete response to subsequent lines of chemotherapy and prolonged overall survival (OS) in the HRD group. This is in keeping with previous data suggesting superior outcomes in patients with HGSOC with *BRCA1/2* mutations, who likely have an HRD phenotype [63].

4.6.1.2 Breast Cancer

Two studies investigated RAD51 assays in patients with breast cancer undergoing neo-adjuvant chemotherapy. Both studies demonstrated tumours that achieved a complete pathological response (pathCR) with neo-adjuvant chemotherapy had lower RAD51 scores [64, 47]. In those with a high RAD51 score, there was a 97% negative predictive value for failure to achieve pathCR [47].

Waks et al. performed RAD51 foci testing in pre/post-treatment samples in a small cohort of patients with *BRCA1/2* mutant metastatic breast cancer and correlated this with response to PARPi and/or platinum. They demonstrated the absence or presence of RAD51 foci correlated well with response or resistance to DNA damaging agents [59]. For example, three patients acquired RAD51 foci on their post-PARPi biopsy and had subsequent platinum chemotherapy. All demonstrated intrinsic platinum resistance. Though their study was small, it clearly illustrated HRD as a dynamic process within individual patients in this unique study design [59].

4.6.2   RAD51 Assays: Biomarker Development Utilising Phase II Trial Datasets

To validate RAD51 as a predictive biomarker of therapy response, a number of recent studies utilised tumour samples from RCTs and correlated these with clinical outcomes. RAD51 testing was conducted as exploratory analysis within these RCT populations, in a number of tumour types (ovary, breast and prostate). These studies generally demonstrated two key developments. Firstly, they showed feasibility of RAD51 testing in these tumour types, using FFPE material and no requirement for exogenous DNA damage. Secondly, they demonstrated a correlation between RAD51 scores and response to therapy (platinum chemotherapy or PARPi), with a consistent method for RAD51 scoring adopted in a number of these studies.

4.6.2.1 Ovarian Cancer

The CHIVA study investigated the addition of nintedanib to neo-adjuvant platinum chemotherapy in advanced epithelial ovarian cancer. Using FFPE material, testing RAD51 foci by IF was possible in 90% of samples (139/155) [65]. There were 55% of patients with evidence of HRD by RAD51 assay, in keeping with estimated prevalence from TCGA [6]. Tumours were considered HRD is <10% of GMN positive cells had five or more RAD51 foci. There was a higher response rate to neo-adjuvant platinum in the HRD compared with HRP group (37% versus 68%). Furthermore, the PFS in the HRD group was longer (20.8 months versus

14.1 months) [65]. Fifteen percent of tumours had a *BRCA1/2* mutation and of these, 67% were RAD51 deficient. Interestingly, in those with a *BRCA1/2* mutation and high RAD51 score (suggestive of HRP), there was a significantly poorer response rate to neo-adjuvant chemotherapy (17% versus 75%). Whether RAD51 assay could prospectively predict response to PARPi (as opposed to platinum chemotherapy) in HGSOC is an important subsequent question.

4.6.2.2 Breast Cancer

PARP inhibitors are licensed in metastatic (HER2 negative) breast cancer in those with *BRCA1/2* mutations and there is significant interest in expanding their use in this tumour type. This is of particular interest in TNBC, for two main reasons. Firstly, the HRD phenotype in this patient group clearly extends beyond those with BRCA mutations. Between 5 and 20% of patients with TNBC have a g*BRCA1* mutation, whilst HRD rates measured by HRDetect have been reported as high as 59% [66–69]. Secondly, a previously unselected approach with PARPi was unsuccessful, with a previous phase 2 study observing no benefit from PARPi when given to an unselected heavily pre-treated advanced TNBC patient cohort [70]. Three studies (GeparSixto, PEMETRAC, RIO) investigated RAD51 assays in this patient group in relation to response to platinum or PARPi [71–73].

4.6.2.3 GeparSixto

This trial investigated the addition of carboplatin to neo-adjuvant chemotherapy in TNBC. A retrospective blinded biomarker analysis for RAD51 assays was conducted using FFPE samples laid on tissue microarrays. There was high levels of endogenous DNA damage, with high γH2AX levels in all tumours. Using the pre-defined RAD51 score $\leq$10%, they identified 61% of patients with HRD. They investigated concordance between RAD51 score versus genomic HRD score (Myriad MyChoice®) and analysed their relationship to patient outcomes (such as survival, pathCR) [72].

In those with a *BRCA1/2* mutation, 93% had a low RAD51 score suggestive of HRD. In the BRCA wild-type group, 45% had HRD, likely due to defects in other HR related genes or epigenetic silencing. When compared to the Myriad MyChoice® assay, the RAD51 and genomic HRD score were 87% concordant. Reasons for discordance could be due to restoration of HR in tumour evolution or tumour heterogeneity. The pathCR was significantly higher with the addition of carboplatin in the HRD group (66% versus 33%), with no significant difference noted in the HRP group (39% versus 31%). When compared to genomic HRD score or *BRCA* mutation status, the RAD51 test was more sensitive at predicting pathCR [72]. It is widely recognised that pathCR to neo-adjuvant chemotherapy is an important prognostic marker with a strong association with disease free survival and OS, particularly in TNBC or HER2 positive hormone receptor negative tumours [74, 75].

This study was supportive for the clinical validity of RAD51 as a functional HRD marker and predictive biomarker of response to platinum in newly diagnosed TNBC. Given there is significant overlap between platinum sensitivity and PARPi sensitivity, this study provides more evidence towards RAD51 testing as a biomarker for PARPi response.

PETREMAC

The PETREMAC trial included patients with primary TNBC who received olaparib for up to 10 weeks prior to chemotherapy. Tumour biopsies underwent targeted DNA sequencing and IF RAD51 foci testing (pre-defined cut off 10%). There were 16/30 (53.3%) of patients identified as HRD by RAD51 testing. RAD51 scores correlated well with PARPi response, with 14/16 patients having complete or partial response [71].

Rio

This trial aimed to identify biomarkers of PARPi activity in sporadic TNBC, by performing tests including; HRDetect, RAD51 foci and *BRCA1* methylation [60]. Patients (n = 43) with newly diagnosed TNBC were given rucaparib for 2 weeks prior to definitive treatment (surgery or neo-adjuvant chemotherapy). This study used IHC for RAD51 and threshold was RAD51<20% (less than 20% geminin positive cells having RAD51 foci deficiency). Of those identified with absent RAD51 foci (17/22), 61% had a detectable HR defect, such as *BRCA1/2* mutation, *BRCA1* methylation, g*PALB2* mutation or *RAD51C* methylation. Though no clinical outcomes have been reported, this study did demonstrate RAD51 foci deficiency correlated well with HRDetect score [73].

4.6.2.4 Prostate Cancer

In metastatic castration resistant prostate cancer, the RAD51 assay was investigated as a biomarker in the phase II TOPARP-B trial. This trial pre-screened patients (n = 98) for DDR mutations using NGS panel. Patients received olaparib as a single arm study. For 52 patients, they had tumour material from the same biopsy for NGS where they could evaluate RAD51 via IF. RAD51 was evaluable in all samples and 42% had low RAD51 scores (threshold<10% GMN positive cells having ≤5 RAD51 foci), suggestive of HRD. All patients with *BRCA1/2* mutations (n = 16) had low RAD51 score. Tumours with biallelic *PALB2* mutations also had evidence of HRD. There was a superior response rate to PARPis in the HRD group (68% versus 23%). There was also an improvement in PFS (9.3 m versus 2.9 m) and OS (17.4 m versus 9.5 m) in the HRD group compared to HRP [76].

4.7 Final Considerations and Limitations

4.7.1 RAD51 Foci Testing in Other Tumour Types

RAD51 foci assays in FFPE material has been successfully performed without exogenous DNA damage in cohorts of breast, ovary, endometrial and prostate cancer [55, 56, 65, 72, 76]. This is based on the hypothesis that genomic instability in these tumours led to reasonable levels of endogenous DNA damage to allow testing. However, in slowly proliferating tumours, this current method is likely to be ineffective. For example, the recent CHIVA trial included patients with advanced epithelial ovarian cancer and reported a small proportion of tumours (8/155) with low γH2AX scores, which included two of the three grade 1 tumours included in the study [65]. Further testing is required to elucidate how transferable the current testing method would therefore be in other tumour types, depending on their proliferation index and inherent genomic stability.

4.7.2 Accuracy of the RAD51 Foci Test

There are a number of reasons for potential inaccuracy of RAD51 foci in predicting HR status and PARPi sensitivity. RAD51 assays will not detect defects in HR that are further downstream of RAD51 loading to an area of DNA breakage [9]. Also, PARPi sensitivity can occur via mechanisms that do not directly impact on HR, for example ATM alterations or RNASEH2 [77, 78]. There have been RAD51-independent mechanisms of PARPi resistance described such as loss of PARG, mechanisms involving replication fork stabilisation or upregulation of MDR1, that would not be identified using the RAD51 assay [79–81].

4.7.3 Where and When to Sample

A major challenge with all HRD tests is the potential for clonal heterogeneity and subpopulations with different treatment sensitivity within tumours [82]. In the context of functional HRD assays, this was illustrated by Tumiati et al. who took multiple biopsy samples from different site, during the same surgery from a treatment naive patient. One patient was classified overall as having a low HR score but had striking variation of scores between sample sites. For example, the left ovary was classified as HRD, peritoneal disease as HR-low and right ovary as HRP. Clinically, the patient had a complete response to primary chemotherapy following optimal debulking [49].

A similar observation was reported in the PEMETRAC study. As described above, it included patients with primary TNBC treated with PARPi prior to surgery or neoadjuvant chemotherapy. There was one patient with a low RAD51 score on primary biopsy, suggestive of HRD, who had progressive disease (by RECIST score) on a PARP inhibitor. Interestingly, they observed a significant regression of the primary tumour (suggestive of HRD) but progressive appearance of axillary metastasis, which suggested HRP tumour subclones metastasizing to the axilla during PARPi treatment [71]. Overall, this raises questions as to the appropriateness of multi-site testing and interpretation of these results. This concept is especially challenging in patients who are pre-treated with more potential for multiple tumour subpopulations.

Given HR is a dynamic process, having current (as opposed to archival) samples to test is preferable. However, repeat biopsies is not without technical challenges, patient risk and resource implications. The timing of sampling therefore also requires consideration and these factors will likely vary between tumour types.

4.7.4 Alternative Functional HRD Tests

The DNA fibre assay has also been investigated as a functional assay, which demonstrates the replication fork phenotype [41]. Fork protection is mediated by a number of proteins, many of which are also involved in HR (such as BRCA1, BRCA2, RAD51). If there is unrepaired DNA damage and replication forks are not protected from nucleases, the stalled replication forks will degrade. This assay visualises this degradation process by IF, by incorporating labelled nucleoside analogues [41, 58]. Replication fork degradation has been associated with sensitivity to chemotherapy in BRCA-deficient tumours. Furthermore, replication fork protection in *BRCA1* mutated cells has been associated with acquired platinum and PARPi resistance [79]. Pre-clinical work has suggested fork instability may correlate better to platinum sensitivity than PARPi sensitivity [58]. This assay also requires fresh tissue [41].

4.8 Conclusion

Functional HRD assays, via the RAD51 foci assay, present a unique opportunity for real-time readout of current HR status, regardless of underlying aetiology. Identification of HRD is becoming increasingly important with the profound benefits demonstrated from PARPis in multiple tumour types.

Supportive pre-clinical data over the last decade has resulted in the successful development of RAD51 foci assay testing which is possible in FFPE material of specific tumour types, without the requirement for exogenous DNA damage induction. Next steps will likely involve further validation of test performance in larger cohorts and other tumour types. Correlation with prospective clinical data and further comparison with other HRD testing modalities (such as genomic scars or signatures) will be paramount. Other considerations in implementing functional testing include the role of re-biopsy, how to expand testing to other tumour types and how to identify RAD51 independent mechanism of PARPi resistance. Furthermore, PARPi are now often being trialled in combination with other agents, in an attempt to improve response and synergy. The predictive power of any HRD test may vary in these different clinical contexts.

Given the complexity of HRD, it is unlikely one single type of test will provide the definitive answer. Instead, the combination of results produced from genomic data and functional assays, alongside a patient's clinical background, is likely to produce the most robust description of an individual's HR status and likelihood of PARPi sensitivity.

Abbreviations

BRCAmt	BRCA mutant
BRCAwt	BRCA wild-type
CHORD	Classifier of homologous recombination deficiency
DSB	Double strand breaks
FFPE	Formalin-fixed paraffin embedded
GMN	Geminin
GIS	Genomic instability score
HGSOC	High grade serous ovarian cancer
HR	Homologous recombination
HRD	Homologous recombination deficiency
HRP	Homologous recombination proficient
IF	Immunofluorescence
IHC	Immunohistochemistry
LOH	Loss of heterozygosity
NGS	Next generation sequencing
NHEJ	Non-homologous end joining
OS	Overall survival
PARPi	PARP inhibitor
pathCR	Pathological complete response
PDX	Patient derived tumour xenografts
PARP	Poly ADP-Ribose polymerase
PFS	Progression free survival
RECAP	REcombination CAPacity
RPA	Replication protein A
TCGA	The cancer genome atlas
TNBC	Triple negative breast cancer
WGS	Whole genome sequencing

References

1. Gourley C, Balmaña J, Ledermann JA, Serra V, Dent R, Loibl S et al (2019) Moving from poly (ADP-Ribose) polymerase inhibition to targeting DNA repair and DNA damage response in cancer therapy. J Clin Oncol: official journal of the American Society of Clinical Oncology 37(25):2257–2269
2. Konstantinopoulos PA, Ceccaldi R, Shapiro GI, D'Andrea AD (2015) Homologous recombination deficiency: exploiting the fundamental vulnerability of ovarian cancer. Cancer Discov 5(11):1137–1154
3. Nguyen L, Martens WM, Van Hoeck A, Cuppen E (2020) Pan-cancer landscape of homologous recombination deficiency. Nat Commun 11(1):5584
4. Gourley C, Miller RE, Hollis RL, Ledermann JA (2020) Role of Poly (ADP-Ribose) Polymerase inhibitors beyond BReast CAncer gene-mutated ovarian tumours: definition of homologous recombination deficiency? Curr Opin Oncol 32(5):442–450
5. Kanchi KL, Johnson KJ, Lu C, McLellan MD, Leiserson MDM, Wendl MC et al (2014) Integrated analysis of germline and somatic variants in ovarian cancer. Nat Commun 5(1):3156
6. Cancer Genome Atlas Research N (2011) Integrated genomic analyses of ovarian carcinoma. Nature 474(7353):609–15
7. González-Martín A, Pothuri B, Vergote I, DePont CR, Graybill W, Mirza MR et al (2019) Niraparib in patients with newly diagnosed advanced ovarian cancer. N Engl J Med 381(25):2391–2402
8. Mirza MR, Monk BJ, Herrstedt J, Oza AM, Mahner S, Redondo A et al (2016) Niraparib maintenance therapy in platinum-sensitive, recurrent ovarian cancer. N Engl J Med 375(22):2154–2164
9. Miller R, Leary A, Scott C, Serra V, Lord C, Bowtell D et al (2020) ESMO recommendations on predictive biomarker testing for homologous recombination deficiency and PARP inhibitor benefit in ovarian cancer. Ann Oncol 31
10. Dasari S, Tchounwou PB (2014) Cisplatin in cancer therapy: molecular mechanisms of action. Eur J Pharmacol 740:364–378
11. Telli ML, Timms KM, Reid J, Hennessy B, Mills GB, Jensen KC et al (2016) Homologous recombination deficiency (HRD) score predicts response to platinum-containing neoadjuvant chemotherapy in patients with triple-negative breast cancer. Clin Cancer Res: an official journal of the American Association for Cancer Research 22(15):3764–3773
12. McMullen M, Karakasis K, Madariaga A, Oza AM (2020) Overcoming platinum and parp-inhibitor resistance in ovarian cancer. Cancers 12(6):1607
13. Fong PC, Yap TA, Boss DS, Carden CP, Mergui-Roelvink M, Gourley C et al (2010) Poly(ADP)-ribose polymerase inhibition: frequent durable responses in BRCA carrier ovarian cancer correlating with platinum-free interval. J Clin Oncol: official journal of the American Society of Clinical Oncology 28(15):2512–2519
14. McCabe N, Turner NC, Lord CJ, Kluzek K, Bialkowska A, Swift S et al (2006) Deficiency in the repair of DNA damage by homologous recombination and sensitivity to poly(ADP-ribose) polymerase inhibition. Cancer Res 66(16):8109–8115
15. Hodgson DR, Dougherty BA, Lai Z, Fielding A, Grinsted L, Spencer S et al (2018) Candidate biomarkers of PARP inhibitor sensitivity in ovarian cancer beyond the BRCA genes. Br J Cancer 119(11):1401–1409
16. Swisher EM, Kwan TT, Oza AM, Tinker AV, Ray-Coquard I, Oaknin A et al (2021) Molecular and clinical determinants of response and resistance to rucaparib for recurrent ovarian cancer treatment in ARIEL2 (Parts 1 and 2). Nat Commun 12(1):2487
17. Pujade-Lauraine E, Brown J, Barnicle A, Rowe P, Lao-Sirieix P, Criscione S et al (2021) Homologous recombination repair mutation gene panels (excluding BRCA) are not predictive of maintenance olaparib plus bevacizumab efficacy in the first-line PAOLA-1/ENGOT-ov25 trial. Gynecol Oncol 162:S26–S27

18. Mateo J, Porta N, Bianchini D, McGovern U, Elliott T, Jones R et al (2020) Olaparib in patients with metastatic castration-resistant prostate cancer with DNA repair gene aberrations (TOPARP-B): a multicentre, open-label, randomised, phase 2 trial. Lancet Oncol 21(1):162–174

19. Bernards SS, Pennington KP, Harrell MI, Agnew KJ, Garcia RL, Norquist BM et al (2018) Clinical characteristics and outcomes of patients with BRCA1 or RAD51C methylated versus mutated ovarian carcinoma. Gynecol Oncol 148(2):281–285

20. Ruscito I, Dimitrova D, Vasconcelos I, Gellhaus K, Schwachula T, Bellati F et al (2014) BRCA1 gene promoter methylation status in high-grade serous ovarian cancer patients–a study of the tumour Bank ovarian cancer (TOC) and ovarian cancer diagnosis consortium (OVCAD). Eur J Cancer 50(12):2090–2098

21. Cunningham J, Cicek M, Larson N, Davila J, Wang C, Larson M et al (2014) Clinical characteristics of ovarian cancer classified by BRCA1, BRCA2 and RAD51C status. Sci Rep 4(1):1–7

22. Swisher EM, Lin KK, Oza AM, Scott CL, Giordano H, Sun J et al (2017) Rucaparib in relapsed, platinum-sensitive high-grade ovarian carcinoma (ARIEL2 Part 1): an international, multicentre, open-label, phase 2 trial. Lancet Oncol 18(1):75–87

23. Jonsson P, Bandlamudi C, Cheng ML, Srinivasan P, Chavan SS, Friedman ND et al (2019) Tumour lineage shapes BRCA-mediated phenotypes. Nature 571(7766):576–579

24. Ewing A, Meynert A, Churchman M, Grimes G, Hollis RL, Herrington CS et al (2021) Structural variants at the BRCA1/2 loci are a common source of homologous repair deficiency in high grade serous ovarian carcinoma. Clin Cancer Res: clincanres. CCR-20-4068-A.2020

25. Konstantinopoulos PA, Norquist B, Lacchetti C, Armstrong D, Grisham RN, Goodfellow PJ et al (2020) Germline and somatic tumor testing in epithelial ovarian cancer: ASCO guideline. J Clin Oncol 38(11):1222–1245

26. Abkevich V, Timms KM, Hennessy BT, Potter J, Carey MS, Meyer LA et al (2012) Patterns of genomic loss of heterozygosity predict homologous recombination repair defects in epithelial ovarian cancer. Br J Cancer 107(10):1776–1782

27. Marquard AM, Eklund AC, Joshi T, Krzystanek M, Favero F, Wang ZC et al (2015) Pan-cancer analysis of genomic scar signatures associated with homologous recombination deficiency suggests novel indications for existing cancer drugs. Biomark Res. 3:9

28. Watkins JA, Irshad S, Grigoriadis A, Tutt ANJ (2014) Genomic scars as biomarkers of homologous recombination deficiency and drug response in breast and ovarian cancers. Breast Cancer Res 16(3):211

29. Coleman RL, Oza AM, Lorusso D, Aghajanian C, Oaknin A, Dean A et al (2017) Rucaparib maintenance treatment for recurrent ovarian carcinoma after response to platinum therapy (ARIEL3): a randomised, double-blind, placebo-controlled, phase 3 trial. The Lancet 390(10106):1949–1961

30. Ray-Coquard I, Pautier P, Pignata S, Pérol D, González-Martín A, Berger R et al (2019) Olaparib plus Bevacizumab as first-line maintenance in ovarian cancer. N Engl J Med 381(25):2416–2428

31. Colombo N, Ledermann JA (2021) Updated treatment recommendations for newly diagnosed epithelial ovarian carcinoma from the ESMO clinical practice guidelines. Ann Oncol 32(10):1300–1303

32. Davies H, Glodzik D, Morganella S, Yates LR, Staaf J, Zou X et al (2017) HRDetect is a predictor of BRCA1 and BRCA2 deficiency based on mutational signatures. Nat Med 23(4):517–525

33. Zhao EY, Shen Y, Pleasance E, Kasaian K, Leelakumari S, Jones M et al (2017) Homologous recombination deficiency and platinum-based therapy outcomes in advanced breast cancer. Clin Cancer Res 23(24):7521

34. Robbe P, Popitsch N, Knight SJL, Antoniou P, Becq J, He M et al (2018) Clinical whole-genome sequencing from routine formalin-fixed, paraffin-embedded specimens: pilot study for the 100,000 genomes project. Genet Med 20(10):1196–1205

35. Mateo J, Lord CJ, Serra V, Tutt A, Balmaña J, Castroviejo-Bermejo M et al (2019) A decade of clinical development of PARP inhibitors in perspective. Ann Oncol 30(9):1437–1447

36. Kondrashova O, Nguyen M, Shield-Artin K, Tinker AV, Teng NNH, Harrell MI et al (2017) Secondary somatic mutations restoring RAD51C and RAD51D associated with acquired resistance to the PARP inhibitor rucaparib in high-grade ovarian carcinoma. Cancer Discov 7(9):984–998

37. Domchek SM (2017) Reversion mutations with clinical use of PARP inhibitors: many genes, many versions. Cancer Discov 7(9):937

38. Hurley RM, McGehee CD, Nesic K, Correia C, Weiskittel TM, Kelly RL et al (2021) Characterization of a RAD51C-silenced high-grade serous ovarian cancer model during development of PARP inhibitor resistance. NAR Cancer 3(3):zcab028

39. Lord CJ, Ashworth A (2012) The DNA damage response and cancer therapy. Nature 481(7381):287–294

40. Grundy MK, Buckanovich RJ, Bernstein KA (2020) Regulation and pharmacological targeting of RAD51 in cancer. NAR Cancer 2(3)

41. Fuh K, Mullen M, Blachut B, Stover E, Konstantinopoulos P, Liu J et al (2020) Homologous recombination deficiency real-time clinical assays, ready or not? Gynecol Oncol 159(3):877–886

42. Lord CJ, Ashworth A (2016) BRCAness revisited. Nat Rev Cancer 16(2):110–120

43. Ladan MM, van Gent DC, Jager A (2021) Homologous recombination deficiency testing for BRCA-like tumors: the road to clinical validation. Cancers 13(5):1004

44. Orhan E, Velazquez C, Tabet I, Sardet C, Theillet C (2021) Regulation of RAD51 at the transcriptional and functional levels: what prospects for cancer therapy? Cancers 13(12):2930

45. Bonner WM, Redon CE, Dickey JS, Nakamura AJ, Sedelnikova OA, Solier S et al (2008) γH2AX and cancer. Nat Rev Cancer 8(12):957–967

46. Castroviejo-Bermejo M, Cruz C, Llop-Guevara A, Gutiérrez-Enríquez S, Ducy M, Ibrahim YH et al (2018) A RAD51 assay feasible in routine tumor samples calls PARP inhibitor response beyond BRCA mutation. EMBO Mol Med 10(12)

47. Graeser M, McCarthy A, Lord CJ, Savage K, Hills M, Salter J et al (2010) A marker of homologous recombination predicts pathologic complete response to neoadjuvant chemotherapy in primary breast cancer. Clin Cancer Res: an official journal of the American Association for Cancer Research 16(24):6159–6168

48. Gonzalez MA, Tachibana K-eK, Chin S-F, Callagy GM, Madine MA, Vowler SL et al (2004) Geminin predicts adverse clinical outcome in breast cancer by reflecting cell cycle progression. J Pathol 204

49. Tumiati M, Hietanen S, Hynninen J, Pietilä E, Färkkilä A, Kaipio K et al (2018) A functional homologous recombination assay predicts primary chemotherapy response and long-term survival in ovarian cancer patients. Clin Cancer Res: an official journal of the American Association for Cancer Research 24(18):4482–4493

50. Naipal KA, Verkaik NS, Ameziane N, van Deurzen CH, Ter Brugge P, Meijers M et al (2014) Functional ex vivo assay to select homologous recombination-deficient breast tumors for PARP inhibitor treatment. Clin Cancer Res: an official journal of the American Association for Cancer Research. 20(18):4816–4826

51. Farmer H, McCabe N, Lord CJ, Tutt AN, Johnson DA, Richardson TB et al (2005) Targeting the DNA repair defect in BRCA mutant cells as a therapeutic strategy. Nature 434(7035):917–921

52. Cruz C, Castroviejo-Bermejo M, Gutiérrez-Enríquez S, Llop-Guevara A, Ibrahim YH, Gris-Oliver A et al (2018) RAD51 foci as a functional biomarker of homologous recombination repair and PARP inhibitor resistance in germline BRCA-mutated breast cancer. Ann Oncol 29(5):1203–1210

53. Meijer TG, Verkaik NS, Sieuwerts AM, van Riet J, Naipal KAT, van Deurzen CHM et al (2018) Functional ex vivo assay reveals homologous recombination deficiency in breast cancer beyond BRCA gene defects. Clin Cancer Res: an official journal of the American Association for Cancer Research. 24(24):6277–6287

54. van Wijk LM, Vermeulen S, Meijers M, van Diest MF, Ter Haar NT, de Jonge MM et al (2020) The RECAP test rapidly and reliably identifies homologous recombination-deficient ovarian carcinomas. Cancers (Basel) 12(10)
55. de Jonge MM, Auguste A, van Wijk LM, Schouten PC, Meijers M, Ter Haar NT et al (2019) Frequent homologous recombination deficiency in high-grade endometrial carcinomas. Clin Cancer Res: an official journal of the American Association for Cancer Research 25(3):1087–1097
56. van Wijk LM, Kramer CJH, Vermeulen S, Ter Haar NT, de Jonge MM, Kroep JR et al (2021) The RAD51-FFPE test; calibration of a functional homologous recombination deficiency test on diagnostic endometrial and ovarian tumor blocks. Cancers (Basel) 13(12)
57. Mukhopadhyay A, Plummer ER, Elattar A, Soohoo S, Uzir B, Quinn JE et al (2012) Clinicopathological features of homologous recombination-deficient epithelial ovarian cancers: sensitivity to PARP inhibitors, platinum, and survival. Can Res 72(22):5675
58. Hill SJ, Decker B, Roberts EA, Horowitz NS, Muto MG, Worley MJ Jr et al (2018) Prediction of DNA repair inhibitor response in short-term patient-derived ovarian cancer organoids. Cancer Discov 8(11):1404–1421
59. Waks AG, Cohen O, Kochupurakkal B, Kim D, Dunn CE, Buendia Buendia J et al (2020) Reversion and non-reversion mechanisms of resistance to PARP inhibitor or platinum chemotherapy in BRCA1/2-mutant metastatic breast cancer. Ann Oncol 31(5):590–598
60. Chopra N, Tovey H, Pearson A, Cutts R, Toms C, Proszek P et al (2020) Homologous recombination DNA repair deficiency and PARP inhibition activity in primary triple negative breast cancer. Nat Commun 11(1)
61. Mukhopadhyay A, Elattar A, Cerbinskaite A, Wilkinson SJ, Drew Y, Kyle S et al (2010) Development of a functional assay for homologous recombination status in primary cultures of epithelial ovarian tumor and correlation with sensitivity to poly(ADP-ribose) polymerase inhibitors. Clin Cancer Res: an official journal of the American Association for Cancer Research 16(8):2344–2351
62. Patterson MJ, Sutton RE, Forrest I, Sharrock R, Lane M, Kaufmann A et al (2014) Assessing the function of homologous recombination DNA repair in malignant pleural effusion (MPE) samples. Br J Cancer 111(1):94–100
63. Hollis RL, Churchman M, Gourley C (2017) Distinct implications of different BRCA mutations: efficacy of cytotoxic chemotherapy, PARP inhibition and clinical outcome in ovarian cancer. Onco Targets Ther 10:2539–2551
64. Asakawa H, Koizumi H, Koike A, Takahashi M, Wu W, Iwase H et al (2010) Prediction of breast cancer sensitivity to neoadjuvant chemotherapy based on status of DNA damage repair proteins. Breast Cancer Res 12(2):R17
65. Blanc-Durand F, Yaniz E, Genestie C, Rouleau E, Berton D, Lortholary A et al (2021) Evaluation of a RAD51 functional assay in advanced ovarian cancer, a GINECO/GINEGEPS study. J Clin Oncol 39(15_suppl):5513
66. Armstrong N, Ryder S, Forbes C, Ross J, Quek RG (2019) A systematic review of the international prevalence of BRCA mutation in breast cancer. Clin Epidemiol 11:543–561
67. Hartman AR, Kaldate RR, Sailer LM, Painter L, Grier CE, Endsley RR et al (2012) Prevalence of BRCA mutations in an unselected population of triple-negative breast cancer. Cancer 118(11):2787–2795
68. Gonzalez-Angulo AM, Timms KM, Liu S, Chen H, Litton JK, Potter J et al (2011) Incidence and outcome of BRCA mutations in unselected patients with triple receptor-negative breast cancer. Clin Cancer Res: an official journal of the American Association for Cancer Research 17(5):1082–1089
69. Staaf J, Glodzik D, Bosch A, Vallon-Christersson J, Reuterswärd C, Häkkinen J et al (2019) Whole-genome sequencing of triple-negative breast cancers in a population-based clinical study. Nat Med 25(10):1526–1533

70. Gelmon KA, Tischkowitz M, Mackay H, Swenerton K, Robidoux A, Tonkin K et al (2011) Olaparib in patients with recurrent high-grade serous or poorly differentiated ovarian carcinoma or triple-negative breast cancer: a phase 2, multicentre, open-label, non-randomised study. Lancet Oncol 12(9):852–861

71. Eikesdal HP, Yndestad S, Elzawahry A, Llop-Guevara A, Gilje B, Blix ES et al (2021) Olaparib monotherapy as primary treatment in unselected triple negative breast cancer. Ann Oncol 32(2):240–249

72. Llop-Guevara A, Loibl S, Villacampa G, Vladimirova V, Schneeweiss A, Karn T et al (2021) Association of RAD51 with homologous recombination deficiency (HRD) and clinical outcomes in untreated triple-negative breast cancer (TNBC): analysis of the GeparSixto randomized clinical trial. Ann Oncol 32(12):1590–1596

73. Chopra N, Tovey H, Pearson A, Cutts R, Toms C, Proszek P et al (2020) Homologous recombination DNA repair deficiency and PARP inhibition activity in primary triple negative breast cancer. Nat Commun 11(1):2662

74. Broglio KR, Quintana M, Foster M, Olinger M, McGlothlin A, Berry SM et al (2016) Association of pathologic complete response to neoadjuvant therapy in HER2-positive breast cancer with long-term outcomes: a meta-analysis. JAMA Oncol 2(6):751–760

75. Cortazar P, Zhang L, Untch M, Mehta K, Costantino JP, Wolmark N et al (2014) Pathological complete response and long-term clinical benefit in breast cancer: the CTNeoBC pooled analysis. Lancet 384(9938):164–172

76. Carreira S, Porta N, Arce-Gallego S, Seed G, Llop-Guevara A, Bianchini D et al (2021) Biomarkers associating with PARP inhibitor benefit in prostate cancer in the TOPARP-B trial. Cancer Discov 11(11):2812–2827

77. Balmus G, Pilger D, Coates J, Demir M, Sczaniecka-Clift M, Barros AC et al (2019) ATM orchestrates the DNA-damage response to counter toxic non-homologous end-joining at broken replication forks. Nat Commun 10(1):87

78. Zimmermann M, Murina O, Reijns MAM, Agathanggelou A, Challis R, Tarnauskaitė Ž et al (2018) CRISPR screens identify genomic ribonucleotides as a source of PARP-trapping lesions. Nature 559(7713):285–289

79. Ray Chaudhuri A, Callen E, Ding X, Gogola E, Duarte AA, Lee JE et al (2016) Replication fork stability confers chemoresistance in BRCA-deficient cells. Nature 535(7612):382–387

80. Gogola E, Duarte AA, de Ruiter JR, Wiegant WW, Schmid JA, de Bruijn R et al (2018) Selective loss of PARG restores PARylation and counteracts PARP inhibitor-mediated synthetic lethality. Cancer Cell 33(6):1078–93.e12

81. Vaidyanathan A, Sawers L, Gannon A-L, Chakravarty P, Scott AL, Bray SE et al (2016) ABCB1 (MDR1) induction defines a common resistance mechanism in paclitaxel- and olaparib-resistant ovarian cancer cells. Br J Cancer 115(4):431–441

82. Patch AM, Christie EL, Etemadmoghadam D, Garsed DW, George J, Fereday S et al (2015) Whole-genome characterization of chemoresistant ovarian cancer. Nature 521(7553):489–494

Clinical Application of Poly(ADP-Ribose) Polymerase (PARP) Inhibitors in Ovarian Cancer

5

Melissa M. Pham, Monica Avila, Emily Hinchcliff, and Shannon N. Westin

5.1 Epithelial Ovarian Cancer

Epithelial ovarian cancer (EOC), which includes primary peritoneal and fallopian tube carcinomas, is the fifth leading cause of cancer-related death in women and the most lethal among all gynecologic cancers [1]. Women are often diagnosed at an advanced stage with higher disease burden, thus leading to significant morbidity and mortality [2]. While EOC is initially responsive to platinum-based chemotherapy, with response rates exceeding 80% when combined with optimal cytoreductive surgery, over 70% of women will face relapse within three years [2, 3]. Moreover, the majority of these women will ultimately die from their disease despite multiple lines of treatment [4]. Reported outcomes for patients with

M. M. Pham · M. Avila · S. N. Westin (✉)
Department of Gynecologic Oncology and Reproductive Medicine, University of Texas, M.D. Anderson Cancer Center, 1155 Herman Pressler Dr. CPB 6.3279, Houston, TX 77030, USA
e-mail: swestin@mdanderson.org

M. M. Pham
e-mail: MMPham@mdanderson.org

M. Avila
e-mail: MAvila21@mdanderson.org

M. Avila
Department of Gynecologic Oncology, H. Lee Moffitt Center and Research Institute, Tampa, USA

E. Hinchcliff
Division of Gynecologic Oncology, Department of Obstetrics and Gynecology, Northwestern University Feinberg School of Medicine and the Robert H. Lurie Comprehensive Cancer Center, Chicago, IL, USA
e-mail: emily.hinchcliff@nm.org

© The Author(s), under exclusive license to Springer Nature Switzerland AG 2023
T. A. Yap and G. I. Shapiro (eds.), *Targeting the DNA Damage Response for Cancer Therapy*, Cancer Treatment and Research 186,
https://doi.org/10.1007/978-3-031-30065-3_5

advanced disease include a median progression free survival (PFS) of between 16 and 21 months and a median overall survival (OS) between 32 and 57 months [5].

Deficiencies in the homologous recombination (HRD) DNA repair pathway are relevant in approximately half of high grade serous ovarian carcinomas (HGSOC) and 20% of HGSOC tumors harbor *BRCA1/2* mutations, including both germline and somatic aberrations [6]. Patients with *BRCA1/2*-mutated or HRD-associated tumors have been shown to have exquisite sensitivity to poly(ADP-ribose) polymerase inhibitor (PARPi) treatment, with clinically relevant survival benefit [7, 8]. The use of PARPi has brought about practice-changing results in different treatment settings—frontline maintenance therapy, maintenance therapy for patients with recurrent platinum-sensitive disease, and treatment in the recurrent setting [9].

5.2 Frontline Maintenance

The efficacy of PARPi as maintenance therapy in the upfront setting has been established based on clinically significant progression free survival benefit demonstrated in newly diagnosed ovarian cancer patients in multiple randomized phase III trials (Table 5.1) [4, 9, 10]. Following the survival benefit demonstrated in SOLO1, olaparib received FDA approval in 2018 for use as frontline maintenance therapy in *BRCA*-mutated ovarian cancers [4]. Niraparib showed progression free survival benefit in the PRIMA clinical trial regardless of *BRCA1/2* mutation or HRD status and was thus approved for use as frontline maintenance in all comers in April 2020 [11]. After results from the PAOLA-1 trial, the combination of bevacizumab and olaparib was FDA approved for use in the frontline maintenance setting only for patients with HRD ovarian cancer [12].

5.2.1 SOLO1

Moore et al. explored the utility of olaparib in the maintenance setting of newly diagnosed advanced ovarian cancer in SOLO1, an international, randomized, double-blind phase III clinical trial. The study population included women with germline or somatic *BRCA1/2*-mutant FIGO stage III or IV high grade serous or endometrioid ovarian, primary peritoneal, or fallopian tube cancers with partial response (PR) or complete response (CR) after platinum-based chemotherapy [4]. Trial participants were randomly assigned in a 2:1 fashion to receive olaparib tablets (300 mg twice daily) versus placebo until investigator-assessed disease progression by Response Evaluation Criteria in Solid Tumors (RECIST) version 1.1, or treatment-related toxicity. Treatment was otherwise discontinued at 24 months unless there was ongoing clinical benefit with approved appeal to the medical monitor [4].

A total of 391 patients underwent treatment randomization, with 260 participants assigned to the olaparib treatment arm and 131 participants to the placebo

Table 5.1 Clinical trials evaluating PARPi for frontline maintenance therapy

Trial	Eligibility criteria	Treatment arms	Results
SOLO1	High-grade serous or endometrioid histology	1. Olaparib (300 mg BID)	Median PFS
	Stage III or IV disease	2. Placebo	**Germline or somatic BRCA1/2 mutation**:
	Complete or partial response to chemotherapy		HR for disease progression or death 0.30; 95% CI: 0.23–0.41, P < 0.001
	Received platinum-based chemotherapy without bevacizumab		
	Deleterious or suspected deleterious germline or somatic *BRCA1/2* mutation		
	Primary endpoint: PFS		
	Secondary endpoint: second PFS, OS, TFST, TSST, health related QOL		
PRIMA/ ENGOT-OV26	High-grade serous or endometrioid histology	1. Niraparib (300 mg daily)	Median PFS
	Stage III or IV disease	2. Placebo	**HRD cohort**:
	Patients required to have inoperable disease, residual disease after surgery, or received NACT if stage III disease		21.9 v 10.4 months (HR 0.43; 95% CI: 0.31–0.59, P < 0.001)
	Complete or partial response to chemotherapy		**Overall cohort**:
	Received 6–9 cycles of chemotherapy		13.8 v 8.2 months (HR 0.62; 95% CI: 0.50–0.76, P < 0.001)
	Subgroup analysis: HRD (*BRCA1/2* mutation or score > 42 on Myriad myChoice test), HRP or HR unknown		

(continued)

Table 5.1 (continued)

Trial	Eligibility criteria	Treatment arms	Results
	Primary endpoint: PFS		
	Secondary endpoint: OS, TFST, second PFS, patient-reported outcomes		
PAOLA-1/ ENGOT-OV25	High-grade serous or endometrioid histology; or other nonmucinous epithelial histology with g*BRCA* mutation	1. Olaparib (300 mg BID) + bevacizumab maintenance	Median PFS
	Stage III or IV disease	2. Placebo + bevacizumab maintenance	**Overall cohort:**
	Complete or partial response to chemotherapy		22.1 v 16.6 months (HR 0.59; 95% CI: 0.49–0.72, P < 0.001)
	Received bevacizumab as part of treatment		***sBRCA1/2* mutant cohort**
	HRD and *BRCA1/2* testing		37.2 v 21.7 months (HR 0.31; 95% CI: 0.20–0.47)
			***BRCA1/2* wildtype cohort**
			18.9 v 16.0 months (HR 0.71; 95% CI: 0.58–0.88)
			HRD cohort
			37.2 v 17.7 months (HR 0.33; 95% CI: 0.25–0.45)
			HRD positive, *BRCA1/2* wildtype cohort
			28.1. v 16.6 months (HR 0.43; 95% CI: 0.28–0.66)
	Primary endpoint: PFS		
	Secondary endpoint: time to progression, patient-reported outcomes		
VELIA/ GOG-3005	High-grade serous histology	1. Carboplatin, paclitaxel + veliparib, followed by veliparib maintenance	Median PFS
	Stage III or IV disease	2. Carboplatin, paclitaxel + veliparib, followed by placebo maintenance	**Overall cohort**

(continued)

Table 5.1   (continued)

Trial	Eligibility criteria	Treatment arms	Results
	Patients enrolled before treatment; required 6 cycles of treatment	3. Carboplatin, paclitaxel + placebo, followed by placebo maintenance	23.5 v 17.3 months (HR 0.68; 95% CI: 0.56–0.83, P < 0.001)
	Patient s/p tumor debulking surgery		**gBRCA1/2 mutant cohort**
	HRD and BRCA1/2 testing		34.7 v 22.0 months (HR 0.44; 95% CI: 0.28–0.68, P < 0.001)
			HRD cohort
			31.9 v 20.5 months (HR 0.57; 95% CI: 0.43–0.76, P < 0.001)
	Primary endpoint: PFS in veliparib throughout group v control analyzed sequentially (*BRCA*-mutant, HRD, ITT cohorts)		
	Secondary endpoint: OS in veliparib throughout v control, PFS/OS in veliparib combo group v control, disease related symptom score		

Abbreviations gBRCA1/2 (germline *BRCA1/2*); sBRCA1/2 (somatic *BRCA1/2*); NACT (neoadjuvant chemotherapy); TFST (time to first subsequent therapy), TSST (time to second subsequent therapy); ITT (intention to treat)

arm. Germline *BRCA1/2* (*gBRCA1/2*) mutations were present in 388 patients and somatic mutations were found in 2 patients. At a median follow up of 41 months, treatment with olaparib in the maintenance setting provided profound clinical benefit to women with newly diagnosed *BRCA1/2*-mutated advanced ovarian cancer. With the primary analysis, the Kaplan–Meier estimate of freedom from disease progression and death at 3 years was 60% in the olaparib group compared to 27% in the placebo group (HR 0.30; 95% CI: 0.23 to 0.41; P < 0.001) [4]. The point estimate of PFS in the olaparib treatment arm was nearly 36 months longer than the placebo arm [4]. In a five-year post-hoc follow up analysis, the median PFS for the olaparib arm was 56.0 months (95% CI; 41.9-not reached) v 13.8 months (11.1–18.2 months) in the placebo group (HR 0.33; 95% CI: 0.25–0.43), further supporting olaparib maintenance therapy as the standard of care for newly diagnosed, *BRCA1/2* mutated advanced ovarian cancer [13].

5.2.2   PRIMA/ENGOT-OV26

PRIMA/ENGOT-OV26/GOG-3012 evaluated the use of niraparib as maintenance therapy following platinum-based chemotherapy in a phase III, multicenter, randomized trial [11]. Patients with stage IV or unresectable or sub-optimally debulked stage III disease with high grade serous or endometrioid histology and response to platinum-based chemotherapy were included, representing a higher risk and poor prognostic cohort than the SOLO1 population. Patients were included regardless of HRD status, with HRD positivity defined as harboring a *BRCA1/2* mutation or a score of greater than or equal to 42 on the Myriad myChoice test (encompassing loss of heterozygosity (LOH), telomeric allelic imbalance (TAI), and large-scale state genomic transitions (LSST)). Participants were randomized to receive niraparib (300 mg daily) or placebo for 36 months or disease progression. In response to increased rates of grade 3 and 4 thrombocytopenia associated with potential markers of toxicity, the trial was ultimately amended to allow for an individualized starting dose of niraparib 200 mg daily for patients meeting criteria of platelets below 150,000/μL or total body weight below 77 kg.

About half of the 733 total patients who underwent treatment randomization met criteria for HRD. Those with HRD tumors saw a PFS benefit of 21.9 months with niraparib compared to 10.4 months with placebo (HR 0.43; 95% CI: 0.31 to 0.59; P < 0.001). However, a PFS benefit was also present in the overall population, regardless of HRD status, with a PFS of 13.8 months associated with niraparib use compared to 8.2 months with placebo (HR 0.62, 95% CI: 0.50–0.76; P < 0.001). While patients with *BRCA*-associated disease experienced more benefit from niraparib maintenance therapy, the homologous recombination proficient (HRP) associated survival benefit is notable and established the rationale for subsequent FDA approval of maintenance treatment in all patients with advanced ovarian cancers after a response to first line platinum-based chemotherapy [11].

5.2.3 PAOLA-1/ENGOT-OV25

PAOLA-1 is a randomized, double-blind, phase III international trial evaluating the utility of combining two previously FDA approved maintenance therapies, bevacizumab and olaparib [12]. Eligible patients had stage III–IV high grade serous or endometrioid ovarian cancer with response after first-line platinum-based chemotherapy with bevacizumab. Patients were included regardless of surgical outcome or *BRCA1/2* status; HRD positivity status was determined by Myriad myChoice test (score ≥ 42). All patients received bevacizumab at the standard 15 mg/kg dose every 3 weeks for up to 15 months. Patients were randomized in a 2:1 fashion to receive olaparib (300 mg twice daily) or placebo for up to 24 months or disease progression. The primary end point was time from randomization to disease progression or death. The median follow up was 22.9 months [12].

A total of 806 patients underwent randomization, with 537 patients in the olaparib and 269 patients in the placebo arms. In the intention to treat analysis, patients receiving olaparib plus bevacizumab experienced improved PFS compared to those receiving placebo plus bevacizumab (22.1 months v 16.6 months, HR 0.59; 95% CI: 0.49–0.72; P < 0.001). In the exploratory analysis, the greatest PFS benefit was demonstrated in patients with HRD and *BRCA1/2*-mutated tumors receiving olaparib plus bevacizumab (HR 0.33; 95% CI: 0.25–0.45). The median PFS for *BRCA1/2*-associated patients receiving combination treatment was 37.2 v 21.7 months with placebo (HR 0.31; 95% CI: 0.20–0.47). Similarly, patients with

HRD tumors saw a PFS benefit of 37.2 months v 17.7 months (HR 0.33; 95% CI: 0.25–0.45). Of note, the study design did not include an olaparib only arm to allow head to head comparison of olaparib alone versus combination with bevacizumab nor exploration of the concept of switch maintenance. This raises questions as to whether bevacizumab added to olaparib provides additional clinical benefit, or if the improved PFS observed in the *BRCA1/2* and HRD subgroups can be attributed to PARP inhibition alone rather than synergistic effect. Regardless, no new safety signals were seen with combination maintenance treatment [12].

5.2.4   VELIA/GOG-3005

The VELIA international, placebo-controlled, phase III trial is unique in that it was the first trial to safely evaluate the efficacy of adding a PARPi to primary platinum-based chemotherapy, followed by PARPi maintenance [10]. Eligible patients had untreated stage III-IV high grade serous ovarian cancer and were randomized in a 1:1:1 ratio to one of three arms: (1) control (carboplatin and paclitaxel plus placebo followed by placebo maintenance), (2) veliparib combination (carboplatin and paclitaxel plus veliparib followed by placebo maintenance), and (3) veliparib throughout (carboplatin and paclitaxel plus veliparib followed by veliparib maintenance). A lower dose of veliparib (150 mg twice daily) was used in combination with chemotherapy than in the maintenance setting (300 mg twice daily). Patients could undergo primary or interval cytoreductive surgery. Chemotherapy was administered for 6 cycles and maintenance was continued for 30 cycles. The primary endpoint of PFS was compared between the veliparib throughout and control arms and was analyzed sequentially among *BRCA1/2*-mutated tumors, HRD associated tumors (score $\geq$ 33 on Myriad myChoice), and the ITT population. Comparison of the veliparib combination with placebo was included as a secondary endpoint [10].

A total of 1140 patients underwent randomization. Patients with *BRCA1/2*-mutated disease treated with the veliparib throughout regimen demonstrated a median PFS of 34.7 months compared to 22.0 months seen among the control group (HR 0.44, 95% CI: 0.28–0.68, p < 0.001). Those with HRD tumors receiving veliparib throughout had a median PFS of 31.9 months compared to 20.5 months in the control group (HR 0.57, 95% CI: 0.43–0.76, p < 0.001). PFS benefit was also seen in the intention to treat analysis (23.5 months v 17.3 month, HR 0.68, 95% CI: 0.56–0.83, <0.001). HR proficient patients did not show PFS benefit in the exploratory analysis (15 months v 11.5 months, HR 0.81, 95% CI: 0.60–1.09) [10]. Adding veliparib to primary chemotherapy and continuing the PARPi as maintenance therapy provided PFS benefit compared to primary platinum-based chemotherapy alone; however, there was no veliparib maintenance arm alone, thus the benefit of veliparib in conjunction with chemotherapy remains unclear. Moreover, further evaluation of HRD score and PFS benefit with veliparib has yet to establish a cutoff range, though low scores showed benefit with veliparib compared to chemotherapy alone [14].

As shown in Table 5.2, robust phase III clinical trials have demonstrated PFS benefit with the use of PARPi in the frontline maintenance setting, leading to FDA approval of olaparib, niraparib, and the combination of olaparib and bevacizumab for maintenance therapy in *BRCA1/2*-mutated, all-comers, and HRD-associated disease, respectively. Most recently, the ATHENA-MONO phase III clinical evaluated the efficacy of rucaparib as frontline maintenance therapy in advanced ovarian cancer. The study authors have reported that the primary outcome of PFS has been reached and is significantly improved in the rucaparib arm compared to placebo, regardless of biomarker status **(ASCO2022 abstract citation)**. Given the compelling findings from these practice-changing trials, many more women will now be treated with PARPi in the frontline setting. Data for the reported trials have not yet matured however, and overall survival outcomes are pending.

Table 5.2 Clinical trials evaluating PARPi for maintenance therapy in platinum-sensitive disease

Trial	Eligibility criteria	Treatment arms	Results
Study 19 (NCT00753545)	High-grade serous histology	1. Olaparib (400 mg BID)	Median PFS
	Received at least 2 prior lines of platinum-based chemotherapy and were platinum sensitive	2. Placebo	**Overall cohort**
	Complete or partial response to chemotherapy		HR 0.35; 95% CI: 0.25–0.49, P < 0.0001
			BRCA1/2 mutant cohort
			HR 0.18; 95% CI: 0.10–0.31, P < 0.0001
			non BRCA1/2 mutant cohort
			HR 0.54; 95% CI: 0.34–0.85, P = 0.0075
	Primary endpoint: PFS		
	Secondary endpoint: time to progression, ORR, disease control rate, OS		
SOLO2/ ENGOT-Ov21	High-grade serous or endometrioid histology	1. Olaparib (300 mg BID)	Median PFS
	Received at least 2 prior lines of platinum-based chemotherapy	2. Placebo	**Overall cohort**

(continued)

Table 5.2 (continued)

Trial	Eligibility criteria	Treatment arms	Results
	Complete or partial response to chemotherapy		19.1 v 5.5 months (HR 0.30; 95% CI: 0.22–0.41, P < 0.0001)
	Predicted or suspected deleterious *BRCA1/2* mutation		***BRCA1/2* mutant subgroup**
			19.3 v 5.5 months (HR 0.33; 95% CI: 0.24–0.44, P < 0.0001)
	Primary endpoint: PFS		
	Secondary endpoint: OS, time to progression, TFST, TSST		
NOVA/ NCT01847274	High-grade serous histology	1. Niraparib (300 mg daily)	Median PFS
	Received at least 2 prior lines of platinum-based chemotherapy and were platinum sensitive	2. Placebo	***gBRCA1/2* mutant cohort:**
	Complete or partial response to chemotherapy		21.0 v 5.5 months (HR 0.27; 95% CI: 0.17–0.41, P < 0.001)
	***BRCA1/2* testing with Myriad Genetics**		**non g*BRCA1/2* mutant, HRD positive cohort:**
			12.9 v 3.8 months (HR 0.38; 95% CI: 0.24–0.59, P < 0.001)
			non g*BRCA1/2* mutant cohort:
			9.3 v 3.9 months (HR 0.45; 95% CI: 0.34–0.61, P < 0.001)
	Primary endpoint: PFS		
	Secondary endpoint: patient reported outcomes, chemo-free interval, TFST, TSST, OS		
ARIEL3	High-grade serous or endometrioid histology	1. Rucaparib (600 mg BID)	Median PFS
	Received at least 2 prior lines of platinum-based chemotherapy	2. Placebo	**Intention-to-treat population**

(continued)

Table 5.2 (continued)

Trial	Eligibility criteria	Treatment arms	Results
	Complete or partial response to chemotherapy		10.8 v 5.4 months (HR 0.36; 95% CI: 0.30–0.45, P < 0.0001)
			BRCA1/2 mutant cohort:
			16.6 v 5.4 months (HR 0.23; 95% CI: 0.16–0.34, P < 0.0001)
			HRD positive cohort:
			13.6 v 5.4 months (HR 0.32; 95% CI: 0.24–0.42, P < 0.0001)
	Primary endpoint: PFS		
	Secondary endpoint: time to progression, OS		

Abbreviations ORR (objective response rate), BICR (blind independent central review), ITT (intention to treat), OR (overall response), TFST (time to first subsequent therapy), TSST (time to second subsequent therapy)

5.3 Recurrent, Platinum Sensitive Maintenance

After complete (CR) or partial response (PR) to platinum-based chemotherapy, PARP inhibitors have shown clinical benefit in the second-line maintenance setting [1]. Olaparib, niraparib and rucaparib have thus gained FDA approval for use as maintenance therapy in the platinum-sensitive setting based on data derived from the clinical trials shown in Table 5.2.

Ledermann et al. first evaluated the efficacy of olaparib as maintenance in the recurrent setting in Study 19, a randomized, phase II trial (NCT00753545) comparing olaparib (400 mg capsule formation BID) to placebo in patients with platinum-sensitive, recurrent high grade serous ovarian cancer after at least two prior lines of platinum-based chemotherapy, regardless of *BRCA1/2* status [3]. The primary endpoint of PFS was significantly improved in the olaparib arm with median PFS 8.4 months compared to 4.8 months in the placebo group (HR 0.35; 95% CI: 0.25–0.49; P < 0.001). PFS benefit was even more pronounced in patients with a *BRCA1/2* mutation (HR 0.11; 95% CI: 0.03–0.26) [3]. Furthermore, SOLO2/ENGOT-Ov21 confirmed PFS benefit of olaparib in *BRCA1/2*-associated, recurrent ovarian cancer. In this phase III trial, patients with platinum-sensitive, recurrent ovarian cancer and *BRCA1/2* mutation were randomized 2:1 to receive either olaparib (300 mg twice daily) or placebo. Median PFS was significantly longer in the olaparib arm compared to placebo (10.1 months v 5.5 months, HR 0.30; 95% CI: 0.22–0.41; P < 0.001). The most common toxicities reported were low grade and manageable, including anemia, abdominal pain, and constipation [15].

The NOVA phase III clinical trial evaluated the utility of niraparib as maintenance therapy for patients with recurrent, platinum-sensitive high grade serous ovarian cancer. Patients were randomized 2:1 to receive niraparib (300 mg daily) v placebo. Patients who received niraparib had a significantly longer median PFS than seen in the placebo group and were analyzed in subgroups based on *BRCA/HRD* status. In this study, HRD was defined as presence of either loss of heterozygosity (LOH), large scale state transitions (LSST), or telomeric-allelic imbalance (TAI) [16]. PFS benefit was most notable in patients with *gBRCA1/2* mutations (21.0 v 5.5 months, HR 0.27; 95% CI: 0.17–0.41, P < 0.001). Patients without *BRCA1/2* mutations but with HRD tumors also demonstrated PFS benefit (12.9 v 3.8 months, HR 0.38; 95% CI: 0.24–0.59, P < 0.001). Moreover, HRP patients without *BRCA1/2* mutations also maintained a PFS benefit with use of niraparib maintenance (9.3 months v 3.9 months, HR 0.45; 95% CI: 0.34–0.61, P < 0.001) [16].

Lastly, in the ARIEL3 phase III clinical trial, rucaparib was evaluated as maintenance therapy again in platinum-sensitive, recurrent ovarian cancer. Eligible patients were randomized 2:1 to receive either rucaparib (600 mg BID) or placebo. The use of rucaparib provided significant PFS benefit in all patient subgroups, where study authors defined HRD as loss of heterozygosity >16% [17]. Patients with *BRCA1/2* mutation (16.6 months v 5.4 months, HR 0.23; 95% CI: 0.16–0.34; P < 0.0001) or HRD tumors (13.6 months v 5.4 months, HR 0.32; 95% CI: 0.24–0.42; P < 0.0001) demonstrated the most significant clinical benefit, but there was also benefit in the intent to treat population (10.8 months v 5.4 months, HR 0.36; 95% CI: 0.30–0.45, P < 0.0001) [17].

5.4   Treatment in the Recurrent Setting

As shown in Table 5.3, olaparib, niraparib, and rucaparib have been FDA approved for use as treatment in the recurrent setting of ovarian, fallopian tube, and primary peritoneal cancer [14]. In patients with germline or somatic *BRCA1/2* mutations or genomic instability, platinum sensitivity is a predictor of response to single-agent PARPi.

The SOLO3 phase III clinical trial compared olaparib to non-platinum-based chemotherapy in patients with *gBRCA1/2* mutations. A total of 266 patients were randomized 2:1 to receive olaparib (300 mg daily) or physician's choice single-agent non-platinum-based chemotherapy (pegylated liposomal doxorubicin, weekly paclitaxel, gemcitabine, or topotecan). Olaparib demonstrated superior objective response rate (ORR) and PFS benefit in patients with *gBRCA1/2*-mutated platinum sensitive, recurrent ovarian cancer after receiving at least 2 prior lines of treatment [18].

Niraparib monotherapy was evaluated as treatment in the late recurrent setting of ovarian cancer in the multicenter, open-label, single-arm QUADRA phase II

Table 5.3 Clinical trials evaluating PARPi for treatment in the recurrent setting

Trial	Eligibility criteria	Treatment arms	Results
SOLO3	High-grade serous or endometrioid histology	1. Olaparib (300 mg BID)	ORR
	Evaluable disease (1 lesion) by CT or MRI	2. Physician's choice single-agent chemotherapy	72.2% v 51.4% (OR 2.53; 95%CI: 1.40–4.58, P = 0.002)
	Received at least 2 prior lines of platinum-based chemotherapy and were platinum sensitive		**Subgroup receiving 2 prior lines of treatment**
	Confirmed gBRCA1/2 mutation		84.6% v 61.5% (OR 3.44; 95% CI: 1.42–8.54)
			Median PFS
			13.4 v 9.2 months (HR 0.62; 95% CI: 0.43–0.91, P = 0.013)
	Primary endpoint: ORR by BICR in measurable disease		
	Secondary endpoint: PFS in ITT population		
QUADRA	High-grade serous histology	1. Niraparib (300 mg daily)	Investigator-assessed confirmed OR
	Received at least 3 prior lines of platinum-based chemotherapy		**HRD-positive, platinum-sensitive cohort**
	All patients underwent HRD testing with Myriad myChoice and *BRCA1/2* testing		28% (13/47) achieved OR (95% CI: 15.6–42.6, p = 0.00053);; median DOR 9.2 months (95% CI: 5.9-not estimable)
			Response evaluable cohort
			10% (38/387) achieved OR
			Modified per-protocol cohort
			8% (38/456) achieved OR; DOR 9.4 months (95% CI: 6.6–18.3)
			Median OS
			BRCA1/2-**mutated subgroup**: 26.0 months (95% CI: 18.1-not estimable)
			HRD-positive subgroup: 19.0 months (95% CI: 14.5–24.6)
			HRP subgroup: 15.5 months (95% CI: 11.6–19.0)

(continued)

Table 5.3 (continued)

Trial	Eligibility criteria	Treatment arms	Results
	Primary endpoint: investigator-assessed confirmed OR		
	Secondary endpoints: OR, DOR, disease control, PFS, OS		
ARIEL2	High-grade serous or endometrioid histology	1. Rucaparib (600 mg BID)	Median PFS
	Received at least 2 prior lines of platinum-based chemotherapy		**BRCA1/2-mutated subgroup**
	Platinum-sensitive to last line of platinum-based therapy		12.8 months (HR 0.27: 95% CI: 0.16–0.44, P < 0.0001)
	Measurable disease per RECIST v 1.1		**LOH high subgroup**
			5.7 months (HR 0.62; 95% CI: 0.42–0.90, P = 0.011)
			LOH low subgroup
			5.2 months
	Primary endpoint: PFS		
	Exploratory analysis: comparison of LOH classification, CA 125 response		

Abbreviations ORR (objective response rate), BICR (blind independent central review), ITT (intention to treat), OR (overall response)

study. Eligible patients had relapsed, high grade serous ovarian cancer and were platinum sensitive to their last line of treatment (patients must have had at least 3 prior lines). All patients underwent HRD testing with Myriad myChoice and germline *BRCA1/2* testing. A total of 463 patients were enrolled and received oral niraparib (300 mg daily) until disease progression. The median follow up for OS was 12.2 months. HRD-positive tumors, including *gBRCA1/2*-mutated, *sBRCA1/2*-mutated, and *BRCA1/2* wild-type/HRD-positive, comprised 48% of the study population; 87/463 or 19% of patients had a germline or somatic *BRCA1/2* mutation. Of the 47 patients who were HRD-positive, platinum-sensitive, and PARP naïve, the median PFS was 5.5 months (95% CI: 3.5–8.2), median duration of response (DOR) 9.2 months (5.9-not estimable), and 68% achieved disease control. The number of patients achieving an overall response was most significant in *BRCA1/2*-mutated and HRD associated tumors. The median OS was 26.0 months in the *BRCA1/2*-mutated group (95% CI: 18.1-not estimable), 19.0 months in HRD group (95% CI: 14.5–24.6), and 15.5 months in the HRD-negative group (95% CI: 11.6–19.0) [19]. This led to the FDA approval of niraparib in patients with HRD-associated recurrent ovarian cancer with 3 or more prior lines of therapy.

In the ARIEL2 phase II trial evaluating rucaparib in the treatment of recurrent, platinum-sensitive high grade ovarian cancer, HRD status (defined by LOH) was explored as a potential predictor of treatment response. Of the 206 patients enrolled, 192 patients were classified into one of three predefined HRD subgroups:

(1) deleterious somatic or germline *BRCA1/2* mutation, (2) *BRCA1/2* wild-type, LOH high, and (3) *BRCA1/2* wild-type LOH low. Median PFS was longer with rucaparib treatment in the *BRCA1/2* mutant (12.8 months, HR 0.27; 95% CI: 0.16–0.44, P < 0.0001) and LOH high subgroups (5.7 months, HR 0.62; 95% CI: 0.42–0.90, P = 0.011) compared to LOH low subgroup (5.2 months) [20]. Data from this study, in combination with early phase data in ovarian cancer, were utilized to yield an FDA approval for rucaparib in recurrent *BRCA* mutant ovarian cancer after 2 or more prior lines of therapy. In post-hoc analysis of tumor samples from ARIEL2, mutations in *RAD51C* and *RAD51D*, as well as HRD status predicted better treatment response [21]. ASCO Guidelines thus recommend using either of the approved PARPi as a treatment strategy in patients who are *BRCA1/2*-mutated or HRD with platinum sensitive, recurrent ovarian cancer [22].

5.5 Treatment Considerations and Management of Common Toxicities

Given the PFS benefit demonstrated in the previously reviewed clinical trials and FDA approval of the use of olaparib, niraparib, and rucaparib in different treatment settings, many more patients will be treated with a PARPi early in their cancer course. To optimize the efficacy and clinical benefit, however, consideration must be made based on predictors of response, including *BRCA1/2* mutation, HRD status, and platinum sensitivity. Ease of administration may also be taken into account, with olaparib and rucaparib requiring twice daily dosing compared to once daily dosing of niraparib. Moreover, a balance of efficacy and toxicities must also be measured. The most common toxicities associated with PARPi include hematologic toxicities, gastrointestinal (GI) toxicities, renal toxicities, and fatigue.

5.5.1 Managing Hematologic Toxicities

Anemia and thrombocytopenia are the most common toxicities reported in clinical trials of PARPi [9, 15, 17, 23]. Fortunately, the cytopenias occur early in treatment initiation and recover after a few cycles of therapy. In the ARIEL3 trial evaluating rucaparib maintenance therapy, 139/372 or 37% of patients experienced anemia [17]. Of the 195 patients treated with olaparib in the SOLO2 trial, 44% had any grade anemia [15]. Niraparib has demonstrated the greatest anemia toxicity, with 50% of patients having any grade and 25% having grade 3 or 4 anemia [16]. Blood transfusions are indicated in the setting of symptomatic anemia, or hemoglobin (Hgb) values <7.0 g/dL. Using the Common Terminology Criteria of Adverse Events, v5.0, if grade 2 or higher anemia is noted, treatment hold and consideration of transfusion if indicated is recommended. Restarting treatment at a reduced dose or discontinuing completely if counts do not recover appropriately are additional strategies to consider [23].

Niraparib is also associated with higher rates of thrombocytopenia, including grade 3 or 4 toxicity occurring in 34% of patients receiving niraparib maintenance [16]. Rates of thrombocytopenia are less frequent with use of olaparib (14%) and rucaparib (28%), including grade 3–4 toxicities at 1 and 5%, respectively [15, 17]. In a subsequent study of patients treated with niraparib 300 mg daily, bodyweight and total platelet counts were noted to be reliable predictors of requiring dose reduction. Grade 3 or 4 thrombocytopenias were more common in patients with bodyweight less than 77 kg or platelet counts less than 150,000 cells/μL (35% v 12%) compared to their counterparts [24]. It is thus clinically recommended that the starting dose of niraparib be adjusted to 200 mg daily for patients meeting these criteria. Grade 2 or greater toxicity warrants treatment hold and consideration of dose reduction or discontinuation if counts do not recover. Dose reduction down to 100 mg was allowable. Monthly complete blood counts (CBC) with differential should be utilized to monitor bone marrow toxicity in patients starting treatment with PARPi. Weekly laboratory testing may be necessary to monitor counts within the first month of initiating niraparib, or after dose modification of any PARPi [23].

5.5.2 Managing GI and Renal Toxicities

The most common GI toxicity demonstrated in clinical trials with PARPi include mild nausea, with only 3–4% of patients experiencing grade 3 or 4 nausea [15–17, 23]. Olaparib (75%), niraparib (74%), and rucaparib (75%) demonstrated similar rates of nausea and management was similar that of chemotherapy-induced emesis [15–17]. Common strategies include daily anti-emetics such as 5-HT3 antagonists, antihistamines as well as recommendation of a light meal prior to PARPi administration [23]. Low grade vomiting, constipation, and diarrhea were reported by up to 40% of patients in clinical trials. Symptoms were often relieved with common over the counter medications, including senna and polyethylene glycol for constipation, loperamide for diarrhea, and anti-emetics for vomiting [23]. Grade 3 or 4 adverse events were rare.

Higher rates of elevated creatinine were reported with rucaparib use compared to placebo (15% v 2%) in ARIEL3 [17]. Similarly, grade 1 or 2 elevated creatinine was seen in 11% (21/195 patients) of patients receiving olaparib maintenance compared to 1% in the placebo group in SOLO2 [15]. The creatinine abnormalities reported in clinical trials were not necessarily associated with dysfunctional glomerular filtration rate (GFR). Rucaparib and olaparib are known to inhibit the poly-specific transporter proteins MATE1 and MATE2-K in the renal tubules and thus affect creatinine secretion. If renal insufficiency is suspected, further interrogation with imaging and radionucleotide scan may be warranted. Otherwise, elevated creatinine has been observed within the first weeks of treatment and recovery with continued treatment. Dose reductions and treatment holds may be avoided if GFR remains within normal limits [23, 25]. Of note, renal toxicity has not been associated with niraparib.

5.5.3 Managing Fatigue

Mild fatigue is a common toxicity seen with all PARPi and typically managed with supportive care measures. Fatigue of any grade was reported in up to 70% of patients in clinical trials evaluating PARPi maintenance. Grade 3 or 4 fatigue was noted in less than 10% of patients [15–17]. First line management of fatigue generally involves exercise and massage or behavioral therapy. Pharmacologic intervention with methylphenidate may be required for refractory, higher grade fatigue [23].

5.5.4 Managing Secondary Malignancies

Secondary malignancies, specifically myelodysplastic syndrome (MDS) and acute myeloid leukemia (AML), have been reported as long-term risks associated with use of PARPi, attributed to PARPi-induced alterations of cellular DNA damage repair pathways [26]. These fatal events have been found to occur 10–15 years after exposure to cytotoxic agents. A meta-analysis of randomized trials exploring use of PARPi in solid tumors reported an increased risk of MDS/AML with use of PARPI in the front-line setting, with a pooled incidence rate ration (IRR) of 5.43 (95% CI: 1.51–19.60) [27]. Interestingly, incidence of MDS/AML was not statistically different in trials that incorporated PARPi in the recurrent setting, despite the large proportion of heavily pretreated patients [27]. For further context, the ovarian cancer-specific clinical trials described in this chapter reported MDS/AML as a rare AE (incidence 0.5–1.4%) [15–17]. Regardless, it is important to discuss these risks given the increasing use of and expanding indications for PARPi. Moreover, as the utility of PARPi after PARPi use is further delineated, the duration of use could be significantly increased and thus potentially increase risk.

In heavily pre-treated ovarian cancer patients, it may be difficult to determine the etiology of secondary malignancies. A thorough workup is warranted for any patient with a history of PARPi use presenting with pancytopenia. Nutritional deficiencies, viral infections, bone marrow dysplasias, and other causes should be ruled out. Referral to Hematology/Oncology and consideration of bone marrow aspiration may be indicated. In the extremely rare event that MDS/AML is observed during treatment, the PARPi should be discontinued immediately [23].

5.6 Future Directions

PARP inhibitors have changed the landscape of the treatment of ovarian cancer with improved PFS and durable responses. The FDA has approved the use of olaparib, niraparib in the frontline maintenance, maintenance of recurrent platinum-sensitive disease, and treatment in the recurrent setting. Rucaparib is pending approval for frontline maintenance but is currently approved for maintenance of recurrent platinum-sensitive disease and treatment in the recurrent setting.

We still face clinical challenges, however, in managing toxicities and extending benefit beyond presumed resistance to PARPi.

The OReO/ENGOT Ov-38 study is a phase III clinical trial evaluating the efficacy of olaparib in platinum-sensitive, recurrent ovarian cancer with at least 1 prior line of PARPi maintenance. Two cohorts of patients were enrolled (*BRCA1/2*-mutant and *BRCA1/2* wildtype) and randomized 2:1 to receive either olaparib 300 mg daily or placebo. The majority of patients had received 3 or more prior lines of therapy. Of the *BRCA1/2* wildtype patients, 40% were HRD positive. Data reported at the recent 2021 ESMO conference demonstrated PFS benefit with re-challenge of olaparib despite *BRCA1/2* mutation status. The PFS of *BRCA1/2*-mutant patients receiving olaparib was 4.3 months compared to 2.8 months in the placebo arm (HR 0.57; 95% CI: 0.37–0.87; P < 0.022). For *BRCA1/2* wildtype patients, a PFS benefit of 5.3 months was demonstrated compared to 2.8 months with placebo (HR 0.43; 95% CI: 0.26–0.71; P = 0.0023) [25]. Unfortunately, due to the high number of prior lines of chemotherapy, the question of whether to use a PARPi after progression during upfront PARPi maintenance cannot be answered by the results of the OReO trial. Further, identification of biomarkers which may predict response and resistance to PARPi re-treatment is critical. While circulating tumor DNA (ctDNA) and liquid biopsy are being utilized to explore the incidence of *BRCA1/2* reversion mutations in early phase clinical trials, this technology has yet to reach the clinical stage and become standard of care due to many different factors, including cost.

To further optimize efficacy of PARPi and overcome resistance, current clinical trials are evaluating combination treatment with other therapies targeting the DNA damage repair pathway, chemotherapy, immunotherapy, and radiation therapy.

References

1. Siegel RL, Miller KD, Fuchs HE, Jemal A (2021) Cancer statistics, 2021. CA Cancer J Clin 71(1):7–33
2. Peres LC, Sinha S, Townsend MK, Fridley BL, Karlan BY, Lutgendorf SK et al (2021) Predictors of survival trajectories among women with epithelial ovarian cancer. Gynecol Oncol 156(2):459–466
3. Ledermann J, Harter P, Gourley C et al (2012) Olaparib maintenance therapy in platinum-sensitive relapsed ovarian cancer. N Engl J Med 366:1382–1392
4. Moore K, Colombo N, Scambia G, Kim BG, Oaknin A, Friedlander M et al (2018) Maintenance olaparib in patients with newly diagnosed advanced ovarian cancer. N Engl J Med 379(26):2495–2505
5. Paoletti X, Lewsley L, Daniele G, Cook A, Yanaihara N et al (2020) Assessment of progression-free survival as a surrogate end point of overall survival in first-line treatment of ovarian cancer. JAMA Netw Open
6. Bell D, Berchuck A, Birrer M et al (2011) Integrated genomic analyses of ovarian carcinoma. Nature 474:609–615
7. McCabe N, Turner N, Lord C et al (2006) Deficiency in the repair of DNA damage by homologous recombination and sensitivity to poly(ADP-ribose) polymerase inhibition. Cancer Res 66(16):8109–8115

8. Lheureux S, Lai Z, Dougherty B, Runswick S et al (2017) Long-term responders on olaparib maintenance in high-grade serous ovarian cancer: clinical and molecular characterization. Clin Cancer Res 23(15):4086–4094

9. Mirza M, Coleman R, Gonzalez-Martin A, Moore K, Colombo N, Ray-Coquard I et al (2020) The forefront of ovarian cancer therapy: update on PARP inhibitors. Ann Oncol S0923–7534(20):39891–39894

10. Coleman RL, Fleming GF, Brady MF, Swisher EM, Steffensen KD, Friedlander M et al (2019) Veliparib with first-line chemotherapy and as maintenance therapy in ovarian cancer. N Engl J Med 381(25):2403–2415

11. Gonzalez-Martin A, Bhavana P, Vergote I et al (2019) Niraparib in patients with newly diagnosed advanced ovarian cancer. N Engl J Med 381:2391–2402

12. Ray-Coquard I, Pautier P, Pignata S, Pérol D, González-Martín A, Berger R et al (2019) Olaparib plus Bevacizumab as First-Line Maintenance in Ovarian Cancer. N Engl J Med 381(25):2416–2428

13. Banerjee S, Moore K, Colombo N, Scambia G, Kim B, Oaknin A et al (2021) Maintenance olaparib for patients with newly diagnosed advanced ovarian cancer and a BRCA mutation (SOLO1/GOG 3004): 5-year follow-up of a randomised, double-blind, placebo-controlled, phase 3 trial. Lancet Oncol 22(1):1721–1731

14. Swisher E, Birrer M, Moore K, Coleman R et al (2020) Exploring the relationship between homologous recombination score and progression-free survival in BRCA wildtype ovarian carcinoma. In: Analysis of veliparib plus carboplatin/paclitaxel in the velia study, Abstract LBA6 presented at proceedings of the society

15. Pujade-Lauraine E, Ledermann J, Selle F, Gebski V, Penson R, Oza A et al (2017) Olaparib tablets as maintenance therapy in patients with platinum-sensitive, relapsed ovarian cancer and a BRCA1/2 mutation (SOLO2/ENGOT-Ov21): a double-blind, randomised, placebo-controlled, phase 3 trial. Lancet Oncol 18(9):1274–1284

16. Mirza MR, Monk BJ, Herrstedt J, Oza AM, Mahner S, Redondo A et al (2016) Niraparib maintenance therapy in platinum-sensitive, recurrent ovarian cancer. N Engl J Med 375(22):2154–2164

17. Coleman R, Oza A, Lorusso D et al (2017) Rucaparib maintenance treatment for recurrent ovarian carcinoma after response to platinum therapy (ARIEL3): a randomised, double-blind, placebo-controlled, phase 3 trial. Lancet 390:1949–1961

18. Penson R, Valencia R, Cibula D, Colombo N, Leath C et al (2020) Olaparib versus nonplatinum chemotherapy in patients with platinum-sensitive relapsed ovarian cancer and a germline BRCA1/2 mutation (SOLO3): a randomized phase III trial. J Clin Oncol 38(11):1164–1174

19. Moore K, Secord A, Geller M et al (2019) Niraparib monotherapy for late-line treatment of ovarian cancer (QUADRA): a multicenter, open-label, single-arm, phase 2 trial. Lancet Oncol 20(5):636–648

20. Swisher EM, Lin KK, Oza AM, Scott CL, Giordano H et al (2017) Rucaparib in relapsed, platinum-sensitive high-grade ovarian carcinoma (ARIEL2 Part 1): an international, multicentre, open-label, phase 2 trial. Lancet Oncol 18(1):75–87

21. Swisher E, Kwan T, Oza A, Tinker A, Ray-Coquard I et al (2021) Molecular and clinical determinants of response and resistance to rucaparib for recurrent ovarian cancer treatment in ARIEL2 (Parts 1 and 2). Nat Commun 12(1):2487

22. Tew W, Lacchetti C, Ellis A, Maxian K, Banerjee S, Bookman M et al (2020) PARP inhibitors in the management of ovarian cancer: ASCO guideline. J Clin Oncol 38(30):3468–3493

23. LaFargue C, Dal Molin G, Sood A, Coleman R (2019) Exploring and comparing adverse events between PARP inhibitors. Lancet Oncol 20(1):15–28

24. Berek J, Matulonis U, Peen U et al (2018) Safety and dose modification for patients receiving niraparib. Ann Oncol 29(8):1784–1792

25. Dal Molin G, Westin S, Msaouel P, Gomes L et al (2020) Discrepancy in calculated and measured glomerular filtration rates in patients treated with PARP inhibitors. Int J Gynecol Cancer 30(1):89–93

26. Shenolikar R, Durden E, Meyer N, Lenhart G, Moore K (2018) Incidence of secondary myelodysplastic syndrome (MDS) and acute myeloid leukemia (AML) in patients with ovarian or breast cancer in a real-world setting in the United States. Gynecol Oncol 151:190–195
27. Nitecki R, Melamed A, Gockley A et al (2021) Incidence of myelodysplastic syndrome and acute myeloid leukemia in patients receiving poly-ADP ribose polymerase inhibitors for the treatment of solid tumors: a meta-analysis of randomized trials. Gynecol Oncol 161(3):653–659

Clinical Use of PARP Inhibitors in BRCA Mutant and Non-BRCA Mutant Breast Cancer

6

Filipa Lynce and Mark Robson

6.1 Introduction

Patients with germline BRCA mutation (gBRCAm)-associated breast cancers tend to occur in younger women compared to those who do not have a germline mutation. In addition, patients with a *BRCA1* deleterious mutation more often develop triple-negative breast cancer (TNBC), a subtype associated with reduced treatment options, while patients with *BRCA2*-associated tumors develop breast cancers that replicate the distribution of subtypes seen in sporadic breast cancers.

The use of poly(ADP-ribose) polymerase (PARP) inhibitors for the treatment of patients with gBRCAm and breast cancer is a success of genomically-directed treatment [1], both in the early and advanced settings. The observations of single-agent activity of PARP inhibitors in BRCA-deficient cancer cells, published in Nature in 2005 by two independent research groups, opened the doors to multiple clinical trials evaluating PARP inhibitors as monotherapy and in combination with other agents [2, 3]. The enthusiasm around PARP inhibitors was initially tampered by the negative results of a phase III trial evaluating the role of iniparib combined with carboplatin and gemcitabine for the treatment of TNBC, following positive randomized phase II results [4, 5]. Subsequent data suggested that iniparib is structurally distinct from PARP inhibitors and a poor inhibitor of PARP activity [6, 7],

F. Lynce (✉)
Harvard Medical School, Medical Oncology, Dana-Farber Cancer Institute, Dana-Farber Brigham Cancer Institute, 450 Brookline Avenue, Boston, MA 02215, USA
e-mail: filipa_lynce@dfci.harvard.edu

M. Robson
Breast Medicine and Clinical Genetics Services, Memorial Sloan Kettering Cancer Center, Weill Cornell Medical College, 300 East 66th Street, Room 813, New York, NY 10065, USA
e-mail: robsonm@mskcc.org

T. A. Yap and G. I. Shapiro (eds.), *Targeting the DNA Damage Response for Cancer Therapy*, Cancer Treatment and Research 186,
https://doi.org/10.1007/978-3-031-30065-3_6

rekindling interest in this drug class for the treatment of BRCA-associated breast cancers.

In this chapter we review the results of trials that have defined the clinical landscape of PARP inhibitor utilization in breast cancer and present ongoing trials that have the potential to impact clinical practice.

6.2 Clinical Use of PARP Inhibitors for Advanced BRCA-Mutant Breast Cancer

6.2.1 Monotherapy

Two large, randomized phase III trials have demonstrated the efficacy of olaparib and talazoparib for the treatment of patients with BRCA-associated breast cancer (Table 6.1). In the phase III OlympiAD trial, 302 patients with a gBRCA mutation and HER2-negative metastatic breast cancer were randomized to receive olaparib or standard therapy in a 2:1 ratio [8]. Standard therapy regimens included one of the following three prespecified chemotherapy regimens: capecitabine, eribulin, or vinorelbine. In terms of platinum exposure, receipt of platinum in the (neo)adjuvant setting was allowed if at least 12 months had elapsed since the last dose, and in the metastatic setting if there was no evidence of disease progression while being treated with a platinum.

Table 6.1 Summary of the randomized phase III studies with PARP inhibitors in BRCA-associated advanced breast cancer

Trial	N	Experimental arm	Control arm	Prior lines of therapy	Prior platinum	Primary endpoint
OlympiAD [8–10]	302	Olaparib	Capecitabine, eribulin, or vinorelbine	≤ 2 previous chemotherapy regimens for metastatic disease Required anthracycline (unless contraindicated) and a taxane in the neoadjuvant, adjuvant or metastatic setting	Previous neoadjuvant or adjuvant platinum was allowed if ≥ 12 months had elapsed since the last dose Previous platinum for metastatic disease was allowed if no evidence of disease progression during treatment	PFS 7.0 versus 4.2 months favoring olaparib; HR 0.58; 95% CI 0.43–0.80; P < 0.001)

(continued)

Table 6.1 (continued)

Trial	N	Experimental arm	Control arm	Prior lines of therapy	Prior platinum	Primary endpoint
EMBRACA [11–13]	431	Talazoparib	Capecitabine, eribulin, gemcitabine, or vinorelbine	≤ 3 previous cytotoxic regimens for advanced breast cancer Required previous treatment with a taxane, an anthracycline, or both, unless this treatment was contraindicated	Previous neoadjuvant or adjuvant platinum-based therapy was permitted, provided the patient had a DFI of ≥ 6 months after the last dose Patients with objective disease progression while receiving platinum chemotherapy for advanced breast cancer were excluded	PFS 8.6 versus 5.6 months favoring talazoparib; HR 0.54; 95% CI 0.41–0.71, p < 0.001
BROCADE [14]	513	Paclitaxel, carboplatin and veliparib	Paclitaxel, carboplatin	≤ 2 previous cytotoxic chemotherapy regimens for metastatic breast cancer Patients could have received a previous taxane as neoadjuvant or adjuvant therapy or to treat locally advanced disease, if given more than 6 months before study start	≤ 1 previous line of platinum therapy without progression within 12 months of completing treatment	PFS 14.5 versus 12.6 months favoring veliparib arm, HR 0.71, CI 0.57–0.88, p 0.002

CI: confidence interval; DFI: disease-free interval; HR: hazard ratio; PFS: progression-free survival

Median progression-free survival (PFS), which was the primary endpoint of the study, was significantly longer for patients treated with olaparib compared to those treated with standard therapy (7.0 months vs. 4.2 months; hazard ratio [HR] for disease progression or death 0.58; 95% confidence interval [CI] 0.43–0.80; $p < 0.001$). The overall response rate (ORR) was 59.9% in the olaparib group and 28.8% in the standard therapy arm. Grade 3 or higher adverse events were lower in the olaparib arm (36.6% vs. 50.5%) and there were no cases of myelodysplastic syndrome (MDS) or acute myeloid leukemia (AML) reported in either arm [9] Health-related quality of life, assessed by patient-completed European Organization for Research and Treatment of Cancer Quality of Life Questionnaire Core 30-item module (EORTC QLQ-C30), was consistently improved for patients treated with olaparib compared with standard therapy [10].

An ad hoc subset analysis of extended follow-up for overall survival (OS) of the OlympiAD study showed that, in the first-line setting, the median OS was longer for olaparib compared to standard therapy (22.6 vs. 14.7 months; HR 0.55; 95% CI 0.33–0.95), with 3-year survival of 40% for olaparib versus 12.8% for standard therapy, suggesting the possibility of meaningful long-term survival with olaparib when used early [9].

In the phase III EMBRACA trial, a similar study design was used to compare talazoparib to physicians' treatment of choice [11]. This was a randomized open-label study where 431 patients with HER2-negative advanced breast cancer carrying a g*BRCA1/2* mutation were assigned, in a 2:1 ratio, to receive talazoparib 1 mg once daily or the physician's choice of chemotherapy (capecitabine, eribulin, gemcitabine, or vinorelbine). The primary endpoint was PFS assessed by blinded independent central review.

Talazoparib demonstrated a statistically significant improvement in PFS compared to standard therapy (8.6 vs. 5.6 months; HR for disease progression or death 0.54; 95% CI 0.41–0.71; p < 0.001). Like what was observed in the OlympiAD trial, the ORR was higher in the talazoparib group compared to the standard-therapy group (62.6% vs. 27.2%; odds ratio 5.0; 95% CI 2.9–8.8; P < 0.001). Hematologic grade 3–4 adverse events (primarily anemia) occurred in 55% of the patients who received talazoparib and in 38% of the patients who received the physician's choice of therapy. There were no confirmed cases of MDS. One case of AML occurred in each arm. Patients assigned to the talazoparib arm had significant overall improvements and significant delays in the time to clinically meaningful deterioration in multiple cancer-related and breast cancer-specific symptoms scales [12]. Similar to the OlympiAD trial, there was no statistically significant differences in OS between arms although subsequent treatments may have impacted analysis [13].

Based on these results, the U.S. Food and Drug Administration (FDA) approved olaparib and talazoparib in 2018 for the treatment of patients with deleterious or suspected deleterious gBRCA-mutated HER2-negative metastatic breast cancer.

6.2.2   In Combination with Chemotherapy

Given the previously demonstrated sensitivity of BRCA-associated cancers to platinum agents, the BROCADE 3 trial explored the use of veliparib, a PARP inhibitor, in combination with a platinum-containing regimen [14]. This was a double-blind phase III trial that randomized 513 patients with deleterious g*BRCA1/2* mutation-associated advanced HER2-negative breast cancer to receive carboplatin and paclitaxel with veliparib or placebo. If patients discontinued carboplatin and paclitaxel due to toxicity prior to progression, they could continue veliparib or placebo until disease progression. The primary endpoint was investigator-assessed PFS. Overall, 8% of participating patients had received prior platinum and 19% had received chemotherapy for metastatic disease. Median PFS was superior for patients who received veliparib (14.5 vs. 12.6 months; HR 0.71; 95% CI 0.57–0.88; p 0.002). With a median follow up of nearly 36 months, 26% of patients treated with veliparib were alive and progression-free compared to 11% of patients in the placebo-containing arm.

The results of this study were not widely adopted but they provided important insights into the treatment of BRCA-associated breast cancer. Since patients were allowed to continue veliparib (or placebo) after chemotherapy was discontinued and the PFS curves seemed to separate after most patients stopped chemotherapy, the benefit of the PARP inhibitors in this study may reflect maintenance use rather than the benefit of combining it with chemotherapy. Therefore, the question remains if there may be a role for induction chemotherapy in patients with metastatic BRCA-associated breast cancer, similar to the current practice in ovarian cancer, followed by maintenance therapy with a PARP inhibitor given as monotherapy [15, 16].

6.2.3 In Combination with Immunotherapy

Preclinical models have shown that PARP inhibitors and anti-PD1 antibodies show synergistic activity. PARP inhibitors activate the STING pathway leading to T cell recruitment and stimulate antigen presentation via increased T cell cytotoxic activity, creating a tumor microenvironment that may be more susceptible to immunotherapy. The combination of these agents in gBRCA-associated breast cancer was evaluated in three studies: the MEDIOLA [17], TOPACIO [18] and the JAVELIN [19] trials.

The MEDIOLA trial was a multicenter phase I/II basket trial of durvalumab and olaparib in solid tumors. One of the initial cohorts included patients with gBRCA-mutated breast cancer [17]. Patients should have received ≤ 2 lines of chemotherapy for metastatic breast cancer. Overall, 34 patients were enrolled with 30 patients comprising the full-analysis set. Twenty-four out of 30 (80%; 90% CI 64.3–90.9%) patients experienced disease control rate (DCR) at 12 weeks (primary efficacy endpoint) and, at a median follow up of 6.7 months, the median PFS was 8.2 months (95% CI 4.6–11.8). The safety profile was similar to what was previously observed with olaparib and durvalumab monotherapy studies.

The TOPACIO trial was a multicenter, open-label, single-arm, phase II study with a phase I lead-in portion evaluating the safety and efficacy of combination treatment with niraparib and pembrolizumab in patients with metastatic TNBC [18]. The primary objective of the phase II study was ORR and secondary endpoints included PFS, DCR and duration of response (DOR). In the full analysis population (n = 55), the confirmed ORR was 21% (90% CI 12–33%) with a complete response in 5 (11%) patients. In all treated patients, the median PFS was 2.3 months (95% CI 2.1–3.9 months). There was evidence of clinical activity in patients irrespective of BRCA or PD-L1 status; although, not surprisingly, the clinical activity was more pronounced in those patients with BRCA-mutated tumors or PD-L1-positive tumors.

Finally, the JAVELIN BRCA/ATM study was a multicenter, open-label, phase IIb trial that evaluated whether the combination of talazoparib and avelumab was effective in patients with pathogenic *BRCA1/2* or *ATM* alterations, regardless of tumor type [19]. Overall, 57 patients with breast cancer were enrolled and 51 had a *BRCA1/2* mutation. Within the *BRCA1/2* breast cancer cohort, the ORR was 47.1% (24/51), which was generally consistent with what was seen with previous PARP inhibitor monotherapy and/or in combination with immune checkpoint inhibitors.

ETCTN 10020 (NCT02849496) is a randomized phase II trial investigating the role of olaparib with or without atezolizumab for the treatment of advanced BRCA-associated HER2-negative breast cancer. The primary endpoint of this study is PFS. This study has completed accrual and results are eagerly awaited.

6.3 Clinical Use of PARP Inhibitors for Early BRCA-Mutant Breast Cancer

6.3.1 Neoadjuvant Setting

The use of PARP inhibitors in the neoadjuvant setting may allow some patients to achieve a pathological complete response (pCR) without requiring the use of polychemotherapy and its associated toxicity. To estimate tumor responses to PARP inhibitor as monotherapy, a pilot trial of 20 patients with gBRCA mutations and stage I-III breast cancer was initially planned. Patients received 2 months of talazoparib before initiating standard neoadjuvant chemotherapy. Two months of treatment with talazoparib resulted in a median decrease of tumor volume of 88% (range, 30% to 98%) measured by breast ultrasound [20], which led to early interruption of the study. A new pilot study was designed to evaluate the pathologic response of talazoparib given as neoadjuvant monotherapy for 6 months [21]. The primary endpoint was residual cancer burden (RCB). Twenty patients were enrolled, 15 had TNBC and 5 had estrogen receptor (ER)-positive HER2-negative disease. The RCB 0 rate was 53% and the RCB 0/I rate was 63%. This led to the conduct of a single-arm phase II trial evaluating talazoparib for 6 months in patients with stage I-III TNBC and gBRCA mutations, the NeoTALA study [22]. In 48 evaluable patients (received at least 80% of the talazoparib dose), treatment with talazoparib resulted in a pCR rate of 45.8%. These studies have suggested that some patients with BRCA mutations and breast cancer may achieve excellent responses with the use of a non-chemotherapy containing neoadjuvant regimen. Niraparib has also been investigated in this setting. A single arm pilot study (NCT03329937) that enrolled 24 patients with early stage HER2-negative

BRCA1/2 mutated breast cancer recently reported a pCR of 38.1% (8 out of 21 efficacy evaluable patients) with 2–6 cycles of niraparib. Of these 8 patients, 2 received neoadjuvant chemotherapy after niraparib and prior to surgery [23]. Interestingly, high niraparib intratumoral concentration was observed in 10 patients with time-matched plasma/tumor samples collected after 2 cycles of niraparib.

The TBCRC056 study (NCT04584255) and the OlympiaN trial (NCT05498155) are also investigating the benefit of adding immunotherapy to a PARP inhibitor in the neoadjuvant setting. In the TBCRC056 study, patients are currently being accrued to receive preoperative niraparib with dostarlimab in patients with *BRCA1/2* or *PALB2*-mutated breast cancer, while in the OlympiaN trial patients receive olaparib with or without durvalumab.

6.3.2 Adjuvant Setting

The OlympiA trial was a phase III double-blind trial that randomized 1836 patients with early-stage HER2-negative breast cancer patients to receive 1 year of adjuvant olaparib or placebo. All eligible patients had a g*BRCA1* or g*BRCA2* mutation and received neoadjuvant or adjuvant chemotherapy. Patients with TNBC treated with adjuvant chemotherapy were required to have node-positive disease or an invasive primary tumor of at least 2 cm, whereas patients receiving neoadjuvant chemotherapy were required to have residual disease at surgery. Patients with hormone receptor-positive breast cancer receiving adjuvant chemotherapy were required to have at least four pathologically confirmed positive lymph nodes, whereas those receiving neoadjuvant chemotherapy were required to have residual disease and a CPS + EG score of 3 or higher. The primary endpoint was invasive disease-free survival (iDFS). In June 2021, at the first pre-planned interim analysis after a median follow up of 2.5 years, there was significant iDFS improvement, with a 3-year iDFS of 85.9% in the olaparib group and 77.1% in the placebo group (HR for invasive disease or death 0.58; 99.5% CI 0.41–0.82; $p < 0.001$). In March 2022, at the second planned interim analysis after a median follow up of 3.5 years, a significant OS benefit was reported (3-year OS 92.8% with olaparib versus 89.1% with placebo; stratified HR 0.68; 98.5% CI 0.47–0.97; $p = 0.009$) [24, 25].

This led to the U.S. FDA approval, on March 11, 2022, of olaparib for the adjuvant treatment of deleterious or suspected deleterious gBRCA-mutated HER2-negative associated high-risk early breast cancer after treatment with neoadjuvant or adjuvant chemotherapy.

The SUBITO trial (Substantially Improving the Cure Rate of High-risk *BRCA1*-like Breast Cancer trial; NCT02810743) is another clinical trial investigating olaparib in the adjuvant setting in patients with features of homologous recombination deficiency (HRD), defined as either g*BRCA1/2* or *BRCA1*-like copy number profile evaluated on tumor tissue [26]. In this phase III randomized study, 174 patients will be randomized to (neo)adjuvant treatment with 4 cycles of dose dense doxorubicin-cyclophosphamide(ddAC) with autologous stem cell rescue or

4 cycles of ddAC followed by 4 cycles of carboplatin(q3)-paclitaxel(q1) and one year of olaparib. The primary outcome is OS.

6.4 Clinical Use of PARP Inhibitors in Non-BRCA Mutant Breast Cancer

In about 5% of the cases, breast cancers are associated with g*BRCA1/2* mutations, and likely to benefit from PARP inhibitors. Identification of other patients whose tumors may be sensitive to these drugs remains a critical need. Several genes involved in the DNA damage response and homologous recombination pathways to repair DNA double-strand breaks, when mutated, may confer increased cancer susceptibility to PARP inhibitors.

Olaparib Expanded (TBCRC048), an investigator-initiated phase II study [27], evaluated the efficacy of olaparib in patients with advanced HER2-negative breast cancer and germline/somatic mutations in homologous recombination related genes other than *BRCA1/2* (cohort 1) or somatic *BRCA1/2* mutations (cohort 2). The primary endpoint was ORR. Fifty-four patients were enrolled. In cohort 1, the ORR was 33% (90% CI 19–51%) and in cohort 2 was 31% (90% CI 15–49%). Confirmed responses were limited to those with germline *PALB2* (ORR 82%) and somatic *BRCA1/2* (ORR 50%) mutations. These results were considered practice changing by many, significantly expanding the pool of patients with breast cancer likely to benefit from PARP inhibitors. Similarly, the Talazoparib beyond BRCA study (NCT02401347) was an open label phase II trial that evaluated talazoparib in patients with pretreated advanced HER2-negative breast cancer (n = 13) or other solid tumors (n = 7) with mutations in HR pathway genes other than *BRCA1* and *BRCA2* [28]. In the cohort of patients with breast cancer, the ORR was 31% (4/13) and 3 additional patients had stable disease of ≥ 6 months (CBR 54%). All patients with germline mutations in PALB2 had treatment-associated tumor regression, consistent with findings from the Olaparib Expanded trial.

The role of a PARP inhibitor as maintenance strategy in metastatic TNBC was explored in the DORA study (NCT03167619) [29]. This was a phase II non-comparator trial that randomized 45 patients with advanced TNBC to olaparib with or without durvalumab after clinical benefit from platinum chemotherapy. The primary endpoint was PFS. At a medium follow-up of 9.8 months, the median PFS was 3.95 months ($p = 0.0023$; 95% CI 2.55–6.13) with olaparib and the median PFS was 6.1 months ($p = < 0.0001$; 95% CI 3.68–10.11) in the combination arm, with some durable responses seen in non-BRCA carriers.

In the neoadjuvant setting, the efficacy of PARP inhibitors beyond BRCA carriers was evaluated in the BrighTNess and the GeparOLA (HRD) studies [30–33]. The BrighTNess study was a phase III study that randomized 634 patients with stage II-III TNBC to paclitaxel plus (a) carboplatin plus veliparib; (b) carboplatin plus veliparib placebo; or (c) carboplatin placebo plus veliparib placebo. All patients received doxorubicin and cyclophosphamide after. The primary endpoint was pCR and secondary endpoints included event-free survival (EFS) [30].

The proportion of patients who achieved a pCR was higher in the paclitaxel, carboplatin, and veliparib group than in patients receiving paclitaxel with placebo (53% vs. 31%; $p < 0.0001$), but not compared with patients receiving paclitaxel plus carboplatin (58%; $p = 0.36$). With median follow-up of 4.5 years, the HR for EFS for carboplatin plus veliparib with paclitaxel versus paclitaxel was 0.63 (95% CI 0.43–0.92; $P = 0.02$), but 1.12 (95% CI 0.72–1.72; $P = 0.62$) for carboplatin plus veliparib with paclitaxel versus carboplatin with paclitaxel. This study showed that improvement in pCR with the addition of carboplatin was associated with long term EFS benefit, but the addition of veliparib did not impact EFS [31].

In GeparOLA [32], patients with TNBC or breast cancer cT1c and Ki67 > 20% with HRD were randomized to receive paclitaxel with olaparib or paclitaxel with carboplatin, both followed by epirubicin and cyclophosphamide. The primary endpoint was pCR. Of the 107 patients enrolled, 72.6% had TNBC and 56.2% had a gBRCA mutation. The pCR rate in the olaparib arm was 55.1% (90% CI 44.5–65.3%) versus 48.6% (90% CI 34.3–63.2%) in the carboplatin arm. Additional long-term efficacy endpoints included distant disease-free survival (DDFS) and OS. The 4-year DDFS rate with the olaparib containing regimen was 81.2% versus 93.4% with the carboplatin containing regimen (HR 3.03; 95% CI 0.67–13.67; log-rank $P = 0.1290$). The 4-year OS rate was 89.2% with the paclitaxel olaparib versus 96.6% with paclitaxel carboplatin (HR 3.27; 95% CI 0.39–27.20; log-rank $P = 0.2444$) [33]. Stratified subgroup analyses showed higher pCR rates in patients with hormone receptor-positive disease. Of 29 patients with hormone receptor-positive cancers, 10/19 had a pCR with paclitaxel and olaparib (52.6% [90% CI 32.0%-72.6%]) and 2/10 with paclitaxel and carboplatin (20.0% [90% CI 3.7%-50.7%]). The results of GeparOLA confirm that overall olaparib added to paclitaxel does not result in improved clinical outcomes compared to carboplatin and paclitaxel for patients with HRD early breast cancer. The subgroup analysis of patients with g*BRCA1/2* associated hormone receptor-positive breast cancer should only be considered explorative given the small number of patients in these subgroups.

Finally, in the adjuvant setting, a low dose of olaparib is being explored in combination with radiotherapy, compared to radiotherapy alone, for patients with inflammatory breast cancer (NCT03598257), regardless of BRCA status. Locoregional control of inflammatory breast cancer is a critical issue of this disease, and multiple existing inflammatory breast cancer preclinical models showed that low doses of olaparib in combination with radiotherapy led to significant radiosensitization [34].

6.5 Conclusion

There is an ongoing effort to try to identify patients beyond those with *BRCA1/2* mutations who may benefit from PARP inhibitors. To date, except for *PALB2* carriers, there is no definitive evidence of the benefit of PARP inhibitors for patients with non-BRCA associated breast cancer. The identification of mechanisms of primary and acquired resistance to PARP inhibitors is also critical in the clinical development of PARP inhibitors, as we often use these agents after prior exposure to platinum-based chemotherapies and these agents can share mechanisms of resistance. There may also be patients who can be cured with neoadjuvant or adjuvant PARP inhibitors alone, obviating the need for chemotherapy.

There has been substantial excitement about the development of PARP1 selective inhibitors and hope that these agents will allow combination with other drugs given its expected improved tolerability profile.

Conflicts of Interest **FL** reports research grants and personal fees from AstraZeneca, personal fees from Pfizer and Daiichi Sankyo, and research grants from CytomX, Eisai and Incyte. **MR** reports personal fees for advisory/consulting roles from Artios Pharma Limited, Change Healthcare Inc., Clinical Education Alliance, LLC, Foundation Medicine, Genome Quebec, MJH Associates, myMedEd, Inc., Pfizer, Inc., Tempus Labs, Inc, and Zenith Pharmaceuticals; travel reimbursement and editorial services from AstraZeneca; and research funding from Merck, Pfizer, and AstraZeneca.

References

1. Couch FJ, Nathanson KL, Offit K (2014) Two decades after BRCA: setting paradigms in personalized cancer care and prevention. Science 343:1466–1470
2. Bryant HE, Schultz N, Thomas HD, Parker KM, Flower D, Lopez E et al (2005) Specific killing of BRCA2-deficient tumours with inhibitors of poly(ADP-ribose) polymerase. Nature 434:913–917
3. Farmer H, McCabe N, Lord CJ, Tutt AN, Johnson DA, Richardson TB et al (2005) Targeting the DNA repair defect in BRCA mutant cells as a therapeutic strategy. Nature 434:917–921
4. O'Shaughnessy J, Osborne C, Pippen JE, Yoffe M, Patt D, Rocha C et al (2011) Iniparib plus chemotherapy in metastatic triple-negative breast cancer. N Engl J Med 364:205–214
5. O'Shaughnessy J, Schwartzberg L, Danso MA, Miller KD, Rugo HS, Neubauer M et al (2014) Phase III study of iniparib plus gemcitabine and carboplatin versus gemcitabine and carboplatin in patients with metastatic triple-negative breast cancer. J Clin Oncol 32:3840–3847
6. Patel AG, De Lorenzo SB, Flatten KS, Poirier GG, Kaufmann SH (2012) Failure of iniparib to inhibit poly(ADP-Ribose) polymerase in vitro. Clin Cancer Res 18:1655–1662
7. Chuang HC, Kapuriya N, Kulp SK, Chen CS, Shapiro CL (2012) Differential anti-proliferative activities of poly(ADP-ribose) polymerase (PARP) inhibitors in triple-negative breast cancer cells. Breast Cancer Res Treat 134:649–659
8. Robson M, Im SA, Senkus E, Xu B, Domchek SM, Masuda N et al (2017) Olaparib for Metastatic Breast Cancer in Patients with a Germline BRCA Mutation. N Engl J Med 377:523–533
9. Robson ME, Im SA, Senkus E, Xu B, Domchek SM, Masuda N et al (2023) OlympiAD extended follow-up for overall survival and safety: Olaparib versus chemotherapy treatment of physician's choice in patients with a germline BRCA mutation and HER2-negative metastatic breast cancer. Eur J Cancer 184:39–47
10. Robson M, Ruddy KJ, Im SA, Senkus E, Xu B, Domchek SM et al (2019) Patient-reported outcomes in patients with a germline BRCA mutation and HER2-negative metastatic breast cancer receiving olaparib versus chemotherapy in the OlympiAD trial. Eur J Cancer 120:20–30
11. Litton JK, Rugo HS, Ettl J, Hurvitz SA, Goncalves A, Lee KH et al (2018) Talazoparib in Patients with Advanced Breast Cancer and a Germline BRCA Mutation. N Engl J Med 379:753–763
12. Ettl J, Quek RGW, Lee KH, Rugo HS, Hurvitz S, Goncalves A et al (2018) Quality of life with talazoparib versus physician's choice of chemotherapy in patients with advanced breast cancer

and germline BRCA1/2 mutation: patient-reported outcomes from the EMBRACA phase III trial. Ann Oncol 29:1939–1947

13. Litton JK, Hurvitz SA, Mina LA, Rugo HS, Lee KH, Goncalves A et al (2020) Talazoparib versus chemotherapy in patients with germline BRCA1/2-mutated HER2-negative advanced breast cancer: final overall survival results from the EMBRACA trial. Ann Oncol 31:1526–1535

14. Dieras V, Han HS, Kaufman B, Wildiers H, Friedlander M, Ayoub JP et al (2020) Veliparib with carboplatin and paclitaxel in BRCA-mutated advanced breast cancer (BROCADE3): a randomised, double-blind, placebo-controlled, phase 3 trial. Lancet Oncol 21:1269–1282

15. Telli ML (2020) BROCADE3: a challenge to the treatment paradigm in BRCA breast cancer? Lancet Oncol 21:1254–1255

16. Tung N, Garber JE (2022) PARP inhibition in breast cancer: progress made and future hopes. NPJ Breast Cancer. 8:47

17. Domchek SM, Postel-Vinay S, Im SA, Park YH, Delord JP, Italiano A et al (2020) Olaparib and durvalumab in patients with germline BRCA-mutated metastatic breast cancer (MEDIOLA): an open-label, multicentre, phase 1/2, basket study. Lancet Oncol 21:1155–1164

18. Vinayak S, Tolaney SM, Schwartzberg L, Mita M, McCann G, Tan AR et al (2019) Open-label Clinical Trial of Niraparib Combined With Pembrolizumab for Treatment of Advanced or Metastatic Triple-Negative Breast Cancer. JAMA Oncol 5:1132–1140

19. Schram AM, Colombo N, Arrowsmith E, Narayan V, Yonemori K, Scambia G et al (2023) Avelumab Plus Talazoparib in Patients With BRCA1/2- or ATM-Altered Advanced Solid Tumors: Results From JAVELIN BRCA/ATM, an Open-Label, Multicenter, Phase 2b. Tumor-Agnostic Trial. JAMA Oncol. 9:29–39

20. Litton JK, Scoggins M, Ramirez DL, Murthy RK, Whitman GJ, Hess KR et al (2017) A feasibility study of neoadjuvant talazoparib for operable breast cancer patients with a germline BRCA mutation demonstrates marked activity. NPJ Breast Cancer. 3:49

21. Litton JK, Scoggins ME, Hess KR, Adrada BE, Murthy RK, Damodaran S et al (2020) Neoadjuvant Talazoparib for Patients With Operable Breast Cancer With a Germline BRCA Pathogenic Variant. J Clin Oncol 38:388–394

22. Litton JK, Beck JT, Jones JM, Andersen J, Blum JL, Mina LA et al (2021) Neoadjuvant talazoparib in patients with germline BRCA1/2 (gBRCA1/2) mutation-positive, early HER2-negative breast cancer (BC): Results of a phase 2 study [abstract]. J Clin Oncol 39:505

23. Spring LM, Han H, Liu MC, Hamilton E, Irie H, Santa-Maria CA et al (2022) Neoadjuvant study of niraparib in patients with HER2-negative, BRCA-mutated, resectable breast cancer. Nat Cancer. 3:927–931

24. Tutt ANJ, Garber JE, Kaufman B, Viale G, Fumagalli D, Rastogi P et al (2021) Adjuvant Olaparib for Patients with BRCA1- or BRCA2-Mutated Breast Cancer. N Engl J Med 384:2394–2405

25. Geyer CE Jr, Garber JE, Gelber RD, Yothers G, Taboada M, Ross L et al (2022) Overall survival in the OlympiA phase III trial of adjuvant olaparib in patients with germline pathogenic variants in BRCA1/2 and high-risk, early breast cancer. Ann Oncol 33:1250–1268

26. Vliek S, Jager A, Jonge-Lavrencic M, Lotz JP, Goncalves A, Graeser M, et al. Substantially improving the cure rate of high-risk BRCA1-like breast cancer patients with personalized therapy (SUBITO) - an international randomized phase III trial [abstract]. Cancer Res. 2018;78:OT2–07–8.

27. Tung NM, Robson ME, Ventz S, Santa-Maria CA, Nanda R, Marcom PK et al (2020) TBCRC 048: Phase II Study of Olaparib for Metastatic Breast Cancer and Mutations in Homologous Recombination-Related Genes. J Clin Oncol 38:4274–4282

28. Gruber JJ, Afghahi A, Timms K, DeWees A, Gross W, Aushev VN et al (2022) A phase II study of talazoparib monotherapy in patients with wild-type BRCA1 and BRCA2 with a mutation in other homologous recombination genes. Nat Cancer. 3:1181–1191

29. Sammons SL, Tan TJ, Im Y-H, Traina T, Anders C, Renzulli E, et al. PD11–12 DORA: A Phase II, Multicenter, International, Non-Comparator Study of Olaparib (O) +/- Durvalumab (D)

as a chemotherapy-free maintenance strategy in Platinum tReated Advanced Triple-Negative Breast Cancer (aTNBC) [abstract]. Cancer Res. 2023;83:PD11–2.

30. Loibl S, O'Shaughnessy J, Untch M, Sikov WM, Rugo HS, McKee MD et al (2018) Addition of the PARP inhibitor veliparib plus carboplatin or carboplatin alone to standard neoadjuvant chemotherapy in triple-negative breast cancer (BrighTNess): a randomised, phase 3 trial. Lancet Oncol 19:497–509

31. Geyer CE, Sikov WM, Huober J, Rugo HS, Wolmark N, O'Shaughnessy J et al (2022) Long-term efficacy and safety of addition of carboplatin with or without veliparib to standard neoadjuvant chemotherapy in triple-negative breast cancer: 4-year follow-up data from BrighTNess, a randomized phase III trial. Ann Oncol 33:384–394

32. Fasching PA, Link T, Hauke J, Seither F, Jackisch C, Klare P et al (2021) Neoadjuvant paclitaxel/olaparib in comparison to paclitaxel/carboplatinum in patients with HER2-negative breast cancer and homologous recombination deficiency (GeparOLA study). Ann Oncol 32:49–57

33. Fasching PA, Schmatloch S, Hauke J, Rey J, Jackisch C, Klare P, et al. Neoadjuvant paclitaxel/olaparib in comparison to paclitaxel/carboplatinum in patients with HER2-negative breast cancer and homologous recombination deficiency – long-term survival of the GeparOLA study [abstract]. Cancer Res. 2023;83:P4–06–13.

34. Michmerhuizen AR, Pesch AM, Moubadder L, Chandler BC, Wilder-Romans K, Cameron M et al (2019) PARP1 Inhibition Radiosensitizes Models of Inflammatory Breast Cancer to Ionizing Radiation. Mol Cancer Ther 18:2063–2073

Development of PARP Inhibitors in Targeting Castration-Resistant Prostate Cancer

7

Kent W. Mouw and Atish D. Choudhury

7.1 Prostate Cancer and the DNA Damage Response

Prostate cancer is the most common non-cutaneous male cancer in the US and is estimated to be responsible for more than 1.4 million new cancer diagnoses annually worldwide [1]. Although many prostate tumors are localized at diagnosis and can therefore be cured with surgery or radiotherapy, a subset of patients have metastatic disease at diagnosis or develop metastatic disease following initial therapy. The backbone of treatment for metastatic prostate cancer is androgen deprivation therapy, which can be achieved surgically via castration or by systemic therapies that block testosterone production or signaling. Although most prostate tumors respond initially to androgen-targeting therapy, resistance occurs and leads to metastatic castrate-resistant prostate cancer (mCRPC), the terminal disease state responsible for 34,000 deaths annually in the US alone (Fig. 7.1) [2].

Over the past decade, numerous genomic studies have comprehensively mapped the genetic and epigenetic landscape of prostate cancer, resulting in a deeper understanding of prostate cancer biology and yielding important therapeutic insights. One notable finding from these studies has been that germline and somatic alterations in DNA damage response (DDR) genes are relatively common in prostate cancer. Predicted deleterious germline DDR alterations are present in 5–20% of

K. W. Mouw (✉)
Department of Radiation Oncology, Dana-Farber Cancer Institute, Brigham & Women's Hospital, Harvard Medical School, 450 Brookline Ave., HIM 328, Boston, MA 02215, USA
e-mail: kent_mouw@dfci.harvard.edu

A. D. Choudhury
Harvard Medical School, Lank Center for Genitourinary Oncology, Dana-Farber Cancer Institute, 450 Brookline Ave., Dana 930, Boston, MA 02215, USA
e-mail: achoudhury@partners.org

T. A. Yap and G. I. Shapiro (eds.), *Targeting the DNA Damage Response for Cancer Therapy*, Cancer Treatment and Research 186,
https://doi.org/10.1007/978-3-031-30065-3_7

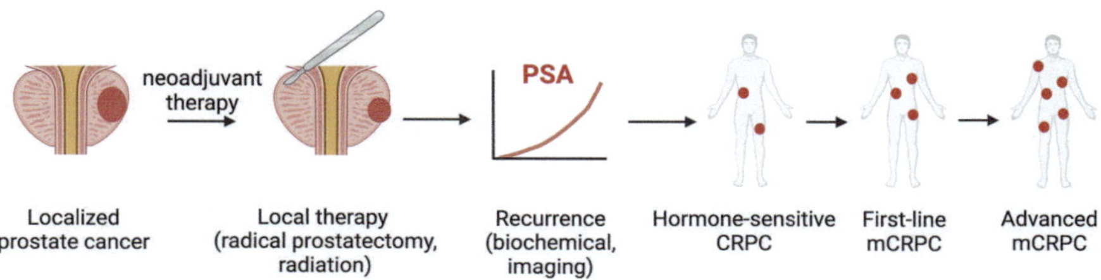

Fig. 7.1 Overview of the prostate cancer disease landscape

men with metastatic prostate cancer unselected for family history, and may be higher in certain ethnic groups or in men with a family history of prostate cancer [3–6]. Somatic DDR gene alterations are present in 10–20% of advanced prostate tumors and appear to be enriched in higher-grade and advanced tumors relative to lower-grade, localized tumors [7–10].

BRCA2 is the most commonly mutated DDR gene in most prostate cancer cohorts, comprising nearly half of the germline and somatic DDR gene alterations in several large cohorts [3, 11]. For reasons that are not understood, and in contrast to other BRCA-associated cancers such as breast and ovarian cancer, BRCA1 alterations are far less common than BRCA2 alterations in prostate cancer. Other commonly mutated genes with known or putative DDR roles are ATM, CHK2, CDK12, and others. In addition, ~3% of advanced prostate tumors have loss of mismatch repair (MMR) function causing microsatellite instability (MSI), and these MMRd/MSI-high prostate tumors can be effectively targeted with immune checkpoint inhibition [12–14].

With the realization that a significant fraction of prostate tumors harbor predicted deleterious DDR gene alterations, several retrospective studies have attempted to identify a relationship between DDR gene alterations and sensitivity to conventional DNA damaging agents used in treatment of advanced prostate cancer. Carboplatin is occasionally used in treatment of patients with metastatic prostate cancer, and patients with germline BRCA2 or ATM alterations may have higher likelihood of response to carboplatin-based therapy [15, 16]. However, the relationship between DDR gene alterations and carboplatin sensitivity has not been prospectively validated and therefore the role of carboplatin in DDR-altered prostate cancer is uncertain. Similarly, although DDR-altered prostate tumors may be more sensitive to ionizing radiation, no studies have clearly demonstrated a relationship between DDR status and radiation sensitivity in the localized or metastatic disease setting. However, attempts to characterize the relationship between DDR status and outcomes following prostate radiation for localized disease are complicated by the observation that DDR-altered tumors may be more likely to harbor locally-advanced or micro-metastatic disease compared to tumors without DDR gene alterations [17].

7.2   The Evolving Role of PARP Inhibitors in Prostate Cancer

PARP inhibitors were first approved for use in homologous recombination (HR)-deficient ovarian cancer and subsequently in HR-deficient breast cancer. Given the relative frequency of DDR gene alterations in prostate cancer, significant attention has turned to studying the activity of PARP inhibition in advanced prostate cancer. One of the first clinical trials to report activity of PARP inhibitors in mCRPC was the TOPARP-A trial published in 2015 (Table 7.1) [18]. TOPARP-A was a Phase 2 trial of olaparib and enrolled 50 mCRPC patients with disease progression despite taxane-based chemotherapy and at least one second-generation androgen receptor (AR)-targeted agent (ARTA). The overall response rate was 33% (16/49); however, 88% (14/16) responders had a predicted deleterious DDR gene alteration with BRCA2 (n = 7) and ATM (n = 4) alterations being the most common. These data demonstrated the activity of PARP inhibition in mCRPC and suggested that patients with DDR-altered tumors may be more likely to respond.

Based on the promising results from the single-arm TOPARP-A trial, TOPARP-B was a randomized Phase 2 trial designed to test the activity of 300 mg versus 400 mg Olaparib in mCRPC patients with DDR alterations (identified by targeted NGS) and disease progression following at least one line of taxane-based chemotherapy [19] The primary endpoint was the composite overall response rate defined as at least one response using radiographic, PSA, or circulating tumor cell (CTC) criteria. Responses were observed in 54% of patients who received 400 mg olaparib and 39% of patients who received 300 mg olaparib. Several exploratory biomarker analyses were also performed and are discussed in detail in the biomarkers section below.

TRITON2 was a Phase II trial of rucaparib in mCRPC patients harboring a tumor alteration in BRCA1/2 or another pre-specified DDR gene (15 genes in total). Outcomes from patients with BRCA1/2 tumor alterations versus those with non-BRCA1/2 alterations were reported separately [21, 31] Among 115 patients with a BRCA1/2 alteration, the overall response rate by independent radiology review was 43% (11% complete response and 32% partial response) and the confirmed PSA response rate was 54.8% (PSA response was defined as $\geq 50\%$ decrease from baseline PSA). Radiographic response rates were similar in patients with BRCA1 versus BRCA2 alterations and in patients with germline versus somatic alterations. PSA responses were more frequently seen with BRCA2 alterations compared to BRCA1 (60% [95% CI, 50% to 69%] v 15% [95% CI, 2% to 45%]). Response rates for the 78 patients with non-BRCA1/2 alterations were significantly lower [21]. ATM was the most commonly altered gene after BRCA2, but the radiographic and PSA response rates for ATM-altered cases were only 10.5% (2/19) and 4.1% (2/49), respectively. CDK12 (n = 15) and CHEK2 (n = 12) were also altered in a subset of patients, but radiographic and PSA response rates were low in both cases (0% and 6.7% for CDK12 and 11% and 17% for CHEK2). Responses were observed in patients with alterations in other, less commonly altered non-BRCA1/2 genes such as FANCA and PALB2, but the number of cases was small (0–4). Based on the results from TRITON2, rucaparib was granted

Table 7.1 Selected completed and on-going prostate cancer PARP inhibitor clinical trials

Disease setting	Trial	Design	Biomarker selection	No. patients	Prior therapies	Treatment(s)	Primary endpoint	Results	Comments	NCT	References
Advanced mCRPC	TOPARP-A	Phase 2	No	50	Docetaxel (100%), abi/enza (98%), cabazi (58%)	Olaparib (400 mg BID)	Objective response rate (PSA, imaging, CTC)	16/49 (33%) ORR; 14/16 (88%) with DDR gene alteration	7/7 patients with BRCA2 and 4/5 patients with ATM alteration had response	NCT01682772	[18]
	TOPARP-B	Rand. Phase 2	Yes; 5 pre-specified groups: BRCA1/2, ATM, CDK12, PALB2, others	529 patients with tissue/161 with DDR gene alteration/98 randomized	Docetaxel (100%), abi/enza (90%), cabazi (38%)	Olaparib (300 mg versus 400 mg)	Objective response rate (PSA, imaging, CTC)	25/46 (54%) ORR in 400 mg arm; 18/46 (39%) in 300 mg arm ($p = 0.14$)	25/30 (88%) ORR for BRCA2; 7/19 (37%) ATM; 5/20 (25%) CDK12; 4/7 (57%) PALB2; 4/20 (20%) others	NCT01682772	[19]
	TRITON-2 (BRCA1/2 cohort)	Phase 2	Yes (BRCA1/2)	115	Taxane-based chemotherapy and 1–2 lines of next-generation anti-androgen therapy	Rucaparib (600 mg BID)	Objective response rate (PSA, imaging)	27/62 (44%) indep rad. review; 33/65 (51%) provider-assessed; 63/115 (55%) PSA response	similar rad. Responses rates for BRCA1 versus BRCA2; higher PSA response rate for BRCA2	NCT02952534	[20]

(continued)

Table 7.1 (continued)

Disease setting	Trial	Design	Biomarker selection	No. patients	Prior therapies	Treatment(s)	Primary endpoint	Results	Comments	NCT	References
	TRITON-2 (non-BRCA1/2 cohort)	Phase 2	Yes (non-BRCA1/2 DDR genes)	78	Taxane-based chemotherapy and 1–2 lines of next-generation anti-androgen therapy	Rucaparib (600 mg BID)	Objective response rate (PSA, imaging)	Rad response: 2/19 ATM, 0/10 CDK12, 1/9 CHEK2, 4/14 other	PSA response: 2/49 ATM, 1/15 CDK12, 2/12 CHEK2, 5/14 other	NCT02952534	[21]
	PROfound	Phase 3	15 DDR genes (Cohort A: BRCA1, BRCA2, ATM; Cohort B: 12 other genes)	245 (Cohort A); 142 (Cohort B)	At least one next-generation anti-androgen (inclusion criteria); at least one taxane (65%)	Olaparib versus enza or abi (2:1)	rPFS in Cohort A	Cohort A rPFS: 7.4 versus 3.6 mo ($p < 0.001$); Cohort A OS: 19.1 versus 14.7 mo ($p = 0.02$); Cohort B OS 14.1 versus 11.5 mo	66% crossover to olaparib in the control arm	NCT02987543	[22]
	GALAHAD	Phase 2	8 DDR genes	289 (142 BRCA1/2 cohort; 81 non-BRCA1/2 cohort)	At least one next-generation anti-androgen and one taxane (inclusion criteria)	Niraparib 300 mg QD	Objective response rate in measurable BRCA1/2 patients	ORR in measurable BRCA1/2 cohort 26/76 (34%);	Composite response rate: 82/142 (55%) BRCA cohort, 12/81/ (15%) non-BRCA cohort	NCT02854436	[23]

(continued)

Table 7.1 (continued)

Disease setting	Trial	Design	Biomarker selection	No. patients	Prior therapies	Treatment(s)	Primary endpoint	Results	Comments	NCT	References
	TALAPRO	Phase 2	11 DDR genes	1425 screened/128 enrolled	1–2 next-generation anti-androgen agents plus 1–2 taxanes (inclusion criteria)	Talazoparib 1 mg QD	Rad. ORR	ORR: 31/104 (30%)	ORR by gene: BRCA1/2 46%, PALB2 25%, ATM 12%, other 0%	NCT03148795	[24]
First-line mCRPC	PROpel	Phase 3	No, but stratified by DDR gene status	796	Primary ADT	Olaparib (300 mg BID)/ abiraterone versus placebo/ abiraterone	rPFS	rPFS: 24.8 versus 16.6 m0 (HR 0.66, $p < 0.0001$); HRR + pts (HR 0.54); HRR- pts (HR 0.76)	HRR status determined by ctDNA analysis; OS endpoint immature	NCT03732820	[25]
	TALAPRO-2	Phase 3	No, but stratified by DDR gene status	19 in dose-finding (completed); 1018 in randomized (on-going)	Primary ADT	Enzalutamide/ talazoparib (0.5 mg QD) versus enzalutamide/ placebo	rPFS	NR	NR	NCT03395197	[26]
	MAGNITUDE	Phase 3	No, but stratified by DDR gene status	423 HRR + (53% BRCA1/2); 233 HRR-	Primary ADT, ≤ 4 mo. abiraterone allowed)	Niraparib (400 mg QD)/ abiraterone versus placebo/ abiraterone	rPFS in BRCA1/ 2-mutant patients	BRCA1/2-mut HR 0.50 ($p =$ 0.0006); HRR + HR 0.64 ($p =$ 0.0022); HRR- HR 1.09 (p = NS)	HRR status determined from tumor tissue	NCT03748641	[27]

(continued)

Table 7.1 (continued)

Disease setting	Trial	Design	Biomarker selection	No. patients	Prior therapies	Treatment(s)	Primary endpoint	Results	Comments	NCT	References
	CASPAR (A031902)	Phase 3	No, but stratified by DDR gene status	984	Primary ADT	Enzalutamide/ rucaparib versus enzalutamide/ placebo	rPFS and OS (co-primary)	NR	NR	NCT04455750	[28]
mCSPC	AMPLITUDE	Phase 3	Yes	788 (planned)	Local therapy, ≤ 6 mo ADT, ≤ 1 mo abiraterone	Abiraterone/ niraparib (200 mg QD) versus abiraterone/ placebo	rPFS	NR	NR	NCT04497844	[29]
	TALAPRO-3	Phase 3	Yes (mutation in ≥ 1 of 12 h/ DDR genes)	550 (planned)	Treatment for localized disease	Enzalutamide/ talazoparib (0.5 mg QD) versus enzalutamide/ placebo	rPFS	NR	NR	NCT04821622	[30]

accelerated approval by the FDA in May 2020 for treatment of mCRPC patients with germline or somatic BRCA1/2 alterations and disease progression despite androgen-directed therapy and taxane chemotherapy. TRITON3 (NCT02975934) is a randomized Phase 3 trial of rucaparib vs. physician's choice (abiraterone acetate or enzalutamide or docetaxel) in HRR gene-altered mCRPC—results from this study (ref: Fizazi K, et al., N Engl J Med. 2023 Feb 23;388(8):719-732) had not yet been reported at the time of this writing.

The PROfound study was a large, multinational Phase 3 randomized trial of olaparib versus physician's choice of either enzalutamide or abiraterone [11]. All participants had mCRPC that had progressed through either enzalutamide or abiraterone as well as a qualifying alteration in one of 15 pre-specified DDR genes. Patients were enrolled in two cohorts: cohort A patients (n = 245) had an alteration in BRCA1, BRCA2, or ATM whereas cohort B patients (n = 142) had an alteration in at least one of 12 other DDR genes (Fig. 7.2). The primary endpoint was imaging-based progression free survival (PFS) in cohort A, which was significantly longer for patients treated with olaparib versus control (7.4 vs. 3.6 mo, p < 0.001). The objective response rate in cohort A was 33% with olaparib versus only 2% with control, and the percentage of patients with $\geq$ 50% decrease from baseline PSA was 43% in the olaparib arm versus 8% in the control arm. With longer follow-up that was reported separately, overall survival was also significantly longer in cohort A patients treated with olaparib versus control (19.1 vs. 14.7 mo, p = 0.02) despite 66% of patients in the control arm crossing over to receive olaparib at the time of progression [20]. When patients from both cohorts A and B were analyzed together, progression-free survival for the overall population was significantly longer with olaparib than control (5.8 vs. 3.5 mo, p < 0.001), but there was no significant difference in overall survival (17.3 vs. 14.0 mo). Gene-level analysis showed that BRCA2 (145 randomized cases) was the most frequently altered DDR gene across both cohorts and BRCA2-altered cases appeared to drive the improved outcomes observed with olaparib in both cohort A as well as the overall (cohorts A + B) population. ATM (cohort A, 92 randomized cases) and CDK12 (cohort B, 99 randomized cases) alterations were also relatively common, but neither gene was significantly associated with olaparib benefit on exploratory analysis (HR for OS 0.93 [95% CI 0.53–1.75] for ATM, 0.97 [0.57–1.71] for CDK12). Based on results from the PROfound trial, olaparib was granted accelerated FDA approval in May 2020 for use in mCRPC patients with HR repair (HRR) gene alterations who experience disease progression following abiraterone or enzalutamide. The approval applies to patients with at least one suspected deleterious mutation in 14 of the 15 genes included in the overall PROfound population (PPP2R2A was excluded) as identified by one of two approved companion diagnostic tests.

GALAHAD was a single-arm Phase 2 trial of the PARP inhibitor niraparib in mCRPC patients with biallelic alterations in a DNA repair gene and disease progression following androgen-directed and taxane-based therapy. Patients with alterations in BRCA1, BRCA2, ATM, FANCA, PALB2, CHEK2, BRIP1, or

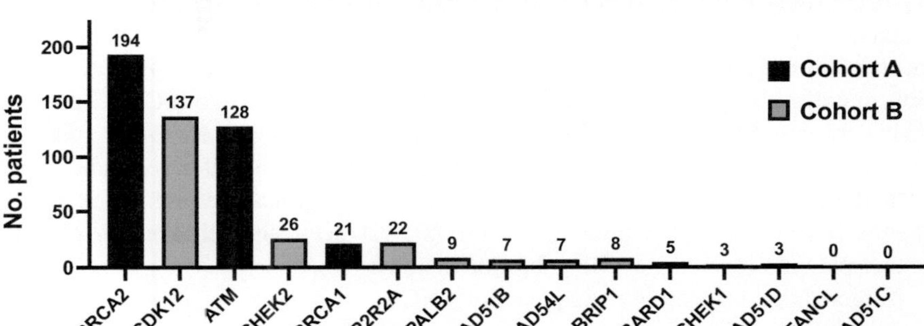

Fig. 7.2 Frequency of DDR gene alterations in randomized patients in the PROfound trial

HDAC2 identified by tissue- or plasma-based sequencing were eligible. The objective response rate in the measurable BRCA1/2 cohort of 76 patients was 34% and the objective response rate in the measurable non-BRCA1/2 cohort of 47 patients was 11% [22]. Sixty-one of 142 patients (43%) in the overall BRCA1/2 cohort had a decrease in PSA of $\geq 50\%$ from baseline while only 4 of 81 patients (5%) in the overall non-BRCA1/2 cohort had a decrease in PSA of $\geq 50\%$ from baseline.

TALAPRO-1 was a single-arm Phase 2 trial of talazoparib in mCRPC patients with one or more predicted deleterious HRD gene mutations who had disease progression following 1–2 lines of taxane-based chemotherapy as well as enzalutamide and/or abiraterone [23]. The list of 11 HRD genes used in the final analysis included: ATM, ATR, BRCA1, BRCA2, CHEK2, FANCA, MLH1, MRE11A, NBN, PALB2, and RAD51C. The primary endpoint was confirmed objective response using radiographic criteria, which was 30% in the total study population. Half of the patients included in the OR analysis had a BRCA2 alteration (52/104), and the OR rate was 46% among BRCA2-altered cases. ATM was the second most frequently altered gene in the cohort, but the OR rate for ATM-altered cases was only 12% (2/17).

7.3 PARP Inhibitor Biomarkers in Prostate Cancer

Targeted and whole exome sequencing of cell-free DNA (cfDNA) from patients enrolled on the TOPARP-A trial were reported separately [24]. There was a significantly greater decrease in cfDNA concentration in responders compared to non-responders. All tumor somatic DNA repair gene alterations were detected in cfDNA and there were sustained decreases in the allele frequency of cfDNA mutations in responders. A $\geq 50\%$ decline in cfDNA concentration at 4 weeks after olaparib initiation was significantly associated with improved rPFS on multivariable analysis and a $\geq 50\%$ decline in cfDNA concentration at 8 weeks after olaparib initiation was significantly associated with improved OS. cfDNA analysis at the time of progression revealed multiple independent (subclonal) reversion mutations in BRCA2 and PALB2, suggesting restoration of HR function as a mechanism of PARP inhibitor resistance in these cases. Multiclonal BRCA2 reversion mutations were also observed from cfDNA analysis of two mCRPC patients with germline BRCA2 alterations at the time of progression on PARP inhibitor therapy [32] Although numerous mechanisms of PARP inhibitor resistance have been described in vitro and in non-prostate cancer clinical settings [33], mechanisms beyond reversion mutations have not yet been characterized in prostate cancer patients receiving PARP inhibitor therapy.

Targeted next-generation sequencing (NGS) was used to screen cases for enrollment in TOPARP-B. In addition, archival hormone-sensitive or fresh castrate-resistant tumor specimens also underwent exploratory biomarker analyses including whole exome sequencing (WES), low-pass whole genome sequencing (lpWGS), ATM immunohistochemistry (IHC), and Rad51 immunofluorescence (IF) to assess homologous recombination function [34] These analyses provided several important insights. Most patients with BRCA1/2 alterations were predicted to have biallelic loss (either a mutation with a detectable second event or homozygous deletion), and these biallelic BRCA1/2-altered patients were most likely to respond to olaparib. Similarly, patients with biallelic (but not monoallelic) PALB2 alterations also were likely to respond to olaparib. Among patients with ATM alterations, biallelic events were present in 57% of cases and were associated with longer PFS (but not OS) than cases with only monoallelic ATM alterations. Loss of ATM protein by IHC was more common in cases with biallelic ATM events, and ATM loss by IHC was associated with longer PFS and OS. Nearly all (18/ 20) CDK12-altered tumors had biallelic events, but despite this, the radiographic and PSA response rate for CDK12-mutant cases was 0%. Finally, tumors with low Rad51 IF scores, indicative of low HR activity, were significantly more likely to respond to olaparib than tumors with high Rad51 IF scores (68% vs. 23%).

Available data demonstrate that PARP inhibitor response varies across different DNA repair genes. BRCA1/2 mutations appear to have the strongest impact on PARP inhibitor response and similar response rates were observed in germline versus somatic alterations in trials such as TOPARP-B, PROfound, GALAHAD, and TRITON2. In all these trials, BRCA2 alterations were more common than BRCA1 alterations, and BRCA2-altered cases may also be more likely to respond than BRCA1-altered cases [35, 36]. The lower likelihood of response in patients with BRCA1 alterations has been attributed to lower frequency of biallelic loss of BRCA1 compared to BRCA2, as well as more frequent co-occurring deleterious alterations in the TP53 gene with BRCA1 alterations [36]. Patients with alterations in other HR genes such as PALB2, BRIP1, and RAD51C also frequently respond, although the frequency of alterations in these genes is significantly lower than BRCA2. Although response rates were higher in cohort A (BRCA1, BRCA2, ATM) than cohort B (12 other genes) in PROfound, this difference was driven primarily by improvements among BRCA1/2 patients. The difference in outcomes in PARPi versus control-treated ATM-altered cases in PROfound was modest, and responses among ATM-altered patients in TRITON2 were rare. Similarly, PARPi response rates in CDK12- or CHEK2-altered cases were also very low across trials. Taken together, these data suggest that BRCA2 is the most common HRR gene alteration in mCRPC and that BRCA2-altered cases appear to be most likely to benefit from PARP inhibition. Mutations in BRCA1 and other less commonly altered HR genes such as PALB2, BRIP1, and RAD51 also may benefit from PARPi. PARPi responses do occur in a minority of ATM altered cases, but are uncommon in CDK12 or CHEK2 altered cases.

Homologous recombination deficiency is associated with unique mutational patterns (signatures) which can be computationally determined using WES/WGS data. These mutational signature-based approaches have been applied in prostate cancer to evaluate the association among specific mutational signatures, HR gene alterations, and clinical properties including PARPi response [37, 38].

7.4 PARP Inhibitor Combinations

7.4.1 Second Generation AR-Targeted Agents (ARTAs)

AR activity promotes HR gene expression and AR signaling is required for efficient HR function in prostate cancer cells [39, 40]. Androgen deprivation therapy upregulates PARP-mediated DNA repair pathways and PARP function is essential for survival following AR blockade. Therefore, co-targeting AR and PARP signaling is an attractive therapeutic strategy. PARP-1 may also have a role in promoting transcription of AR-regulated genes, thereby promoting AR-associated disease progression [41], suggesting that the combination of an second generation ARTA with a PARP inhibitor would have synergistic activity in advanced prostate cancer.

This strategy was tested in a randomized Phase 2 trial of abiraterone plus olaparib versus abiraterone plus placebo in biomarker-unselected mCRPC patients [42]. Eligible patients were those who had previously received docetaxel but had not received a second-generation AR-targeted agent such as abiraterone or enzalutamide. A total of 142 patients were randomized, and rPFS was the primary endpoint. rPFS was significantly longer with abiraterone plus olaparib compared to abiraterone plus placebo (13.8 vs. 8.2 mo, $p = 0.034$). Prespecified subgroup analyses of rPFS suggested no differential benefit based on HRR mutation (HRRm) status.

The PROpel trial is a Phase 3 randomized trial of abiraterone plus olaparib versus abiraterone plus placebo in first-line treatment of mCRPC with or without HRR gene alterations. A planned interim analysis reported in abstract form in February 2022 [25] and published after this writing (ref: Clarke NW et al. NEJM Evidence. 2022 Aug 23;1(9)) showed a significantly prolonged radiographic PFS in the olaparib-containing arm (24.8 vs. 16.6 mo, $p < 0.0001$). A planned subgroup analysis showed rPFS benefit in both HRRm (HR 0.50 [95% CI 0.34–0.73]) and non-HRRm (HR 0.76 [0.60–97]) patients. In PROPEL, HRRm status was determined retrospectively, with patients classified as HRRm if one or more HRR gene mutations was detected by either tumor or ctDNA testing, and as non-HRRm if no HRR gene mutations were detected by either test (18 patients were classified as unknown HRRm because no valid HRR test result from either test was available; these patients were excluded from analysis by HRRm status). Overall survival data remains immature but there is a trend favoring the olaparib arm (HR 0.86).

MAGNITUDE is a Phase 3 randomized trial of abiraterone plus niraparib versus abiraterone plus placebo in first-line mCRPC patients with and without pre-specified HRR gene alterations. In MAGNITUDE, patients were prospectively tested for HRR BM (biomarker) status by plasma, tissue and/or saliva/whole blood—those who were negative by plasma were required to test by tissue to confirm HRR BM− status. Patients were then separately enrolled into parallel studies of HRR BM + (planned N = 400) and HRR BM− (planned N = 600) cohorts. A planned interim analysis reported in February 2022 [27] and published after this writing (Chi KN, et al. J Clin Oncol 2023 Jun 20;41(18):3339-3351) showed a significant radiographic PFS improvement in the niraparib-containing arm for patients with a BRCA1/2 (16.6 vs. 10.9 mo) or any HRR gene alteration (16.5 vs. 13.7 mo). However, the Independent Data Monitoring Committee (IDMC) recommended stopping enrollment in the HRR BM−cohort at the time of prespecified early futility analysis due to no evidence for added benefit in this subgroup based on a HR for composite progression endpoint (radiographic or PSA progression) of 1.09 (95% CI 0.75–1.59).

The reasons why there appeared to be an rPFS benefit in the non-HRRm subgroup in PROpel while enrollment to the HRR BM−subgroup was halted early due to futility in MAGNITUDE are not fully clear. The designs of these studies were different, including that HRRm status was determined retrospectively in PROpel and prospectively in MAGNITUDE. In MAGNITUDE, HRR BM−status determined by ctDNA testing needed to be confirmed by tissue testing whereas this was not formally required in PROpel—as such, there may have been a small number of patients in PROpel without HRR gene alteration detected on ctDNA testing but without confirmatory tissue amenable to analysis who could have been misclassified as non-HRRm. This is unlikely to represent a large number of patients as most who enrolled did have tissue amenable to analysis, and the overall frequency of HRRm vs. non-HRRm patients in the study are similar to previously published mCRPC cohorts. It is also possible that futility in the HRR BM−population at interim analysis of MAGNITUDE was seen due to random chance (and largely driven by PSA progression), and that rPFS difference may have been seen if planned enrollment were completed, but this seems unlikely given entirely overlapping composite progression Kaplan-Meyer curves for niraparib and placebo arms. Another possibility is some differential activity between olaparib and niraparib at the doses tested in these studies, though this has not been reported in other clinical contexts. Any differential activity is unlikely related to the canonical mechanism of synthetic lethality of PARP inhibition with BRCA1/2 loss, since the degree of benefit in the BRCA1/2 loss population was similar between the studies—it cannot be excluded that olaparib has additional activities (including non-specific cytotoxicity) to explain some of the improvement in rPFS compared to placebo in the non-HRRm subgroup. The results from the HRR BM− population of MAGNITUDE do not support the biological hypothesis of abiraterone inducing a "BRCAness" phenotype that sensitizes to PARP inhibitors as a class in the absence of HR gene alterations, at least in the population studied and at clinically relevant doses. The combination of niraparib and abiraterone is being tested in the Phase 3 AMPLITUDE study in metastatic hormone-sensitive prostate cancer (mHSPC) with HR repair gene defects (NCT04497844) [29], in an outcome-adaptive and randomized multi-arm biomarker driven study in mCRPC called ProBio (NCT03903835), as neoadjuvant therapy for high risk localized prostate cancer in the Genomic Biomarker-Selected Umbrella Neoadjuvant Study (GUNS) in DDR-altered patients prior to prostatectomy (NCT04812366), and as adjuvant treatment after radiation for high-risk locoregional prostate cancer in a biomarker-unselected population (NCT04947254).

Combinations of a PARP inhibitor with enzalutamide are also being studied in advanced prostate cancer. CASPAR (Alliance A031902) is a Phase 3 randomized trial of enzalutamide plus rucaparib versus enzalutamide plus placebo in first-line treatment of mCRPC (NCT04455750) [28]. The trial opened in late 2020 and will enroll 984 men with or without HRR gene alterations—prior second generation ARTA (other than enzalutamide) is permitted, and prospective assessment of HRR gene status is required for stratification. TALAPRO-2 is a Phase 3 trial randomizing 1st line mCRPC patients (prior docetaxel and abiraterone permitted in mHSPC) to enzalutamide plus talazoparib versus enzalutamide plus placebo [26] with results published after this writing (Agarwal N et al. Lancet 2023 Jul 22; 402(10398):291-303). Like in CASPAR, enrolled patients are stratified based on the presence or absence of a predicted deleterious DDR gene alteration. The combination of talazoparib with enzalutamide is being studied in mHSPC with DDR gene alterations in the Phase 3 TALAPRO-3 trial (NCT04821622) [30].

7.4.2 Immune Checkpoint Inhibitors (ICIs)

While clinical responses to anti-PD1 and anti-PDL1 ICIs are uncommon in mCRPC, the subset of patients with mismatch repair deficiency/microsatellite-high phenotype (MMRd/MSI-H) can experience deep and durable responses to these agents [43], and it has been suggested that patients whose cancers harbor other DDR gene alterations may be more likely to respond to ICIs compared to non-DDR altered patients as well [44]. PARP inhibition may potentiate DNA damage and inefficient repair in tumors, thus leading to accumulation of mutations that would increase vulnerability to ICIs [45], and lead to increase in cytosolic dsDNAs and micronuclei in tumor cells that activate a STING-dependent antitumor immune response that can be augmented by anti-PD1 ICIs [46].

An early study testing the combination of a PARP inhibitor with an ICI was a trial of durvalumab with olaparib in mCRPC patients previously treated with enzalutamide and/or abiraterone [47]. In this study, 9 of 17 (53%) patients had a radiographic and/or PSA response, though only 2 of the 9 responders had no detected DDR gene biomarker of response. Phase 2 studies of this combination in biochemically recurrent prostate cancer with DDR alterations (NCT03810105) or predicted to have a high neoantigen load (NCT04336943) are currently enrolling. The nivolumab plus rucaparib cohorts of the CheckMate 9KD study demonstrated PSA response rates of 18.2% (95% CI 8.2–32.7%) for HRD + patients and 5.0% (0.6–16.9) for HRD-patients in Cohort A1 (post-chemotherapy mCRPC) [48], and 41.9% (24.5–60.9) for HRD + patients and 14.3% (4.8–30.3) for HRD-patients in Cohort A2 (chemotherapy-naïve mCRPC) [49]. The combination of olaparib with pembrolizumab was studied in biomarker-unselected post-chemotherapy mCRPC in Arm A of the KEYNOTE-365 trial. In this study, the combination showed modest clinical activity with confirmed PSA response rate of 14.7% (95% CI, 8.5–23.1), and radiographic response rate of 6.9% (95% CI, 1.9–16.7) [50] It is not clear in any of these studies that the combination of a PARP inhibitor with ICI leads to synergistic activity beyond what would be expected for the single agents. Results from studies of niraparib plus cetrelimab (NCT03431350) and talazoparib plus avelumab (NCT03330405) have yet to be reported.

The Phase 3 KEYLYNK-010 trial enrolled a biomarker-unselected population of mCRPC patients previously treated with abiraterone or enzalutamide (but not both) and randomized them to receive the combination of pembrolizumab with olaparib vs. switching to the other ARTA. The findings of this study have yet to be presented at the time of this writing, but in a press release (https://www. merck.com/news/merck-announces-keylynk-010-trial-evaluating-keytruda-pembro lizumab-in-combination-with-lynparza-olaparib-in-patients-with-metastatic-cas tration-resistant-prostate-cancer-to-stop-for-f/), Merck announced that the study is being discontinued following the recommendation of the IDMC based on a planned interim analysis demonstrating no rPFS or OS benefit of the experimental arm compared to a relatively inactive control arm of switching ARTA. As such, the proposed mechanism of synergy between PARP inhibitors and ICIs has not yet been demonstrated in unselected mCRPC patients. These disappointing results suggest that beyond limited biomarker-selected subsets of patients, alternative approaches to stimulating an immune response are needed. One promising approach is through bispecific antibodies that simultaneously target both immune checkpoint receptors PD-1 and CTLA-4; Cohort C of a Phase 2 trial of the bispecific antibody XmAb20717 is testing this agent in combination with olaparib in patients with HRD/CDK12 mutation positive tumors not previously treated with PARP inhibitors (NCT05005728).

7.4.3 Radiopharmaceuticals

The radiopharmaceuticals radium-223 [51] and 177Lu-PSMA-617 [52] have both demonstrated overall survival benefit in mCRPC. Inhibition of PARP-mediated DNA damage repair through PARP inhibition has been proposed to help sensitize cells to radiation by prolonging strand breaks and by leading to a cell-death signaling pathway, among other mechanisms [53]. In a phase 1b trial of niraparib with radium-223 [54], the maximally tolerated dose of niraparib with radium-223 was determined to be 100 mg in chemo-exposed patients and 200 mg in chemo-naïve patients; PSA50 responses were seen in 0/15 chemo exposed patients and 3/15 (20%) of chemo-naïve patients. The combination of olaparib with radium-223 is being studied in the COMRADE trial (NCT03317392). In the Phase 1 part [55], the recommended Phase 2 dose of olaparib was determined to be 200 mg BID when combined with radium-223; the Phase 2 part of COMRADE of radium-223 ± olaparib is currently enrolling. A phase 1 dose-escalation and dose-expansion study of olaparib + 177Lu-PSMA-617 (NCT03874884) is also currently enrolling.

7.4.4 PI3K/AKT/mTOR Inhibitors

Multiple pre-clinical studies have suggested synergistic activity of inhibitors of the PI3K/AKT/mTOR signaling pathway with PARP inhibition. For example, the pan-PI3K inhibitor buparlisib (BKM120) has been reported to increase DNA damage (as assessed by increase in γ-H2AX staining) in both *BRCA1*-deficient [56] and HR-proficient [57] models. In HR-proficient models of triple-negative breast cancer, buparlisib decreased the expression of BRCA1/2 and impaired DNA damage repair, thus sensitizing to olaparib treatment [57, 58]. A recent study [58] suggests that olaparib treatment leads to upregulation of forkhead box M1 (FOXM1) and Exonuclease 1 (Exo1) to increase HRR function; as FOXM1 and Exo1 are downstream of AKT signaling, co-treatment with buparlisib abrogated upregulation of these genes and thus synergized with olaparib to promote cell death. Similar results were seen with the mTOR inhibitor everolimus, where everolimus treatment downregulated expression of genes involved in DDR including SUV39H1 in both HR-proficient [59] and *BRCA2*-deficient [60] breast cancer models, leading to synergy with PARP inhibition.

There are multiple studies of the combination of a PARP inhibitor with an inhibitor of the PI3K/AKT/mTOR pathway currently in progress. For example, rucaparib is being studied in combination with the AKT inhibitor ipatasertib in advanced breast, ovarian, and prostate cancers in the dose escalation part of a phase 1b study (NCT03840200); the dose expansion phase of this study will only enroll advanced mCRPC patients previously treated with second generation ARTA. Olaparib is being studied in combination with the novel p110α isoform-specific PI3K inhibitor CYH33 in multiple tumor types (NCT04586335), and the combination of rucaparib with the p110α/p110δ inhibitor copanlisib is being studied in mCRPC (NCT04253262), where the Phase 2 part is for HRRm patients [20]. Given pre-clinical evidence of synergy of PARP inhibitors with both PI3K inhibitors and ICIs, a phase 1b study of the triplet combination of olaparib, copanlisib, and durvalumab is being undertaken in solid tumors with germline or somatic mutations in DDR genes, actionable alterations in *PTEN*, or hotspot mutations (E542, E545 or H1047) in *PIK3CA* (NCT03842228).

7.4.5 Epigenetic Modifiers

The epigenetic modifier Enhancer of Zeste Homolog 2 (EZH2) is overexpressed in mCRPC and is involved in cancer progression and therapeutic resistance – partially through its canonical role in mediating trimethylation of histone H3 lysine 27 (H3K27me3) as part of the polycomb repressive complex 2 (PRC2), [61] as well as non-canonical roles in activating AR signaling [62] and in driving lineage plasticity [63, 64]. In pre-clinical mCRPC models, EZH2 directly regulates the expression of a number of genes involved in DNA damage repair (DDR), particularly base excision repair; EZH2 inhibition leads to downregulation of these genes and thus heightened sensitivity to genotoxic stress, such as that induced by PARP inhibitors [65] Synergy between PARP inhibitors and EZH2 inhibitors was also demonstrated in breast [66] and ovarian [67] cancer models. Importantly, in these models, the mechanism of synergy of EZH2 inhibition and PARP inhibition does not require underlying defects in the DNA damage response in the treated cancer cells. A Phase 1 trial of the PARP inhibitor talazoparib with the EZH2 inhibitor tazemetostat in biomarker-unselected mCRPC is currently in progress (NCT04846478).

Bromodomain-containing protein 4 (BRD4) is a member of the Bromodomain and Extraterminal (BET) protein family, and acts as an epigenetic reader that recognizes histone proteins and acts as a transcriptional regulator to trigger tumor growth. In pre-clinical mCRPC models, BET inhibition was demonstrated to disrupt the physical interaction of BRD4 with AR, thus disrupting AR recruitment to target gene loci and leading to anti-tumor activity in CRPC xenograft mouse models [68]. In pre-clinical models of BET inhibitor resistance, increased DNA damage associated with PRC2-mediated transcriptional silencing of DDR genes was observed, leading to PARP inhibitor sensitivity [68]. These studies suggest the potential for combinatorial activity of BET inhibitors with PARP inhibitors, and trials of olaparib in combination with the BET inhibitor PLX2853 (NCT04556617) and the BD2-selective BET inhibitor NUV-868 (NCT05252390) are in progress.

7.5 Targeting the DNA Damage Response in Prostate Cancer: Beyond PARP Inhibitors

ATR (ataxia-telangiectasia and Rad3-related) is a serine/threonine kinase that plays a critical role in sensing and responding to DNA damage and replication stress (RS). ATR is activated by single-stranded DNA (ssDNA) and phosphorylates numerous targets including the DDR kinase CHK1 to coordinate repair activities with cell cycle checkpoints and other cellular processes [69]. Tumors frequently have high levels of DNA damage, and RS and may therefore have increased dependence on ATR-mediated signaling to avoid toxic levels of genomic instability. Several ATR inhibitors are being tested alone and in combination with either DNA damaging agents or with other DDR-targeted agents in a variety of tumor contexts [70]. Recently, a randomized Phase II trial showing a benefit of addition of the ATR inhibitor berzosertib to gemcitabine compared to gemcitabine alone in platinum-resistant ovarian cancer was published [71], the first randomized trial to show a benefit of ATR inhibition. However, studies of berzosertib in combination with cisplatin and gemcitabine in urothelial cancer [72] and in combination with carboplatin in prostate cancer [73] failed to demonstrate benefit compared to the control chemotherapy regimens.

The TRAP study (NCT03787680) is a Phase II trial that combines the ATR inhibitor ceralasertib (AZD6738) with olaparib in mCRPC patients with disease progression through at least one second-generation anti-androgen therapy. Preclinical evidence suggests that addition of ATR inhibition may sensitize homologous recombination (HR) proficient cells to PARP inhibition and may also increase the depth and duration of PARP inhibitor response in HR-deficient (HRD) tumors [74]. Therefore, patients with and without tumor HRD (defined as mono- or biallelic ATM loss or biallelic BRCA1/2 loss) were enrolled on the TRAP trial. The primary endpoint was response rate (defined as radiographic response by RECIST criteria and/or a $\geq 50\%$ decrease in PSA) in patients without predicted tumor HRD. Early results from the TRAP trial were recently presented in abstract format and showed a response in 4 of 12 HRD + patients and 4 of 35 HRD-patients [75].

Several other small molecule inhibitors of DDR proteins are in various phases of preclinical and clinical development, including inhibitors of ATM, CHK1, CHK2, DNA-PK, and WEE1. However, none of these agents have yet been tested in a prostate cancer specific clinical trial. On-going preclinical efforts are focused on defining the therapeutic activity of these agents in prostate cancer models and identifying prostate cancer molecular features that are associated with sensitivity to specific DDR-targeted agents.

7.6 Summary and Conclusions

The treatment landscape for advanced prostate cancer is rapidly evolving and multiple novel approaches to target prostate tumor biology beyond AR signaling are under clinical investigation. Genomic and functional studies have revealed that DDR pathway alterations occur in a subset of advanced prostate tumors, and evidence from multiple clinical trials has demonstrated that PARP inhibition can provide clinical benefit for patients with homologous recombination deficient prostate cancer. To date, the clearest signal for PARP inhibitor activity is in patients with germline or somatic BRCA2 alteration; however, patients with tumor homologous recombination deficiency conferred by other, less commonly altered HR genes such as PALB2 also appear likely to benefit. PARP inhibitor response rates for patients with alterations in DDR genes such as ATM or CDK12 appear less likely to benefit from PARP inhibition, and numerous efforts are underway to investigate combination approaches that will increase response rates in these patients as well as in patients who lack alterations in DDR genes. The future is promising, and it is likely that the role for PARP inhibitors and perhaps other DDR targeted agents will continue to expand across the prostate cancer disease spectrum.

Disclosures

Kent Mouw
Advisory/Consulting: EMD Serono, Pfizer, UroGen

Research Funding: Pfizer, Novo Nordisk

Writing/editor fees: UpToDate

Speaking fees: OncLive

Patents: Institutional patent filed on mutational signatures of DNA repair deficiency.

Atish Choudhury
Advisory/Consulting: Clovis, Dendreon, Bayer, Eli Lilly, Blackstone, AstraZeneca, Astellas, Blue Earth, Janssen, Sanofi Aventis, Color Health

Research Funding: Bayer, Pfizer
Speaking fees: Bayer, Pfizer, Lantheus

References

1. Sung H, Ferlay J, Siegel RL et al (2021) Global cancer statistics 2020: GLOBOCAN estimates of incidence and mortality worldwide for 36 cancers in 185 countries. CA Cancer J Clin 71(3):209–249
2. Siegel RL, Miller KD, Fuchs HE et al (2021) Cancer statistics, 2021. CA Cancer J Clin 71(1):7–33
3. Cheng HH, Pritchard CC, Boyd T et al (2016) Biallelic inactivation of BRCA2 in platinum-sensitive metastatic castration-resistant prostate cancer. Eur Urol 69(6):992–995. 4909531
4. Castro E, Romero-Laorden N, Del Pozo A, et al (2019) PROREPAIR-B: a prospective cohort study of the impact of germline DNA repair mutations on the outcomes of patients with metastatic castration-resistant prostate cancer. J Clin Oncol, p JCO1800358
5. Nicolosi P, Ledet E, Yang S et al (2019) Prevalence of germline variants in prostate cancer and implications for current genetic testing guidelines. JAMA Oncol 5(4):523–528. PMC6459112
6. Bree KK, Henley PJ, Pettaway CA (2021) Germline predisposition to prostate cancer in diverse populations. Urol Clin North Am 48(3):411–423
7. Robinson D, Van Allen EM, Wu YM et al (2015) Integrative clinical genomics of advanced prostate cancer. Cell 161(5):1215–1228. PMC4484602
8. Abida W, Cyrta J, Heller G et al (2019) Genomic correlates of clinical outcome in advanced prostate cancer. Proc Natl Acad Sci U S A 116(23):11428–11436. PMC6561293
9. Armenia J, Wankowicz SAM, Liu D et al (2018) The long tail of oncogenic drivers in prostate cancer. Nat Genet 50(5):645–651. PMC6107367
10. Lee DJ, Hausler R, Le AN et al (2021) Association of inherited mutations in DNA repair genes with localized prostate cancer. Eur Urol

11. de Bono J, Mateo J, Fizazi K et al (2020) Olaparib for metastatic castration-resistant prostate cancer. N Engl J Med 382(22):2091–2102

12. Antonarakis ES, Shaukat F, Isaacsson Velho P et al (2019) Clinical features and therapeutic outcomes in men with advanced prostate cancer and DNA mismatch repair gene mutations. Eur Urol 75(3):378–382. PMC6377812

13. Le DT, Uram JN, Wang H et al (2015) PD-1 blockade in tumors with mismatch-repair deficiency. N Engl J Med 372(26):2509–2520. PMC4481136

14. Nava Rodrigues D, Rescigno P, Liu D et al (2018) Immunogenomic analyses associate immunological alterations with mismatch repair defects in prostate cancer. J Clin Invest 128(10):4441–4453. PMC6159966

15. Zafeiriou Z, Bianchini D, Chandler R, et al (2019) Genomic analysis of three metastatic prostate cancer patients with exceptional responses to carboplatin indicating different types of DNA repair deficiency. Eur Urol 75(1):184–192. PMC6291437

16. Pomerantz MM, Spisak S, Jia L et al (2017) The association between germline BRCA2 variants and sensitivity to platinum-based chemotherapy among men with metastatic prostate cancer. Cancer 123(18):3532–3539. PMC5802871

17. Taylor RA, Fraser M, Livingstone J et al (2017) Germline BRCA2 mutations drive prostate cancers with distinct evolutionary trajectories. Nat Commun 8:13671. PMC5227331 financial interests

18. Mateo J, Carreira S, Sandhu S et al (2015) DNA-repair defects and olaparib in metastatic prostate cancer. N Engl J Med 373(18):1697–1708. PMC5228595

19. Mateo J, Porta N, Bianchini D et al (2020) Olaparib in patients with metastatic castration-resistant prostate cancer with DNA repair gene aberrations (TOPARP-B): a multicentre, open-label, randomised, phase 2 trial. Lancet Oncol 21(1):162–174. PMC6941219

20. Hussain M, Mateo J, Fizazi K et al (2020) Survival with olaparib in metastatic castration-resistant prostate cancer. N Engl J Med 383(24):2345–2357

21. Abida W, Patnaik A, Campbell D et al (2020) Rucaparib in men with metastatic castration-resistant prostate cancer harboring a BRCA1 or BRCA2 gene alteration. J Clin Oncol 38(32):3763–3772. PMC7655021

22. Smith MR, Scher HI, Sandhu S et al (2022) Niraparib in patients with metastatic castration-resistant prostate cancer and DNA repair gene defects (GALAHAD): a multicentre, open-label, phase 2 trial. Lancet Oncol 23(3):362–373

23. de Bono JS, Mehra N, Scagliotti GV et al (2021) Talazoparib monotherapy in metastatic castration-resistant prostate cancer with DNA repair alterations (TALAPRO-1): an open-label, phase 2 trial. Lancet Oncol 22(9):1250–1264

24. Goodall J, Mateo J, Yuan W et al (2017) Circulating cell-free DNA to guide prostate cancer treatment with PARP inhibition. Cancer Discov 7(9):1006–1017. PMC6143169

25. Saad F, Armstrong AJ, Thiery-Vuillemin A et al (2022) PROpel: phase III trial of olaparib (ola) and abiraterone (abi) versus placebo (pbo) and abi as first-line (1L) therapy for patients (pts) with metastatic castration-resistant prostate cancer (mCRPC). J Clin Oncol 40(6_suppl):11

26. Agarwal N, Azad A, Shore ND et al (2021) TALAPRO-2: a phase 3 randomized study of enzalutamide (ENZA) plus talazoparib (TALA) versus placebo in patients with new metastatic castration-resistant prostate cancer (mCRPC). J Clin Oncol 39(15_suppl):TPS5089-TPS5089

27. Chi KN, Rathkopf DE, Smith MR et al (2022) Phase 3 MAGNITUDE study: first results of niraparib (NIRA) with abiraterone acetate and prednisone (AAP) as first-line therapy in patients (pts) with metastatic castration-resistant prostate cancer (mCRPC) with and without homologous recombination repair (HRR) gene alterations. J Clin Oncol 40(6_suppl):12

28. Rao A, Ryan CJ, VanderWeele DJ et al (2021) CASPAR (Alliance A031902): a randomized, phase III trial of enzalutamide (ENZ) with rucaparib (RUCA)/placebo (PBO) as a novel therapy in first-line metastatic castration-resistant prostate cancer (mCRPC). J Clin Oncol 39(6_suppl):TPS181-TPS181

29. Rathkopf DE, Chi KN, Olmos D et al (2021) AMPLITUDE: a study of niraparib in combination with abiraterone acetate plus prednisone (AAP) versus AAP for the treatment of patients with deleterious germline or somatic homologous recombination repair (HRR) gene-altered

metastatic castration-sensitive prostate cancer (mCSPC). J Clin Oncol 39(6_suppl):TPS176-TPS176

30. Agarwal N, Azad A, Fizazi K et al (2022) Talapro-3: a phase 3, double-blind, randomized study of enzalutamide (ENZA) plus talazoparib (TALA) versus placebo plus enza in patients with DDR gene mutated metastatic castration-sensitive prostate cancer (mCSPC). J Clin Oncol 40(6_suppl):TPS221

31. Abida W, Campbell D, Patnaik A et al (2020) Non-BRCA DNA damage repair gene alterations and response to the PARP inhibitor rucaparib in metastatic castration-resistant prostate cancer: analysis from the phase II TRITON2 study. Clin Cancer Res 26(11):2487–2496

32. Quigley D, Alumkal JJ, Wyatt AW et al (2017) Analysis of circulating cell-free DNA identifies multiclonal heterogeneity of BRCA2 reversion mutations associated with resistance to PARP inhibitors. Cancer Discov 7(9):999–1005. PMC5581695

33. D'Andrea AD (2018) Mechanisms of PARP inhibitor sensitivity and resistance. DNA Repair (Amst) 71:172–176

34. Carreira S, Porta N, Arce-Gallego S et al (2021) Biomarkers associating with PARP inhibitor benefit in prostate cancer in the TOPARP-B Trial. Cancer Discov

35. Taza F, Holler AE, Fu W et al (2021) Differential activity of PARP inhibitors in BRCA1— versus BRCA2-altered metastatic castration-resistant prostate cancer. JCO Precis Oncol 5. PMC8575434

36. Markowski MC, Antonarakis ES (2020) BRCA1 versus BRCA2 and PARP inhibitor sensitivity in prostate cancer: more different than alike? J Clin Oncol 38(32):3735–3739. PMC7655018

37. De Sarkar N, Dasgupta S, Chatterjee P et al (2021) Genomic attributes of homology-directed DNA repair deficiency in metastatic prostate cancer. JCI Insight 6(23). PMC8675196

38. Sztupinszki Z, Diossy M, Krzystanek M et al (2020) Detection of molecular signatures of homologous recombination deficiency in prostate cancer with or without BRCA1/2 mutations. Clin Cancer Res 26(11):2673–2680. PMC8387086

39. Asim M, Tarish F, Zecchini HI et al (2017) Synthetic lethality between androgen receptor signalling and the PARP pathway in prostate cancer. Nat Commun 8(1):374. PMC5575038

40. Polkinghorn, W.R., Parker, J.S., Lee, M.X., et al. Androgen receptor signaling regulates DNA repair in prostate cancers. Cancer Discov, 2013. 3(11): p. 1245–53. PMC3888815

41. Schiewer MJ, Goodwin JF, Han S et al (2012) Dual roles of PARP-1 promote cancer growth and progression. Cancer Discov 2(12):1134–1149. PMC3519969

42. Clarke N, Wiechno P, Alekseev B et al (2018) Olaparib combined with abiraterone in patients with metastatic castration-resistant prostate cancer: a randomised, double-blind, placebo-controlled, phase 2 trial. Lancet Oncol 19(7):975–986

43. Abida W, Cheng ML, Armenia J et al (2018) Analysis of the prevalence of microsatellite instability in prostate cancer and response to immune checkpoint blockade. JAMA Oncol

44. Mouw KW, Goldberg MS, Konstantinopoulos PA et al (2017) DNA damage and repair biomarkers of immunotherapy response. Cancer Discov 7(7):675–693. PMC5659200

45. Strickland KC, Howitt BE, Shukla SA et al (2016) Association and prognostic significance of BRCA1/2-mutation status with neoantigen load, number of tumor-infiltrating lymphocytes and expression of PD-1/PD-L1 in high grade serous ovarian cancer. Oncotarget 7(12):13587–13598. PMC4924663

46. Ding L, Kim HJ, Wang Q et al (2018) PARP inhibition elicits STING-dependent antitumor immunity in Brca1-deficient ovarian cancer. Cell Rep 25(11):2972–2980.e5. PMC6366450

47. Karzai F, VanderWeele D, Madan RA et al (2018) Activity of durvalumab plus olaparib in metastatic castration-resistant prostate cancer in men with and without DNA damage repair mutations. J Immunother Cancer 6(1):141

48. Pachynski RK, Retz M, Goh JC et al (2021) CheckMate 9KD cohort A1 final analysis: Nivolumab (NIVO) + rucaparib for post-chemotherapy (CT) metastatic castration-resistant prostate cancer (mCRPC). J Clin Oncol 39(15_suppl):5044

49. Petrylak D, Perez-Gracia J, Lacombe L et al (2021) 579MO CheckMate 9KD cohort A2 final analysis: Nivolumab (NIVO)+ rucaparib for chemotherapy (CT)-naïve metastatic castration-resistant prostate cancer (mCRPC). Ann Oncol 32:S629–S630

50. Yu E, Piulats J, Gravis G et al (2021) 612P Pembrolizumab (pembro) plus olaparib in patients with docetaxel-pretreated metastatic castration-resistant prostate cancer (mCRPC): Update of KEYNOTE-365 cohort A with a minimum of 11 months of follow-up for all patients. Ann Oncol 32:S652–S653

51. Parker C, Nilsson S, Heinrich D et al (2013) Alpha emitter radium-223 and survival in metastatic prostate cancer. N Engl J Med 369(3):213–223

52. Sartor O, de Bono J, Chi KN et al (2021) Lutetium-177-PSMA-617 for metastatic castration-resistant prostate cancer. N Engl J Med 385(12):1091–1103. PMC8446332

53. Lesueur P, Chevalier F, Austry JB et al (2017) Poly-(ADP-ribose)-polymerase inhibitors as radiosensitizers: a systematic review of pre-clinical and clinical human studies. Oncotarget 8(40):69105–69124. PMC5620324

54. Kelly WK, Leiby B, Einstein DJ et al (2020) Radium-223 (Rad) and niraparib (Nira) treatment (tx) in castrate-resistant prostate cancer (CRPC) patients (pts) with and without prior chemotherapy (chemo). J Clin Oncol 38(15_suppl):5540

55. McKay RR, Xie W, Ajmera A et al (2021) A phase 1/2 study of olaparib and radium-223 in men with metastatic castration-resistant prostate cancer (mCRPC) with bone metastases (COMRADE): results of the phase 1 study. J Clin Oncol 39(15_suppl):e17020

56. Juvekar A, Burga LN, Hu H et al (2012) Combining a PI3K inhibitor with a PARP inhibitor provides an effective therapy for BRCA1-related breast cancer. Cancer Discov 2(11):1048–1063

57. Ibrahim YH, García-García C, Serra V et al (2021) PI3K inhibition impairs BRCA1/2 expression and sensitizes BRCA-proficient triple-negative breast cancer to PARP inhibition. Cancer Discov 2(11):1036–1047. PMC5125254

58. Li Y, Wang Y, Zhang W et al (2021) BKM120 sensitizes BRCA-proficient triple negative breast cancer cells to olaparib through regulating FOXM1 and Exo1 expression. Sci Rep 11(1):4774. PMC7910492

59. Mo W, Liu Q, Lin CC-J et al (2016) mTOR inhibitors suppress homologous recombination repair and synergize with PARP inhibitors via regulating SUV39H1 in BRCA-proficient triple-negative breast cancer. Clin Cancer Res 22(7):1699–1712

60. El Botty R, Coussy F, Hatem R et al (2018) Inhibition of mTOR downregulates expression of DNA repair proteins and is highly efficient against BRCA2-mutated breast cancer in combination to PARP inhibition. Oncotarget 9(51):29587–29600. PMC6049870

61. Bracken AP, Dietrich N, Pasini D et al (2006) Genome-wide mapping of Polycomb target genes unravels their roles in cell fate transitions. Genes Dev 20(9):1123–1136. PMC1472472

62. Xu K, Wu ZJ, Groner AC et al (2012) EZH2 oncogenic activity in castration-resistant prostate cancer cells is Polycomb-independent. Science 338(6113):1465–1469. PMC3625962

63. Berger A, Brady NJ, Bareja R et al (2019) N-Myc-mediated epigenetic reprogramming drives lineage plasticity in advanced prostate cancer. J Clin Invest 130

64. Dardenne E, Beltran H, Benelli M et al (2016) N-Myc induces an EZH2-mediated transcriptional program driving neuroendocrine prostate cancer. Cancer Cell 30(4):563–577

65. Liao Y, Chen CH, Xiao T et al (2022) Inhibition of EZH2 transactivation function sensitizes solid tumors to genotoxic stress. Proc Natl Acad Sci U S A 119(3). PMC8784159

66. Yamaguchi H, Du Y, Nakai K et al (2018) EZH2 contributes to the response to PARP inhibitors through its PARP-mediated poly-ADP ribosylation in breast cancer. Oncogene 37(2):208–217. PMC5786281

67. Karakashev S, Fukumoto T, Zhao B et al (2020) EZH2 inhibition sensitizes CARM1-high, homologous recombination proficient ovarian cancers to PARP inhibition. Cancer Cell 37(2):157–167 e6

68. Asangani IA, Dommeti VL, Wang X et al (2014) Therapeutic targeting of BET bromodomain proteins in castration-resistant prostate cancer. Nature 510(7504):278–282. PMC4075966

69. Blackford AN, Jackson SP (2017) ATM, ATR, and DNA-PK: the trinity at the heart of the DNA damage response. Mol Cell 66(6):801–817
70. Barnieh FM, Loadman PM, Falconer RA (2021) Progress towards a clinically-successful ATR inhibitor for cancer therapy. Curr Res Pharmacol Drug Discov 2:100017. PMC8663972
71. Konstantinopoulos PA, Cheng SC, Wahner Hendrickson AE et al (2020) Berzosertib plus gemcitabine versus gemcitabine alone in platinum-resistant high-grade serous ovarian cancer: a multicentre, open-label, randomised, phase 2 trial. Lancet Oncol 21(7):957–968. PMC8023719
72. Pal SK, Frankel PH, Mortazavi A et al (2021) Effect of cisplatin and gemcitabine with or without berzosertib in patients with advanced urothelial carcinoma: a phase 2 randomized clinical trial. JAMA Oncol 7(10):1536–1543
73. Choudhury AD, Xie W, Folefac E et al (2021) A phase 2 study of berzosertib (M6620) in combination with carboplatin compared with docetaxel in combination with carboplatin in metastatic castration-resistant prostate cancer. J Clin Oncol 39(15_suppl):5034
74. Cleary JM, Aguirre AJ, Shapiro GI et al (2020) Biomarker-guided development of DNA repair inhibitors. Mol Cell 78(6):1070–1085. PMC7316088
75. Reichert ZR, Devitt ME, Alumkal JJ et al (2022) Targeting resistant prostate cancer, with or without DNA repair defects, using the combination of ceralasertib (ATR inhibitor) and olaparib (the TRAP trial). J Clin Oncol 40(6_suppl):88

Strategies for the Management of Patients with Pancreatic Cancer with PARP Inhibitors

Talia Golan, Maria Raitses-Gurevich, Tamar Beller, James Carroll, and Jonathan R. Brody

8.1 Pancreatic Cancer is a Rising Threat

Pancreatic cancer is the seventh deadliest cancer in the world, and will soon be the second deadliest in the US despite nearly 50 years of improvements to diagnostic capabilities, surgical techniques, and chemotherapy [1]. The five-year survival rate is around 11% for all stages of pancreatic cancer, but most patients are diagnosed with advanced, metastatic disease and succumb within a year (3% five-year survival rate) due to the limitations of current effective therapies [2–5]. Indeed, over the last twenty years, there have been virtually no major therapeutic advances other than identifying combination chemotherapies, the administration of neoadjuvant therapies, and improving the safety of surgical techniques for this disease.

T. Golan (✉) · M. Raitses-Gurevich · T. Beller
Cancer Center, Chaim Sheba Medical Center and Sackler Faculty of Medicine, Tel Aviv University, Tel Aviv, Israel
e-mail: Talia.Golan@sheba.health.gov.il

M. Raitses-Gurevich
e-mail: Maria.Raitses@sheba.health.gov.il

T. Beller
e-mail: Tamar.Beller@sheba.health.gov.il

J. Carroll · J. R. Brody
Department of Surgery, Brenden Colson Center for Pancreatic Care, Knight Cancer Institute, Oregon Health and Science University, Portland, OR, USA
e-mail: carrolja@ohsu.edu

J. R. Brody
e-mail: brodyj@ohsu.edu

© The Author(s), under exclusive license to Springer Nature Switzerland AG 2023
T. A. Yap and G. I. Shapiro (eds.), *Targeting the DNA Damage Response for Cancer Therapy*, Cancer Treatment and Research 186,
https://doi.org/10.1007/978-3-031-30065-3_8

Pancreatic ductal adenocarcinoma (PDAC) is the most common form of pancreatic cancer and arises through histologically distinct pre-malignant lesions characterized by the accumulation of genetic mutations in four well-described driver genes: oncogenic *KRAS* mutations occur in as much as 95% of lesions, followed by losses of tumor suppressors *TP53* (70–74%), *CDKN2A* (28–35%), and *SMAD4* (23–31%) [6, 7]. Outside of these primary mutations, the prevalence of other alterations falls to around 15% or less. Further, transcriptomic-based subtyping of PDAC identified two robust subtypes termed basal-like and classical that prognosticate patients by outcome but have proven limited for informing therapeutic interventions [8–11]. Yet, large-scale efforts to sequence pancreatic cancers suggest that around half of PDAC lesions harbor targetable alterations, with the largest proportion of these (around 8–18%) occurring in the DNA damage response (DDR) pathways [12–14]. By 2020, as many as 30% (154) of PDAC clinical trials were testing targeted therapeutic interventions against DNA repair and cell cycle control mechanisms; some have since met with modest, promising success [13, 15]. In the remainder of this chapter, we will discuss the current state of targeted therapies against the DNA repair pathway in PDAC.

8.1.1 Targeting the DNA Repair Pathway in PDAC

The accessibility to germline and somatic testing has improved in recent years, and it is now clear that PDACs are heterogeneous within a cohort, with a subset of patients harboring actionable mutations [13]. *KRAS* mutations are the most prevalent genetic aberration in PDACs and are detected in roughly ~95% of tumors. However, the many attempts to target mutated *KRAS* in the clinic have been unsuccessful, with the recent exception of specific low frequency *KRAS G12C* mutations (2%) [16]. For example, adagrasib is an investigational, highly selective, and oral small-molecule inhibitor of *KRAS G12C*, for which preliminary efficacy has been demonstrated in early phase clinical trials (Mirati Therapeutics Press Release). An increased level of interest has emerged in targeting additional low-prevalence, actionable aberrations, such as those involving *BRCA1/2, NTRK1/2/3,* or mismatch repair (MMR) deficiencies [17, 18]. There are several therapies targeted to actionable aberrations already approved by the Food and Drug administration (FDA): TRK inhibitors larotrectinib and entrectinib for patients with NTRK fusion mutation, the PD-1 inhibitor pembrolizumab for mismatch repair-deficient patients, and the poly-ADP-ribose polymerase (PARP) inhibitor olaparib in patients with germline *BRCA1/2* mutations as a maintenance therapy [19–22].

<u>Checkpoint inhibitors in PDAC</u>: Unfortunately, many immunotherapy approaches that are promising in other cancer types have shown little effect in PDAC [23]. These agents include IL-2, oncolytic viruses, checkpoint blockade, TGFb inhibitors, neoantigen vaccines, T_{reg} depletion, and CD47 blockade [24]. PDAC has been considered a non-immunogenic, 'cold' tumor and employs immune evasion. These mechanisms include the recruitment of regulatory immune

cells and the secretion of immunosuppressive chemokines. However, additional studies have shown significant T cell infiltration in PDAC [25].

Early clinical studies investigating PD-1/PDL1 antagonists showed no activity in patients with PDAC, despite remarkable efficacy seen across a wide range of malignancies. Similar findings have been reported with CTLA-4 antagonists and with combining PD-1 blockade with a small molecule inhibitor of indoleamine 2,3-deoxygenase [26–28]. In contrast, response to PD-1/PDL1 antagonists has been observed in PDAC patients with microsatellite instable tumors {Le 2017 #39}. Tumors with microsatellite instability (MSI)/defective DNA mismatch repair (dMMR) harbor germline (Lynch syndrome) or somatic mutations in *MSH2, MSH6, PMS2* and *MLH1* genes accumulate thousands of mutations and are characterized by a hypermutated genome. This leads to increased number of mutation-associated neoantigens [29]. The prevalence of MSI/dMMR tumors among PDAC cases is very low: 1–2% [29]. However, several studies have demonstrated efficacy of check point inhibitors in tumors with dMMR and this led to FDA approval for pembrolizumab in MSI/dMMR tumors [20, 30].

BRCA1/2 mutated tumors can be candidates for treatment with immune checkpoint inhibitors: The unstable genome, one of four subtypes identified by compressive genomic analysis, is associated with genomic alterations in DNA damage repair (DDR) genes and is predominantly enriched in patients harboring germline *BRCA1/2* mutations [31]. Unstable genomes are characterized by high tumor mutational burden and increased neoantigen load [32]. In addition, *BRCA1/2* mutated tumors are known to harbor biallelic inactivation of *BRCA1/2* loci, an allelic state responsive to treatment with platinum-based agents and PARP inhibition. However, this sensitive state may be reversed by introduction of compensatory frameshift reverse mutations, a known resistance mechanism in all BRCA-associated tumors [33, 34]. Occurrence of reversion mutations usually caused by deletions/insertion in the vicinity of the original pathogenic germline mutations introduces novel amino acid sequences, which differ from the original WT protein, which can thus constitute neoantigens [35]. This may open a window of opportunity to treat with alternative treatments such as immunotherapy. Preliminary clinical data have been shown to support this hypothesis (Terrero et al. ASCO GI 2022). Additionally, studies have shown that besides PARP inhibition direct effect on cancer cells death, PARPi can enhance an immune response. PARPi can induce accumulation of cytosolic DNA damage and to trigger the interferon pathways, and activation of immune cells [36, 37]. PARPi can also induce PD-L1 expression [38]. The high mutational load of BRCA mutated tumors and PARPi effect on the tumor microenvironment and priming of the immune system rationalizes for the combination of PARPi and immune checkpoint inhibition. Ongoing clinical efforts assessing the combination of PARPi with immune checkpoint inhibition in pancreatic cancer is currently being performed (NCT: 04548752, 04753879, 03851614, 03637491).

T-Cell Receptor Therapy targeting mutant *KRAS* and TP53 in pancreatic cancer: Even though PDAC employs immune evasion using various mechanisms, recent work has shown that most primary PDAC tumors are infiltrated with tumor-reactive T-cells. Those can be isolated and expanded ex-vivo with similar efficiency as those isolated from melanoma, resulting in reactive T-cell cultures against the autologous tumor [25]. Employing the most abundant alterations in PDAC such as *KRAS* (95%) and p53 (72%) [39, 40]. The immunotherapeutic targeting of driver mutations is conceptually attractive since they are tumor-specific, biologically crucial for tumor progression, and expressed by most tumor cells [41]. This approach is novel yet has not been exploited in PDAC, which may be especially relevant for patients with low tumor burden, like those harboring *BRCA1/2* and other DDR-deficient mutations.

Targeting DNA damage repair deficiency: Recently, the POLO trial demonstrated a progression-free survival (PFS) benefit in metastatic PDAC patients with a germline *BRCA1/2* mutation treated with maintenance olaparib (Lynparza), the poly (ADP-ribose) polymerase (PARP) inhibitor, following platinum-based induction chemotherapy [21]. This was the first phase III randomized trial to establish a biomarker-driven approach in the treatment of PDAC and establishes a precedent for maintenance therapy in PDAC. The POLO trial was eligible for germline *BRCA1/2* carriers only, while these mutations comprise only a small proportion of genes that are involved in DDR, whereas other genes are more common; however, data regarding their role in homology repair deficiency (HRD)/DDR therapy is still lacking. Further insight was shown in a recent study by the application of various HRD classifiers on the whole genome sequencing dataset of 391 PDAC patients. An HRD signature could be attributed to alterations in *BRCA1/2, PALB2, RAD51C/D, XRCC2* and a tandem duplicator phenotype, but not to additional alterations in genes like *ATM, ATR* and *CHEK2*. Of note, in advanced disease, the HRD signature was predictive for platinum response and survival benefit [32, 42].

Despite the great success of POLO trial and its promising results, not all patients with germline *BRCA1/2* mutations will equally benefit from olaparib treatment. Clinical observations of patients with BRCA-associated PDAC demonstrate three diverse types of responses to platinum-based and/or PARP inhibition treatments. It is important to note that cross resistance between cisplatin and PARPi has been demonstrated [43, 44]. The DNA damage response is determined by the type and timing of the damage. Different DDR pathways may compensate in the absence of the optimal or bespoke repair pathway [45]. Many patients demonstrate responses to the combination of platinum-based chemotherapy followed by PARPi maintenance treatment. However, resistance emerges, Golan et. al defined these patients as having "acquired resistance to platinum/PARP-inhibition." A small percentage of patients were refractory to platinum-based therapy and were coined as having "refractory resistance to platinum/PARP-inhibition". Lastly, a subgroup of patients, which have maintained a durable response to the platinum treatment and PARP-inhibition maintenance for more than three years, were defined as "super-responders to platinum/PARP-inhibition [46].

It is of note that sensitivity to treatment, and hence overall survival (OS) in BRCA associated PDAC can be associated with the allelic status of the BRCA genes. Germline mutations in *BRCA1/2* genes are monoallelic, leaving the second wild copy fully functional. However, ~85% of BRCA-associated PDAC tumors have loss of the wild type allele, loss of heterozygosity (LOH) or a second hit mutation in the *BRCA1/2* genes, leading to biallelic inactivation, rendering the tumors deficient in homologous recombination repair, which makes them exquisitely sensitive to platinum drugs and PARPi [32, 47]. Germline BRCA carriers with somatic, tumor biallelic inactivation of *BRCA1/2* gene have superior OS compared to patients who retain BRCA heterozygous tumors [32]. However, clinical observations indicate that such superior OS is limited, and resistance to treatment emerges. Reversion mutations in the mutated *BRCA1/2* allele is one of the most frequent resistance mechanisms employed by BRCA-associated tumors [48]. Golan et al. previously demonstrated occurrence of reversion mutations in biallelic PDAC tumors, leading to restoration of the *BRCA1/2* reading frame, thus potentially restoring the protein functionality and shortening the patient's OS [32, 49]. Targeting DDR pathway remains the most promising personalized therapeutic option in PDAC due to the significant effort spent in understanding the biology of these tumors along with the resistance mechanisms they develop.

8.1.2   Ongoing Clinical Trials

The vulnerability of PDAC tumors harboring mutations in HR to DNA damaging agents has been shown in multiple previous trials. First line platinum treatment followed by PARPi maintenance has shown improved RR and PFS [21, 50] and is now standard of care for germline BRCA PDAC. As described previously, most patients develop resistance to platinum/PARPi treatment. These patients can be identified in the clinic in the state of minimal residual disease with low tumor burden which may facilitate response to next line treatment options. Yet, limited options for treatment are available. There is an ongoing attempt to identify additional treatment options for this unique group of patients. Current clinical trials are now addressing this clinical problem by focusing on PARPi as a single agent or in combination with other agents. Table 8.1 shows active clinical trials examining treatments for HRD-PDAC.

PARPi single agent: In Table 8.1, rows 1–3 describe active trials using single-agent PARPi. Current trials are assessing the efficacy of new PARPi agents or PARP inhibition in tumors harboring mutations in HR beyond *BRCA1/2*.

PARPi combined with chemotherapy: Given the effectiveness of DNA damaging agents such as platinum agents and PARPi it has been hypothesized that combining both treatments may have a synergistic therapeutic efficacy, however overlapping toxicity profiles need to be taken into consideration. Previously reported clinical trials have evaluated this combination. The combination of PARPi with cisplatin and gemcitabine was not superior to chemotherapy alone in a phase II trial [51]. This may be attributed to higher rates of hematologic toxicities and

Table 8.1 Clinical trials targeting DDR in PDAC patients

	Trial identifier	Treatment	Phase	Patient population	Eligibility, exclusion	Status
1	NCT02677038	Olaparib	II	BRCAness Germ line *BRCA1,2* excluded	Stage IV 2nd line of treatment	Active, Not recruiting
2	NCT03140670	Rucaparib	II	Germ line- *BRCA1,2*, PALB2 mut	Stage III-IV No progression on platinum	Active, Not recruiting
3	NCT03601923	Niraparib	II	Germ line or somatic- *BRCA1,2*, PALB2, CHEK2, ATM mut	Stage III-IV Second line	Active, recruiting
4	NCT02890355	FOLFIRI+ Veliparib	II	Unselected	Stage IV Second line	Active, not recruiting
5	NCT03682289	ATR inhibitor ± Olaparib	II	PDAC RCC		Recruiting
6	NCT04890613	CX-5461	Ib	Solid tumor with *BRCA2*, PALB2 mut		Recruiting
7	NCT04548752	Olaparib ± Pembrolizumab	II	*BRCA1/BRCA2*	Maintenance	Recruiting
8	NCT04493060	Dostarlimab + niraparib	II	*BRCA1/2*, PALB2, BARD1, RAD51c/d	≥ 2 line	Recruiting
9	NCT04673448	Niraparib + TSR-042	IB	BRCA mut tumor	Any	Recruiting

need for frequent dose reductions. Additionally, in this clinical trial veliparib, a weaker PARPi was used. Combination of PARPi with topoisomerase inhibitors is also hypothesized to have synergistic effect with increasing of catalytic PARP inhibition. This combination has high toxicity rates as shown in preliminary data from a phase II trial (Table 8.1; row 4).

Targeting DDR: Targeting DNA damage repair pathways beyond PARP inhibition is currently being developed as monotherapy or in combination with other agents. These selective inhibitors include ATRi, ATMi, CHK1/2i, WEE1i and more. Preclinical studies have shown that olaparib-resistant cancer models may be re-sensitized to olaparib when combined with a WEE1 or ATR inhibitors [52, 53]. Several clinical trials are currently underway evaluating these combinations (Table 8.1; rows 5–6).

Immune checkpoint inhibitors: As discussed, the impact of Immune checkpoint inhibitors on PDAC, is limited, with the exception of MMR deficient tumors. There is now growing evidence that HRD tumors may have a unique immune response or there may be an opportunity to take advantage of these tumors from an immune perspective. The genomic instability and increased total mutational load of HRD tumors result in neoantigens which may increase the efficacy of immunotherapy in these tumors [54]. Additionally, preclinical data suggest PARP inhibition may have immunomodulatory potential PARPi treatment on HRD tumors is thought to increase neoantigen and tumor-associated antigen expression and reshape the tumor microenvironment with the potential to restore the antitumor immune response [54]. Based on accumulated preclinical evidence, clinical trials have been designed to address *BRCA1/2* germline mutated PDAC and are currently recruiting (Table 8.1, rows 7–9). Current trials are testing whether the addition of checkpoint inhibition to maintenance PARPi treatment will prolong PFS and possibly OS.

8.1.3 Expanded Targeting of DNA Damage Response Mechanisms

It is important to discriminate between the different mechanisms of actions of the chemotherapeutic agents versus PARPis and additional, emerging targeted DDR drugs in development. These considerations may have a profound clinical impact, since a DDR-deficient tumor may show sensitivity to DDR-related chemotherapy (platinum-based), but not to a specific targeted DDR drug in development (e.g., PARP, WEE1, and ATR inhibitors).

The platinum salts (carboplatin, cisplatin, and oxaliplatin) generate covalent cross-links between DNA bases. The cytotoxic effects are determined by the relative amount and specific structure of DNA adducts [55]. Alkylating agents (e.g., temozolomide) modify DNA bases. Electrophilic alkyl groups covalently bind to cellular nucleophilic sites, including bases in DNA, and these interactions are responsible for cytotoxicity [56]. Topoisomerases are essential for all organisms as they prevent DNA and RNA entanglements and resolve DNA supercoiling during replication and transcription. Inhibitors of topoisomerase 1 (camptothecin, topotecan, and irinotecan) and topoisomerase 2 (etoposide and doxorubicin) generate non-productive topoisomerase-DNA cleavage complexes (so-called TOP-DNA adducts) leading to inefficient re-ligation and ultimately DNA-strand breaks [56]. There are clear similarities and differences between the DNA-damage-inducing chemotherapies irinotecan and platinum agents, which are both part of a standard of care treatment for PDAC.

A more specific approach to targeting the DDR pathway includes biological therapeutics, specifically PARP inhibitors, for tumors with defects in DNA repair. Tumors with compromised ability to repair double-strand breaks (DSBs) by HR are highly sensitive to blockage of the repair of DNA single-strand breaks (SSBs) via the specific and targeted inhibition of PARP. PARP-inhibition causes failure of the repair of SSBs that, when encountered by the replication fork, can stall the fork and lead to its collapse and the formation of DSBs, especially in the absence of HR functional proteins (e.g. *BRCA1/2*). Additional PARP inhibition mechanisms include the "trapping" of PARP-1 protein at the site of DNA damage, which may also interfere with replication fork progression. This therapeutic strategy has demonstrated wide applicability in BRCA-associated ovarian, breast, prostate, and pancreatic cancers. Furthermore, this approach has been seen in the treatment of sporadic cancers with additional HR pathway impairments [57].

The most well described HRD biomarker in PDAC is germline *BRCA1/2* mutations. The global prevalence of germline *BRCA1/2* is around 7% [58]. This subgroup of patients has shown a superior OS when treated with platinum-based chemotherapy in retrospective studies [59]. However, the toxicity profile of platinum treatment including the accumulating neuropathy and hematological toxicity is well described and needs to be considered here [60]. PDAC associated with a germline *BRCA1/2* mutation demonstrate efficacy to platinum treatment. However, the side effects are debilitating, and dose reductions or cessations are usually mandatory, thus limiting the profound therapeutic usefulness in BRCA-associated cancers. Therefore, additional maintenance strategies have been explored. The aim of a maintenance treatment is to provide an alternative treatment approach without compromising the patient's quality of life. The clinical trial design in maintenance studies, include comparison of drugs in the maintenance setting that have a potentially superior therapeutic window. For instance, the aim of the POLO study: Olaparib as Switch Maintenance Therapy after Response to platinum-based treatment of metastatic germline BRCA-mutant pancreatic cancer [58]. Patients had to have received a minimum of 16 weeks of platinum-based first line chemotherapy, and they had to demonstrate stable disease (SD) or partial response (PR) or complete response (CR) in order to be eligible for the clinical trial. Identified patients were randomized in a 2:1 ration olaparib 300 mg twice daily or placebo. The primary endpoint PFS was 7.4 months on olaparib versus 3.8 months in the placebo arm, HR 0.53. (95% CI 0.35, 0.82; P = 0.0038). OS did not demonstrate statistically significant difference between olaparib and placebo (HR 0.83; p = 0.3487). At 3 years: 17.2% of patients remained on olaparib treatment vs 3.3% on placebo; 21.5% of patients in the olaparib arm remained free of subsequent cancer therapy vs 3.6% in the placebo arm (TFST: HR 0.44, nominal p < 0.0001); 33.9% of patients receiving olaparib were alive compared with 17.8% on placebo (Golan et al. ASCO GI 2021). No statistical differences were noted in quality-of-life measurements between the olaparib versus placebo arm. Olaparib-arm patients were more likely to achieve a response to treatment or maintain disease control; responses were durable lasting a median of over 2 years. Of note, this strategic approach of first line platinum-based chemotherapy followed by maintenance PARP inhibitor together has an extended PFS benefit to patients with a germline *BRCA1/2* mutations and metastatic disease. This study is the first Phase III trial to validate a targeted treatment in a biomarker-selected population of pancreatic cancer patients, highlighting the importance of germline BRCA mutations testing in this setting. PARPi in patients with DDR genomic alterations (beyond germline *BRCA1/2*) in advanced PDAC have been assessed in a phase II study with limited efficacy to date [61].

Additional biological agents targeted to DDR pathways (beyond PARPi) are recently emerging, as described above. The rationale behind development of new therapeutic strategies is to expand response to treatment by tackling additional pathways to overcome emerging resistance to PARP inhibition.

Rad-3 related (ATR) is a serine/threonine kinase involved in DDR signaling and plays a key role in maintaining genome integrity during DNA replication through the phosphorylation and activation of Chk1 and regulation of the DNA damage response. Preclinical evidence suggests that targeting ATR can selectively sensitize cancer cells but not normal cells to DNA damage, and this strategy can cause synthetic lethality in ATM-mutant cancer cells [62]. Additionally, targeting ATR in high-grade serous ovarian cancer in combination with PARPi was shown to be synergistic and leading to durable and complete responses in a variety of PDX models that harbor genetic alterations, including *BRCA1* mutations. Of note, all PDX models evaluated exhibited PARPi or platinum resistance [63]. Thus, ATR is among actionable DDR targets [46] and ATR inhibitors are in the early stages of clinical development in patients with solid tumors, including PDAC (NCT03188965, NCT03718091 and NCT04514497).

WEE1 Another actionable DDR target in PDAC, which participates in both the intra-S phase and G2/M checkpoint activities [45, 46]. WEE1 kinase regulates the G2/M checkpoint by phosphorylating CDC2 in response to DNA damage [64, 65]. Previous studies have reported that the highly selective, small molecule WEE1 inhibitor AZD1775 (adavosertib, previously MK-1775) can abrogate the G2/M checkpoint, thereby forcing damaged DNA through mitosis [64, 66]. Inhibition of WEE1 prevents the arrest of damaged DNA, which enhances CDC2 activity and drives cells in S phase to prematurely enter mitosis before repair [65]. In cells with mutated p53 (~75% of all PDCA cases) G1 checkpoint is defected, thus forcing cancer cells to rely primarily on the G2/M checkpoint to repair DNA damage before mitosis. AZD1775 has also been shown to enhance sensitization to chemotherapy and antimetabolites in cancer cells with wild type p53, which indicates the beneficial effects of this compound are not dependent on dysfunctional p53 [67]. Phase 1 clinical data has shown AZD1775 is clinically viable and can safely be combined with chemotherapies (gemcitabine, cisplatin or carboplatin) in advanced solid tumors NCT00648648 demonstrating partial response or stable disease [68]. Preclinical studies using PDAC PDX models with different p53 status showed tumor growth inhibition with combination of AZD1775 and irinotecan or capecitabine in the p53-mutated models [69]. These and other preclinical studies have built the basis for clinical trial design in PDAC patients testing WEE1i (AZD1775) in combination with chemotherapy.

8.1.4 Novel Therapies and Therapeutic Resistance

Virtually all therapies for PDAC have limited disease modifying effect due to therapeutic resistance, which emerges in most cases. And the clinical management of PDAC, with so few active targeted therapeutic options, would certainly benefit from an expansion in druggable targets leveraging DDR defects in particular [70, 71]. Studying resistance mechanisms emerging in response to existing active therapies, like PARPi, offers an opportunity to identify promising therapeutic targets and combination therapies.

For example, data have suggested a role for post-transcriptional gene regulation in rapidly modulating multiple, co-signaling pathways involved in PDAC tumorigenesis and therapeutic resistance. A key protein involved in this mode of gene regulation is the RNA-binding protein HuR (*ELAVL1*) [72]. HuR is overexpressed in PDAC cells where it promotes mRNA stabilization and the expression of specific mRNAs functionally linked to PDAC cell survival. In vivo studies also indicate that the efficacy of clinically relevant therapies (i.e., oxaliplatin and PARPi) is enhanced by HuR inhibition [73–76], suggesting that HuR and/or its downstream mRNA targets may play a role in refractory PDAC. The prioritization of certain HuR targets has aided the discovery of non-canonical targets in these kinds of tumors, including the DNA repair protein poly (ADP-ribose) glycohydrolase (PARG) in PDAC cells [77–79]; cell cycle regulator WEE1 [80, 81]; and the serine threonine kinase PIM1 [73].

Example of an HuR target that may be important for targeting resistance and the DDR pathway: The use of PARG inhibitors in PDAC.

Recent efforts targeting PARG have been promising [78, 79]. PARG is an essential enzyme primarily responsible for the rapid turnover of poly (ADP-ribose) (PAR) created by PARP1/2 in response to DNA damage [82–84]. PARylation, or the creation of PAR polymer chains, at DNA damage sites is thought to represent a flagging system involved in the recruitment of the various components of the repair process. Once repair is underway or completed, PARG removes PAR chains, contributing to the release of PARP from the damaged site and, in the S-phase, aids the restart of the replication fork.

Why target PARG in PDAC? Evidence suggests pro-oncogenic HuR is elevated in PDAC and amplifies PARG expression in cancer cells, and based upon the role PARG plays in DNA damage resolution and replication fork restart [78], there is a strong basis for targeting PARG in combination with other DDR proteins. In a PDAC xenograft mouse model with doxycycline-induced PARG silencing, Jain et al. 2019 revealed that PARG knockdown significantly decreased tumor volume, which was directly ascribed to increased tumor cell killing. This was true especially (but not exclusively) in the context of HR-deficient cells, such as *BRCA1/2*-deficient cells, where the main pathway for double strand DNA break repair is not functional [79]. At the cellular level, PARG inhibition may act in more than one way to add stress and induce death in cancer cells. First, PARG inhibition contributes to DNA damage by limiting replication fork restart in the context of replication stress response; stalled forks increase the probability for double strand breaks, eventually leading to apoptosis. Additionally, PARG inhibition limits the turnover of PAR chains, which are created by PARP-driven oligomerization of NAD+ monomers. NAD+ is an essential cofactor metabolite and cancer cells have unique dependencies on NAD+ metabolic pathways, including those critical for cell survival. PARG inhibition depletes freely available NAD+ by preventing PAR breakdown, resulting in NAD+ sequestration and collapse of metabolic homeostasis leading to cell death [85]. In PDAC, multiple preliminary lines of evidence, from in vitro to in vivo, show that targeting PARG both genetically (i.e., CRISPR and sh/siRNA strategies) and with available small molecule inhibitors can inhibit PDAC cells [77–79]. However, a limited number of compounds exists that target PARG, and in some cases their poor bioavailability prevents in vivo studies. Mechanistically, PARG inhibition can alter DNA repair, the cell cycle, and cause apoptosis [79]. Identifying and characterizing new targets with synthetic lethal potential is critical for the development of novel therapeutic options for PDAC.

Synergistic partners to PARG inhibition. The importance of identifying and investigating novel synergistic approaches cannot be overstated; there is a desperate unmet need to develop new therapy regimens for PDAC, where the outcomes remain dismal and the standard-of-care therapies are combination therapies (i.e., FOLFIRINOX). Synergy is important because the enhanced effect of two (or more) compounds may create a scenario that is detrimental to a cancer cell; and combination therapies may allow for lower doses to be achieved for a desired therapeutic effect, diminishing unwanted side effects. The interest in PARG is further increased by evidence in the literature that PARG inhibition can synergize with a number of molecules [77, 85–87]. Among these:

WEE1: The Brody lab [77, 88] and others [89] have shown synergy by simultaneously targeting PARG and WEE1 (AZD1775), both using inhibitory compounds and with genetic silencing. WEE1 is a protein kinase with the ability to phosphorylate—and therefore inhibit—Cdk1, a protein which is crucial for the cyclin-dependent checkpoint especially at the G2/M transition. Agostini et al. 2020 have demonstrated [77] successful co-targeting of WEE1 (with a WEE1 inhibitor) and PARG (via a CRISPR silencing of the gene) in: (1) an in vivo model of cancer; (2) the synergistic effects of targeting PARG and WEE1 in a colony formation assay in PDAC cells; and (3) how it mechanistically targets PARylation and causes DNA damage.

CF10: Haber et al. 2021 suggested that PARG inhibition could synergize with CF10, targeting PARylation, DNA damage, and cancer cell death [86]. Importantly,

CF10 synergizes with PARG but nor PARP inhibition, suggesting a mechanism of action that might be relevant to patients who develop resistance to PARPi. CF10 is a second generation polymeric fluoropyrimidine, targeting the key enzymes DNA topoisomerase-1 (Top1) and thymidylate synthase (TS), which aims at addressing some of the limitations of 5-FU and Irinotecan, two of the components of the common chemotherapy regimen FOLFIRINOX. The polymeric nature of CF10 allows a more efficient conversion to the TS-inhibitory metabolite FdUMP, and generation of lower levels of ribonucleotide metabolites that are responsible for 5-FU's systemic toxicities. These are frequently serious and even life-threatening in some patients. CF10 also includes a non-native nucleotide (AraC) at the 3'-terminus to limit plasma degradation and enhance anti-cancer activity while PEG5 at the 5'-terminus modulates binding to plasma proteins [90]. Researchers are now looking to leverage these data in preclinical modeling developed with Dr. Gmeiner at Wake Forest University.

Future clinical trials and ex vivo modeling that could target both DDR pathways and therapeutic resistance. At the 2022 American Association of Cancer Research, Dr. Charles Sawyers presented the concept that for targeted therapies there are acquired "on-target" resistance mechanisms and "off-target" resistance mechanisms (see Fig. 8.1). For an updated discussion on broad therapeutic resistance mechanisms (e.g., innate and acquired) please see a review by Tyner J. et al. 2022 [91]. Although DNA damaging agents certainly have on-target resistance events (such as reversion mutations) that induce PDAC cell resistance, off-target resistance (e.g., HuR transcript regulation) is also a significant contributor to poor clinical responses. Although many opportunities present themselves in the

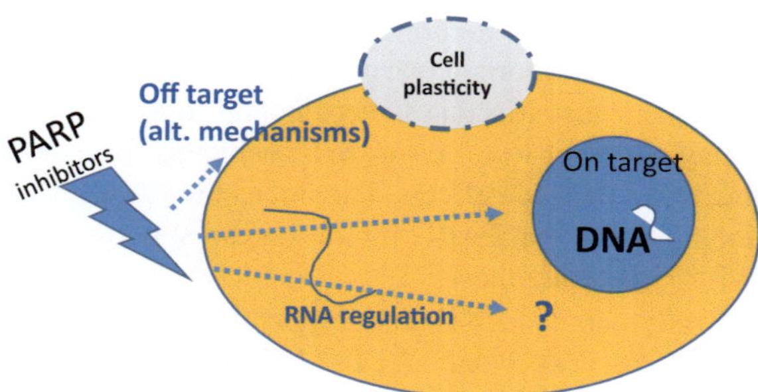

Fig. 8.1 It is helpful to conceptualize two categories of resistance, on target (genomic) and off target (non-genomic). On target resistance is well studied and refers to the acquisition of point mutations or other genomic rearrangements, including whole or partial genome duplications, which alter structural motifs of targeted proteins (loss of drug binding) or lead to increased copy numbers of proteins implicated in resistance or bypass pathways. Off target resistance is less studied and refers to concepts like the non-genomic transformations of cells into subtypes that are more resistant to therapy, or changes in transcript regulation via RNA binding proteins like HuR, among other mechanisms yet to be elucidated. Note: inspired, adapted, and modified from a Preliminary Session talk by Dr. Charles Sawyers (AACR, 2022). Created with Biorender.com

on-target setting; it is worthwhile to evaluate tractable, off-target resistance mechanisms such as PARG. Taking advantage of ongoing, cutting-edge clinical trials such as the SMMART program and/or the COMPASS trials, will allow the community to assess the effect of treatments in "real-time" on the tumor ecosystem. Understanding these changes upon treatment will provide clues to our ability to target the plasticity of off-target pathways [92, 93]. In addition to this modernized clinical trial, the generation and validation of patient derived models from these trials will provide opportunities to test targeting these strategies outside the patient. In the future, once researchers have better mastered the generation of model systems like these, resistance mechanisms may be modeled in real time and used to select rational combinations that are more likely to drive tumors toward extinction.

In conclusion, targeting the DNA damage response in DDR-altered PDAC is the best-in-class personalized approach to the treatment of these patients to date. The key to future clinical success in this arena will be: 1) discovering and evaluating novel targets of DDR and therapeutic resistance; 2) expanding and understanding the role of other DDR-related defective genes in PDAC (e.g., as predictive markers); 3) development of clinical trials that collect longitudinal biopsies to evaluate changes to the tumor ecosystem (including the important tumor microenvironment and the immune system) in real-time; and 4) integrating patient derived models into predictive marker platforms. The field is primed to target the Achilles' heel of DDR-altered PDAC in an effort to dramatically improve patient outcomes.

References

1. Rahib L, Wehner MR, Matrisian LM, Nead KT (2021) Estimated projection of US cancer incidence and death to 2040. JAMA Network Open 4(4):e214708. %U https://doi.org/10.1001/jamanetworkopen.2021.4708
2. Global Burden of Disease Cancer C (2022) Cancer Incidence, Mortality, Years of Life Lost, Years Lived With Disability, and Disability-Adjusted Life Years for 29 Cancer Groups From 2010 to 2019: a systematic analysis for the global burden of disease study 2019. JAMA Oncology 8(3):420–44. %U https://doi.org/10.1001/jamaoncol.2021.6987
3. Ushio J, Kanno A, Ikeda E, Ando K, Nagai H, Miwata T et al (2021) Pancreatic ductal adenocarcinoma: epidemiology and risk factors. Diagnostics (Basel, Switzerland) 11(3):562
4. Cancer of the Pancreas—Cancer Stat Facts %U https://seer.cancer.gov/statfacts/html/pancreas.html.SEER
5. Survival Rates for Pancreatic Cancer %U https://www.cancer.org/cancer/pancreatic-cancer/detection-diagnosis-staging/survival-rates.html
6. Waddell N, Pajic M, Patch A-M, Chang DK, Kassahn KS, Bailey P, et al. (2015) Whole genomes redefine the mutational landscape of pancreatic cancer. Nature 518(7540):495–501. %U https://www.ncbi.nlm.nih.gov/pmc/articles/PMC4523082/
7. Zhang X, Mao T, Zhang B, Xu H, Cui J, Jiao F, et al. (2022) Characterization of the genomic landscape in large-scale Chinese patients with pancreatic cancer. eBioMedicine 77. %U https://www.thelancet.com/journals/ebiom/article/PIIS2352-3964(22)00081-0/fulltext
8. Puleo F, Nicolle R, Blum Y, Cros J, Marisa L, Demetter P, et al. (2018) Stratification of pancreatic ductal adenocarcinomas based on tumor and microenvironment features. Gastroenterology 155(6):1999–2013.e3 %U https://linkinghub.elsevier.com/retrieve/pii/S0016508518349199

9. Collisson EA, Sadanandam A, Olson P, Gibb WJ, Truitt M, Gu S, et al. (2011) Subtypes of pancreatic ductal adenocarcinoma and their differing responses to therapy. Nature Med 17(4):500–3. %U http://www.nature.com/articles/nm.2344

10. Moffitt RA, Marayati R, Flate EL, Volmar KE, Loeza SGH, Hoadley KA, et al. (2015) Virtual microdissection identifies distinct tumor- and stroma-specific subtypes of pancreatic ductal adenocarcinoma. Nature Genetics 47(10):1168–78. %* 2015 Nature Publishing Group, a division of Macmillan Publishers Limited. All Rights Reserved. %U https://www.nature.com/articles/ng.3398

11. Bailey P, Chang DK, Nones K, Johns AL, Patch AM, Gingras MC et al (2016) Genomic analyses identify molecular subtypes of pancreatic cancer. Nature 531(7592):47–52

12. Pishvaian MJ, Bender RJ, Halverson D, Rahib L, Hendifar AE, Mikhail S et al (2018) Molecular profiling of patients with pancreatic cancer: initial results from the know your tumor initiative. Clin Cancer Res 24(20):5018–5027

13. Pishvaian MJ, Blais EM, Brody JR, Lyons E, DeArbeloa P, Hendifar A et al (2020) Overall survival in patients with pancreatic cancer receiving matched therapies following molecular profiling: a retrospective analysis of the know your tumor registry trial. Lancet Oncol 21(4):508–518

14. Perkhofer L, Gout J, Roger E, de Almeida FK, Simões CB, Wiesmüller L et al (2021) DNA damage repair as a target in pancreatic cancer: state-of-the-art and future perspectives. Gut 70(3):606–617

15. Katayama ES, Hue JJ, Bajor DL, Ocuin LM, Ammori JB, Hardacre JM, et al. (2020) A comprehensive analysis of clinical trials in pancreatic cancer: what is coming down the pike? Oncotarget 11(38):3489–501. %U https://www.ncbi.nlm.nih.gov/pmc/articles/PMC7517959/

16. Nollmann FI, Ruess DA (2020) Targeting mutant KRAS in pancreatic cancer: futile or promising? Biomedicines 8(8)

17. Nevala-Plagemann C, Hidalgo M, Garrido-Laguna I (2020) From state-of-the-art treatments to novel therapies for advanced-stage pancreatic cancer. Nat Rev Clin Oncol 17(2):108–123

18. Dreyer SB, Chang DK, Bailey P, Biankin AV (2017) Pancreatic cancer genomes: implications for clinical management and therapeutic development. Clin Cancer Res 23(7):1638–1646

19. Drilon A, Laetsch TW, Kummar S, DuBois SG, Lassen UN, Demetri GD et al (2018) Efficacy of Larotrectinib in trk fusion-positive cancers in adults and children. N Engl J Med 378(8):731–739

20. Le DT, Durham JN, Smith KN, Wang H, Bartlett BR, Aulakh LK et al (2017) Mismatch repair deficiency predicts response of solid tumors to PD-1 blockade. Science 357(6349):409–413

21. Golan T, Hammel P, Reni M, Van Cutsem E, Macarulla T, Hall MJ et al (2019) Maintenance Olaparib for germline BRCA-mutated metastatic pancreatic cancer. N Engl J Med 381(4):317–327

22. Crowley F, Park W, O'Reilly EM (2021) Targeting DNA damage repair pathways in pancreas cancer. Cancer Metastasis Rev 40(3):891–908

23. Beatty GL, Gladney WL (2015) Immune escape mechanisms as a guide for cancer immunotherapy. Clin Cancer Res 21(4):687–692

24. Balachandran VP, Beatty GL, Dougan SK (2019) Broadening the impact of immunotherapy to pancreatic cancer: challenges and opportunities. Gastroenterology 156(7):2056–2072

25. Poschke I, Faryna M, Bergmann F, Flossdorf M, Lauenstein C, Hermes J et al (2016) Identification of a tumor-reactive T-cell repertoire in the immune infiltrate of patients with resectable pancreatic ductal adenocarcinoma. Oncoimmunology. 5(12):e1240859

26. Naing A, Powderly JD, Falchook G, Creelan B, Nemunaitis J, Lutzky J, et al. (2018) Abstract CT177: epacadostat plus durvalumab in patients with advanced solid tumors: preliminary results of the ongoing, open-label, phase I/II ECHO-203 study. Cancer Res 78(13_Supplement):CT177-CT

27. Topalian SL, Hodi FS, Brahmer JR, Gettinger SN, Smith DC, McDermott DF et al (2012) Safety, activity, and immune correlates of anti-PD-1 antibody in cancer. N Engl J Med 366(26):2443–2454

28. Royal RE, Levy C, Turner K, Mathur A, Hughes M, Kammula US et al (2010) Phase 2 trial of single agent Ipilimumab (anti-CTLA-4) for locally advanced or metastatic pancreatic adenocarcinoma. J Immunother 33(8):828–833
29. Luchini C, Brosens LAA, Wood LD, Chatterjee D, Shin JI, Sciammarella C et al (2021) Comprehensive characterisation of pancreatic ductal adenocarcinoma with microsatellite instability: histology, molecular pathology and clinical implications. Gut 70(1):148–156
30. Le DT, Uram JN, Wang H, Bartlett BR, Kemberling H, Eyring AD et al (2015) PD-1 blockade in tumors with mismatch-repair deficiency. N Engl J Med 372(26):2509–2520
31. Waddell N, Pajic M, Patch AM, Chang DK, Kassahn KS, Bailey P et al (2015) Whole genomes redefine the mutational landscape of pancreatic cancer. Nature 518(7540):495–501
32. Golan T, O'Kane GM, Denroche RE, Raitses-Gurevich M, Grant RC, Holter S et al (2021) Genomic features and classification of homologous recombination deficient pancreatic ductal adenocarcinoma. Gastroenterology 160(6):2119–32.e9
33. Li H, Liu ZY, Wu N, Chen YC, Cheng Q, Wang J (2020) PARP inhibitor resistance: the underlying mechanisms and clinical implications. Mol Cancer 19(1):107
34. Lin KK, Harrell MI, Oza AM, Oaknin A, Ray-Coquard I, Tinker AV et al (2019) BRCA reversion mutations in circulating tumor DNA predict primary and acquired resistance to the PARP inhibitor rucaparib in high-grade ovarian carcinoma. Cancer Discov 9(2):210–219
35. Pettitt SJ, Frankum JR, Punta M, Lise S, Alexander J, Chen Y et al (2020) Clinical BRCA1/2 reversion analysis identifies hotspot mutations and predicted Neoantigens associated with therapy resistance. Cancer Discov 10(10):1475–1488
36. Bakhoum SF, Ngo B, Laughney AM, Cavallo JA, Murphy CJ, Ly P et al (2018) Chromosomal instability drives metastasis through a cytosolic DNA response. Nature 553(7689):467–472
37. Shen J, Zhao W, Ju Z, Wang L, Peng Y, Labrie M et al (2019) PARPi triggers the STING-dependent immune response and enhances the therapeutic efficacy of immune checkpoint blockade independent of BRCAness. Cancer Res 79(2):311–319
38. Jiao S, Xia W, Yamaguchi H, Wei Y, Chen MK, Hsu JM et al (2017) PARP inhibitor upregulates PD-L1 expression and enhances cancer-associated immunosuppression. Clin Cancer Res 23(14):3711–3720
39. (2017) Integrated Genomic Characterization of Pancreatic Ductal Adenocarcinoma. Cancer Cell 32(2):185-203.e13
40. Tran E, Robbins PF, Lu YC, Prickett TD, Gartner JJ, Jia L et al (2016) T-cell transfer therapy targeting mutant KRAS in cancer. N Engl J Med 375(23):2255–2262
41. Cafri G, Yossef R, Pasetto A, Deniger DC, Lu YC, Parkhurst M et al (2019) Memory T cells targeting oncogenic mutations detected in peripheral blood of epithelial cancer patients. Nat Commun 10(1):449
42. Armstrong SA, Schultz CW, Azimi-Sadjadi A, Brody JR, Pishvaian MJ (2019) ATM dysfunction in pancreatic adenocarcinoma and associated therapeutic implications. Mol Cancer Ther 18(11):1899–1908
43. Fong PC, Yap TA, Boss DS, Carden CP, Mergui-Roelvink M, Gourley C et al (2010) Poly(ADP)-ribose polymerase inhibition: frequent durable responses in BRCA carrier ovarian cancer correlating with platinum-free interval. J Clin Oncol 28(15):2512–2519
44. McMullen M, Karakasis K, Madariaga A, Oza AM (2020) Overcoming platinum and PARP-inhibitor resistance in ovarian cancer. Cancers (Basel) 12(6)
45. O'Connor MJ (2015) Targeting the DNA damage response in cancer. Mol Cell 60(4):547–560
46. Golan T, Atias D, Stossel C, Raitses-Gurevich M (2021) Patient-derived xenograft models of BRCA-associated pancreatic cancers. Adv Drug Deliv Rev 171:257–265
47. Wang Y, Park JYP, Pacis A, Denroche RE, Jang GH, Zhang A et al (2020) A preclinical trial and molecularly annotated patient cohort identify predictive biomarkers in homologous recombination-deficient pancreatic cancer. Clin Cancer Res 26(20):5462–5476
48. Rose M, Burgess JT, O'Byrne K, Richard DJ, Bolderson E (2020) PARP inhibitors: clinical relevance, mechanisms of action and tumor resistance. Front Cell Dev Biol. 8:564601
49. Stossel C, Raitses-Gurevich M, Atias D, Beller T, Glick Gorman Y, Halperin S, Peer E, Denroche RE, Zhang A, Notta F, Wilson JM, O'Kane GM, Haimov Talmoud E, Amison N,

Schvimer M, Salpeter SJ, Bar V, Zundelevich A, Tirosh I, Tal R, Dinstag G, Kinar Y, Eliezer Y, Ben-David U, Gavert NS, Straussman R, Gallinger SJ, Berger R, Golan T (2023) Spectrum of response to platinum and parp inhibitors in germline BRCA-associated pancreatic cancer in the clinical and preclinical setting. Cancer Discov 13(8):1826–1843. https://doi.org/10.1158/2159-8290.CD-22-0412

50. Wattenberg MM, Asch D, Yu S, O'Dwyer PJ, Domchek SM, Nathanson KL et al (2020) Platinum response characteristics of patients with pancreatic ductal adenocarcinoma and a germline BRCA1, BRCA2 or PALB2 mutation. Br J Cancer 122(3):333–339

51. O'Reilly EM, Lee JW, Zalupski M, Capanu M, Park J, Golan T et al (2020) Randomized, multicenter, phase II trial of gemcitabine and cisplatin with or without veliparib in patients with pancreas adenocarcinoma and a germline BRCA/PALB2 mutation. J Clin Oncol 38(13):1378–1388

52. Yazinski SA, Comaills V, Buisson R, Genois M-M, Nguyen HD, Ho CK et al (2017) ATR inhibition disrupts rewired homologous recombination and fork protection pathways in PARP inhibitor-resistant BRCA-deficient cancer cells. Genes Dev 31(3):318–332

53. Kim H, George E, Ragland R, Rafail S, Zhang R, Krepler C et al (2017) Targeting the ATR/CHK1 axis with PARP inhibition results in tumor regression in BRCA-mutant ovarian cancer models. Clin Cancer Res 23(12):3097–3108

54. Samstein RM, Krishna C, Ma X, Pei X, Lee K-W, Makarov V et al (2021) Mutations in BRCA1 and BRCA2 differentially affect the tumor microenvironment and response to checkpoint blockade immunotherapy. Nat Cancer 1(12):1188–1203

55. Johnstone TC, Suntharalingam K, Lippard SJ (2016) The next generation of platinum drugs: targeted Pt(II) agents, nanoparticle delivery, and Pt(IV) prodrugs. Chem Rev 116(5):3436–3486

56. Agarwala SS, Kirkwood JM (2000) Temozolomide, a novel alkylating agent with activity in the central nervous system, may improve the treatment of advanced metastatic melanoma. Oncologist 5(2):144–151

57. Lord CJ, Ashworth A (2017) PARP inhibitors: synthetic lethality in the clinic. Science 355(6330):1152–1158

58. Golan T, Kindler HL, Park JO, Reni M, Mercade TM, Hammel P, et al. (2018) Geographic and ethnic heterogeneity in the BRCA1/2 pre-screening population for the randomized phase III POLO study of olaparib maintenance in metastatic pancreatic cancer (mPC). J Clinical Oncol 36(15_suppl):4115

59. Golan T, Kanji ZS, Epelbaum R, Devaud N, Dagan E, Holter S et al (2014) Overall survival and clinical characteristics of pancreatic cancer in BRCA mutation carriers. Br J Cancer 111(6):1132–1138

60. Oun R, Moussa YE, Wheate NJ (2018) The side effects of platinum-based chemotherapy drugs: a review for chemists. Dalton Trans 47(19):6645–6653

61. Javle M, Shacham-Shmueli E, Xiao L, Varadhachary G, Halpern N, Fogelman D et al (2021) Olaparib monotherapy for previously treated pancreatic cancer with DNA damage repair genetic alterations other than germline BRCA variants: findings from 2 phase 2 nonrandomized clinical trials. JAMA Oncol 7(5):693–699

62. Fokas E, Prevo R, Hammond EM, Brunner TB, McKenna WG, Muschel RJ (2014) Targeting ATR in DNA damage response and cancer therapeutics. Cancer Treat Rev 40(1):109–117

63. Kim H, Xu H, George E, Hallberg D, Kumar S, Jagannathan V et al (2020) Combining PARP with ATR inhibition overcomes PARP inhibitor and platinum resistance in ovarian cancer models. Nat Commun 11(1):3726

64. Dobbelstein M, Sørensen CS (2015) Exploiting replicative stress to treat cancer. Nat Rev Drug Discov 14(6):405–423

65. Aarts M, Sharpe R, Garcia-Murillas I, Gevensleben H, Hurd MS, Shumway SD et al (2012) Forced mitotic entry of S-phase cells as a therapeutic strategy induced by inhibition of WEE1. Cancer Discov 2(6):524–539

66. Hirai H, Iwasawa Y, Okada M, Arai T, Nishibata T, Kobayashi M et al (2009) Small-molecule inhibition of Wee1 kinase by MK-1775 selectively sensitizes p53-deficient tumor cells to DNA-damaging agents. Mol Cancer Ther 8(11):2992–3000

67. Van Linden AA, Baturin D, Ford JB, Fosmire SP, Gardner L, Korch C et al (2013) Inhibition of Wee1 sensitizes cancer cells to antimetabolite chemotherapeutics in vitro and in vivo, independent of p53 functionality. Mol Cancer Ther 12(12):2675–2684

68. Leijen S, van Geel RMJM, Pavlick AC, Tibes R, Rosen L, Razak ARA et al (2016) Phase I study evaluating WEE1 inhibitor AZD1775 as monotherapy and in combination with gemcitabine, cisplatin, or carboplatin in patients with advanced solid tumors. J Clin Oncol 34(36):4371–4380

69. Hartman SJ, Bagby SM, Yacob BW, Simmons DM, MacBeth M, Lieu CH et al (2021) WEE1 inhibition in combination with targeted agents and standard chemotherapy in preclinical models of pancreatic ductal adenocarcinoma. Front Oncol 11:642328

70. Zeng S, Pöttler M, Lan B, Grützmann R, Pilarsky C, Yang H (2019) Chemoresistance in pancreatic cancer. Int J Mol Sci 20(18)

71. Quiñonero F, Mesas C, Doello K, Cabeza L, Perazzoli G, Jimenez-Luna C et al (2019) The challenge of drug resistance in pancreatic ductal adenocarcinoma: a current overview. Cancer Biol Med 16(4):688–699

72. Schultz CW, Preet R, Dhir T, Dixon DA, Brody JR (2020) Understanding and targeting the disease-related RNA binding protein human antigen R (HuR). Wiley Interdiscip Rev RNA 11(3):e1581

73. Blanco FF, Jimbo M, Wulfkuhle J, Gallagher I, Deng J, Enyenihi L et al (2016) The mRNA-binding protein HuR promotes hypoxia-induced chemoresistance through posttranscriptional regulation of the proto-oncogene PIM1 in pancreatic cancer cells. Oncogene 35(19):2529–2541

74. Blanco FF, Preet R, Aguado A, Vishwakarma V, Stevens LE, Vyas A et al (2016) Impact of HuR inhibition by the small molecule MS-444 on colorectal cancer cell tumorigenesis. Oncotarget 7(45):74043–74058

75. Cai J, Wang H, Jiao X, Huang R, Qin Q, Zhang J et al (2019) The RNA-binding protein HuR confers oxaliplatin resistance of colorectal cancer by upregulating CDC6. Mol Cancer Ther 18(7):1243–1254

76. Zarei M, Lal S, Parker SJ, Nevler A, Vaziri-Gohar A, Dukleska K et al (2017) Posttranscriptional upregulation of IDH1 by HuR establishes a powerful survival phenotype in pancreatic cancer cells. Cancer Res 77(16):4460–4471

77. Agostini LC, Jain A, Shupp A, Nevler A, McCarthy G, Bussard KM, et al. (2020) Combined targeting of PARG and Wee1 causes decreased cell survival and DNA damage in an S-phase dependent manner. Mol Cancer Res

78. Chand SN, Zarei M, Schiewer MJ, Kamath AR, Romeo C, Lal S et al (2017) Posttranscriptional regulation of PARG mRNA by HuR facilitates DNA repair and resistance to PARP inhibitors. Cancer Res 77(18):5011–5025

79. Jain A, Agostini LC, McCarthy GA, Chand SN, Ramirez A, Nevler A et al (2019) Poly (ADP) ribose glycohydrolase can be effectively targeted in pancreatic cancer. Cancer Res 79(17):4491–4502

80. Lal S, Zarei M, Chand SN, Dylgjeri E, Mambelli-Lisboa NC, Pishvaian MJ et al (2016) WEE1 inhibition in pancreatic cancer cells is dependent on DNA repair status in a context dependent manner. Sci Rep 6(1):33323

81. Agostini LC, Jain A, Shupp A, Nevler A, McCarthy G, Bussard KM et al (2021) Combined targeting of PARG and Wee1 causes decreased cell survival and DNA damage in an S-phase–dependent manner. Mol Cancer Res 19(2):207–214

82. Gogola E, Duarte AA, de Ruiter JR, Wiegant WW, Schmid JA, de Bruijn R et al (2019) Selective loss of PARG restores PARylation and counteracts PARP inhibitor-mediated synthetic lethality. Cancer Cell 35(6):950–952

83. Houl JH, Ye Z, Brosey CA, Balapiti-Modarage LPF, Namjoshi S, Bacolla A et al (2019) Selective small molecule PARG inhibitor causes replication fork stalling and cancer cell death. Nat Commun 10(1):5654
84. Marques M, Jangal M, Wang LC, Kazanets A, da Silva SD, Zhao T et al (2019) Oncogenic activity of poly (ADP-ribose) glycohydrolase. Oncogene 38(12):2177–2191
85. Nagashima H, Lee CK, Tateishi K, Higuchi F, Subramanian M, Rafferty S et al (2020) Poly(ADP-ribose) glycohydrolase inhibition sequesters NAD(+) to potentiate the metabolic lethality of alkylating chemotherapy in IDH-Mutant tumor cells. Cancer Discov 10(11):1672–1689
86. Haber AO, Jain A, Mani C, Nevler A, Agostini LC, Golan T, et al. (2020) AraC-FdUMP[10] (CF10) is a next generation fluoropyrimidine with potent antitumor activity in PDAC and is synergistic with a novel small molecule inhibitor of PARG. Under Rev
87. Slade D (2020) PARP and PARG inhibitors in cancer treatment. Genes Dev 34(5–6):360–394
88. Lal S, Burkhart RA, Beeharry N, Bhattacharjee V, Londin ER, Cozzitorto JA et al (2014) HuR posttranscriptionally regulates WEE1: implications for the DNA damage response in pancreatic cancer cells. Cancer Res 74(4):1128–1140
89. Pillay N, Tighe A, Nelson L, Littler S, Coulson-Gilmer C, Bah N, et al. (2019) DNA replication vulnerabilities render ovarian cancer cells sensitive to poly(ADP-Ribose) glycohydrolase inhibitors. Cancer Cell 35(3):519–33 e8
90. Gupta V, Bhavanasi S, Quadir M, Singh K, Ghosh G, Vasamreddy K et al (2019) Protein PEGylation for cancer therapy: bench to bedside. J Cell Commun Signal 13(3):319–330
91. Tyner JW, Haderk F, Kumaraswamy A, Baughn LB, Van Ness B, Liu S et al (2022) Understanding drug sensitivity and tackling resistance in cancer. Can Res 82(8):1448–1460
92. Aung KL, Fischer SE, Denroche RE, Jang GH, Dodd A, Creighton S et al (2018) Genomics-driven precision medicine for advanced pancreatic cancer: early results from the COMPASS trial. Clin Cancer Res 24(6):1344–1354
93. Mitri ZI, Parmar S, Johnson B, Kolodzie A, Keck JM, Morris M et al (2018) Implementing a comprehensive translational oncology platform: from molecular testing to actionability. J Transl Med 16(1):358

Combining Poly (ADP-Ribose) Polymerase (PARP) Inhibitors with Chemotherapeutic Agents: Promise and Challenges

9

Kyaw Zin Thein, Rajat Thawani, and Shivaani Kummar

9.1 Introduction

Better understanding of molecular drivers and dysregulated pathways has furthered the concept of precision oncology and rational drug development. The role of DNA damage response (DDR) pathways has been extensively studied in carcinogenesis and as potential therapeutic targets to improve response to chemotherapy or overcome resistance [1–3]. The integrity of DNA is maintained by the repair processes; subtle damage such as damage at DNA base pair or single-strand breaks (SSBs) are repaired by base excision repair (BER) or nucleotide excision repair (NER) whereas large-scale double-strand breaks (DSBs) or clustered lesions require homologous recombination repair (HR) and non-homologous end joining repair (NHEJ) [4–6]. BReast CAncer genes 1 and 2 (BRCA1/2), RAD51 and Partner and localizer of BRCA2 (PALB2) genes are important key players in HR [7]. Genomic instability, which is one of the hallmarks and characteristics of most cancers, can occur where there are errors in the DDR pathway. HR-deficient

K. Z. Thein · R. Thawani
Comprehensive Cancer Centers of Nevada, Las Vegas, NV, USA
e-mail: kyaw.thein@usoncology.com

R. Thawani
e-mail: thawani@ohsu.edu

S. Kummar (✉)
DeArmond Endowed Chair of Cancer Research, Division of Hematology and Medical Oncology, Clinical and Translational Research, Knight Cancer Institute (KCI), Center for Experimental Therapeutics (KCI), Oregon Health and Science University, 3181 SW Sam Jackson Park Rd, OC14HO, Portland, OR 97239, USA
e-mail: kummar@ohsu.edu

cancer cells such as those harboring germline mutations in BRCA 1/2 (gBR-CAm), are dependent upon lower-fidelity SSB repair mechanisms and patients with gBRCAm was known to be predisposed to ovarian, breast, prostate, and other cancers [8, 9]. PARP1, one of the most prominent proteins among 17 PARP family enzymes, binds to the single-strand DNA break sites and PARP complexes then lead to auto-PARylation and downstream recruitement of the SSB repair effectors [5, 10, 11].

Treatment with small molecule inhibitors of PARP has resulted in clinical response and conferred survival benefit to patients with ovarian cancer, BRCA-mutant breast cancer, HRD-deficient prostate cancer and BRCA-mutant pancreatic cancer, leading to US Food and Drug Administration (FDA) approvals [12–21]. However, the observed clinical benefit with single agent PARP inhibitors is limited to few tumor types within the relevant genetic context. Since DDR pathways are essential for repair of damage caused by cytotoxic agents, PARP inhibitors have been evaluated in combination with various chemotherapeutic agents to broaden the therapeutic application of this class of drugs. Resistance mechanisms to PARP inhibitors are upregulation of drug efflux pump ATP-binding cassette (ABC) transporter protein ABCB1 transporter, Homologous recombination (HR) repair restoration via re-expression of BRCA1/2 mutations or BRCA1-independent or restoration of DNA replication fork stability/ protection, and various target factors such as mutations in PARP1 or loss of poly (ADP-ribose) glycohydrolase (PARG) [2]. In this chapter, we discuss the combination of PARP inhibitors with different chemotherapeutics agents, clinical experience to date, lessons learnt, and future directions for this approach.

9.2 Clinical Development of Poly (ADP-Ribose) Polymerase (PARP) Inhibitors

Four PARP inhibitors (olaparib, rucaparib, niraparib and talazoparib), are currently approved by the US FDA. The potent molecule AZD2281 (olaparib) enhances its potency and stability via a fluorine atom where another potent, small molecule rucaparib (AGO14699) suppresses phosphorylated signal transducer and transcription 3 (STAT 3) activation and helps in sensitizing tumor cells [22, 23]. Veliparib (ABT-888), a small potent oral PARP 1/2 inhibitor, has demonstrated broad activity in sensitizing cancer cells to different anticancer treatments (radiation therapy and chemotherapy) [24]. Although ABT-888 has less activity in stabilizing PARP-DNA complex in preclinical models compared to olaparib and has shown modest tumor suppression as a single agent, ABT-888 was studied more in CNS malignancies due to higher CNS penetration capability [25, 26]. In contrast, talazoparib (BMN 673), another PARP inhibitor which was shown to trap more PARP-DNA complexes and be 100 times more potent in cytotoxicity assays compared to olaparib and rucaparib [27]. Similarly, niraparib (MK-4827), another potent oral small molecule PARP 1/2 inhibitor, also has stronger PARP trapping activity than olaparib and veliparib [28]. Currently, the approvals of PARP inhibitors are for the treatment of ovarian cancer, BRCA-mutant breast cancer, HRD-deficient prostate cancer and BRCA-mutant pancreatic cancer. Although EMBRACA study showed improvement in PFS and talazoparib got approved in BRCA-mutant breast cancer, the PFS benefit did not translate into OS benefit [12, 29]. Moreover, Golan and group presented the updated final results from the POLO trial, which led to the approval of olaparib in gBRCA-mutant metastatic pancreatic adenocarcinoma after the study demonstrated significant PFS benefit, at the ASCO gastrointestinal cancers meeting in 2021 and showed that study arm failed to confer statistically significantly better OS compared to control arm [30]. Single agent PARP inhibitors are overall well tolerated but have limited clinical activity in a few tumor types. Hence identifying an optimal combination regimen has become an important focus of ongoing investigations.

9.3 Combination of PARP with Cytotoxic Chemotherapeutic Agents

Cytotoxic chemotherapeutic agents, such as platinum-based compounds or alkylating agents, cause DNA damage in rapidly-proliferating cancer cells through formation of platinum-associated crosslinks or alkylated nucleobases [1]. Damage caused by chemotherapy is repaired by the following main processes; BER or NER for the subtle damage, such as damage at the DNA base pair SSBs, and HR and NHEJ for large-scale DSBs [4–6]. Hence targeting DNA repair pathways to improve efficacy of chemotherapeutic agents, concept of chemopotentiation, has been actively pursued in the clinic [1]. PARP-1 accounts for the majority (75%) of PARP activity and increased expression has been shown to confer resistance to chemotherapeutic agents in both in vitro and in vivo studies [1]. High PARP-1 expression has been shown to be associated with poor response to platinum therapy in lung cancer cell lines while low PARP activity conferred higher response to chemotherapy in pancreatic cancer cell lines [31, 32]. Preclinical studies have also demonstrated synergy between PARP inhibitors and chemotherapy, prompting multiple trials (Table 9.1).

9.4 Early Phase Combination Trials in Advanced Solid Tumors

Early phase studies were conducted utilizing different PARP inhibitors with various chemotherapies to evaluate safety, tolerability, and overall efficacy of the regimen (Table 9.1) [33–37]. A study led by National Cancer Institute first demonstrated the tolerability and promising activity of oral veliparib, a small molecule inhibitor of PARP, in combination with metronomic cyclophosphamide especially in BRCA-mutant tumors [38]. Of 35 patients, 7 achieved partial response (PR) while 6 had stable disease (SD) for at least 6 cycles. Grade 2 myelosuppression

Table 9.1 Selected published early phase clinical trials with PARP inhibitors and chemotherapy in different solid malignancies

First author/study name	Cancer types	Treatments rendered (PARPi and chemotherapy)	Study phase/ number of patients	ORR	PFS (months) and OS (months)	Toxicities/ DLT	References
Advanced solid tumors							
Kummar et al.	Refractory solid tumors and lymphomas	Veliparib + metronomic cyclophosphamide	Phase I 35	20%	NA	G2 myelosuppression (MC) 2 DLTs	[38]
LoRusso et al.	Advanced solid tumors	Veliparib + irinotecan	Phase I 35	19%	NA	Diarrhea (63%), fatigue (60%), nausea (60%), neutropenia (49%) and leukopenia (49%) 4 DLTs	[39]
Del Conte et al.	Advanced solid tumors	Olaparib + liposomal doxorubicin	Phase I 44 (28 OC, 13 BC)	33% (13 out of 14 had OC, and 11 gBRCAm)	NA	G ≥ 3 AEs (61%) SAEs (27%) 2 DLTs	[41]
Appleman et al.	Advanced solid tumors	Veliparib + carboplatin + paclitaxel	Phase I 73	40% (9/13 had BC, and 7/16 had LC)	NA	Neutropenia G3 (19%) and G4 (31%), and FN 7% 8 DLTs	[40]
Balmana et al.	Advanced breast, ovarian and other solid tumors	Olaparib + cisplatin	Phase I 54 (42 BC, 10 OC, 29 BRCAm)	41% (43% in BRCAm OC, 71% in BRCAm BC)	NA	Neutropenia G ≥ 3 (16.7%) Anemia G ≥ 3 (9.3%) Leucopenia G ≥ 3 (9.3%) 4 DLTs	[33]

(continued)

Table 9.1 (continued)

First author/study name	Cancer types	Treatments rendered (PARPi and chemotherapy)	Study phase/ number of patients	ORR	PFS (months) and OS (months)	Toxicities/ DLT	References
Khan et al.	Advanced solid tumors	Olaparib + dacarbazine	Phase I 40 (33 melanoma)	5% (2 PR—melanoma)	NA	$G \geq 3$ AEs (72.5%) Neutropenia $G \geq 3$ (22.5%) Lymphopenia $G \geq 3$ (15%) Leukopenia $G \geq 3$ (12.5%) 3 DLTs	[44]
Wilson et al.	Advanced solid tumors	IV Rucaparib + carboplatin (A) IV Rucaparib + carboplatin/ paclitaxel (B) IV Rucaparib + cisplatin/ pemetrexed (C) IV Rucaparib + eribulin/ cyclophosphamide (D) Oral rucaparib + carboplatin (A-Oral)	Phase I 85 (22 BC, 15 O/PC, and others)	11.8% (1 CR, 9 PR)	NA	$G \geq 3$ AEs (75.3%) Neutropenia $G \geq 3$ (27.1%) Thrombocytopenia $G \geq 3$ (18.8%) Fatigue $G \geq 3$ (12.9%) Anemia $G \geq 3$ (11.8%) 3 DLTs in A-Oral	[45]

(continued)

Table 9.1 (continued)

First author/study name	Cancer types	Treatments rendered (PARPi and chemotherapy)	Study phase/ number of patients	ORR	PFS (months) and OS (months)	Toxicities/ DLT	References
Gynecological malignancies							
Kummar et al.	HGSOC, primary peritoneal, or fallopian tube cancers, or BRCAm OC	Cyclophosphamide alone (C) Versus Veliparib + cyclophosphamide combination (V + C combo)	Phase II C (38) Versus V + C combo (37)	C (19.4%) V + C combo (11.8%)	PFS C (2.3 mo) V + C combo (2.1 mo)	Leucopenia G2/3; C (6/0) versus V + C combo (10/2) Lymphopenia G2/3; C (13/3) versus V + C combo (11/13) 1 each with G4 lymphopenia and thrombocytopenia in combo	[34]
Gray et al.	Advanced OC and other solid malignancies	Veliparib + carboplatin + gemcitabine	Phase I 75 (54 OC, 12 BC)	49.2% (CR 15.3%) BRCA + OC (69%, CR 24.1%) BRCA w/uk (42.9%, CR 7.1%)	PFS—7 mo BRCA + OC (8.6 mo) versus BRCA w/uk (5.9 mo)	Thrombocytopenia G3/4 (53%) Neutropenia G3/4 (56%) 6 DLTs	[51]
Thaker et al. (NRG Oncology Study)	Recurrent cervical cancer	Veliparib + cisplatin + paclitaxel	Phase I 34	34% (CR 7%)	PFS—6.2 mo OS—14.5 mo	Neutropenia G3/4 (65%) Anemia G3/4 (34%) 1 DLT	[55]

(continued)

Table 9.1 (continued)

First author/study name	Cancer types	Treatments rendered (PARPi and chemotherapy)	Study phase/ number of patients	ORR	PFS (months) and OS (months)	Toxicities/ DLT	References
Lee et al.	BRCAm breast or ovarian cancer	Olaparib + carboplatin	Phase I/Ib 45 (37 OC/8 BC)	52.4% (1 CR/6 PR—BC)	NA	Neutropenia G3/4 (42.2%) Thrombocytopenia G3/4 (20%) Anemia G3/4 (15.6%)	[35]
Perez-Fidalgo et al. (ROLANDO study)	Platinum-resistant OC regardless of BRCA status	Olaparib + pegylated liposomal doxorubicin	GEICO Phase II 31	29%	PFS—5.8 mo (BRCAm– 6.5 mo) OS—14.5 mo (BRCAm– 21.3 mo)	Grade $\geq$ 3 TRAE (74%) Neutropenia G $\geq$ 3 (48%) 3 FN Anemia G $\geq$ 3 (23%)	[52]
Oza et al.	Platinum-sensitive, recurrent, HGSOC	Olaparib + carboplatin + paclitaxel Versus Carboplatin + paclitaxel	Phase II 81 versus 81	64% (CR 10%) 58% (CR 7%)	PFS—12.2 mo versus 9.6 mo (HR 0.51; p = 0.0012) BRCAm—HR 0.21; p = 0.0015) OS—33.8 mo versus 37.6 mo (HR 1.17; p = 0.44) BRCAm—HR 1.28; p = 0.69)	Any TRAE (100% vs 97%) Grade $\geq$ 3 TRAE (65% vs 57%) Neutropenia Grade $\geq$ 3 (43% vs 35%) Anemia Grade $\geq$ 3 (9% vs 7%) SAEs (15% vs 21%)	[53]

(continued)

Table 9.1 (continued)

First author/study name	Cancer types	Treatments rendered (PARPi and chemotherapy)	Study phase/ number of patients	ORR	PFS (months) and OS (months)	Toxicities/ DLT	References
Breast cancer							
Kummar et al.	Recurrent advanced TNBC	Cyclophosphamide alone (C) Versus Veliparib + cyclophosphamide combination (V + C combo)	Phase II 45 (18 vs 21)	C (1 PR) V + C combo (2 PR)	PFS C (1.9 mo) V + C combo (2.1 mo)	Lymphopenia G2/3; C (2/18) versus V + C combo (7/21) Leucopenia G2/3 (0 vs 4) G4 lymphopenia in combo (0 vs 2)	[36]
Dent et al.	Metastatic TNBC	Olaparib + paclitaxel	Phase I 19 (10—cohort 2- GCSF)	37%	PFS 6.3 mo -cohort 1, 5.2 mo -cohort 2	G ≥ 3 AEs (68%) Neutropenia G ≥ 3 (44% in cohort 1, 20% in cohort 2)	[47]
Rodler et al.	Advanced TNBC and/or BRCAm BC	Veliparib + cisplatin + vinorelbine	Phase I 50 (gBRCAm 28)	35% (2 CR)	PFS—5.5 mo 6 mo PFS on gBRCAm—71% versus 30% (p = 0.01)	Neutropenia G3/4 (36%, 3 FN) Anemia G3/4 (30%) Thrombocytopenia G3/4 (12%) 1 DLT	[46]

(continued)

Table 9.1 (continued)

First author/study name	Cancer types	Treatments rendered (PARPi and chemotherapy)	Study phase/ number of patients	ORR	PFS (months) and OS (months)	Toxicities/ DLT	References
Xu et al.	Metastatic BC with and without BRCA1/2 mutations	Veliparib + temozolomide	Phase II 62 (BRCAm 48%)	12% (1 CR) BRCAm (7/30, 23%)	PFS—2.1 mo BRCAm – 3.3 mo versus 1.8 mo (HR 0.48; $p = 0.006$)	Thrombocytopenia G3/4 (50%) Neutropenia G3/4 (27%) Anemia G3/4 (8%) 3 FN	[37]
Han et al. (BROCADE)	gBRCAm locally recurrent or metastatic BC	Veliparib + carboplatin + paclitaxel (VCP) Versus Veliparib + temozolomide (VT) Versus Carboplatin + paclitaxel (CP)	Phase II 97 versus 94 versus 99	VCP versus CP—78% versus 61.3% ($p = 0.027$) VT (28.6%)	PFS (VCP vs CP)—14.1 mo versus 12.3 mo (HR 0.789, $p = 0.227$) OS (VCP vs CP)—28.3 mo vs 25.9 mo (HR 0.75, $p = 0.156$) VT (PFS 7.4 mo, OS 19.1 mo)	Neutropenia G3/4 (55.9% vs 36.6% vs 55.2%) Thrombocytopenia G3/4 (31.2% vs 48.4% vs 26%) Anemia G3/4 (17.2% vs 7.5% vs 17.7%) FN G3/4 (8.6% vs 1.1% vs 3.1%)	[49]

(continued)

Table 9.1 (continued)

First author/study name	Cancer types	Treatments rendered (PARPi and chemotherapy)	Study phase/ number of patients	ORR	PFS (months) and OS (months)	Toxicities/ DLT	References
Lung cancer							
Ramalingam et al.	Advanced metastatic NSCLC	Veliparib + carboplatin + paclitaxel Versus Carboplatin + paclitaxel	Phase II 105 versus 53	32.4% versus 32.1%	PFS—5.8 mo versus 4.2 mo (HR 0.72, p = 0.17) OS—11.7 mo versus 9.1 mo (HR 0.80, p = 0.27)	Grade ≥ 3 TRAE (69% vs 58%) Neutropenia G ≥ 3 (19% vs 23%) Anemia G ≥ 3 (10% vs 10%) Thrombocytopenia G ≥ 3 (5% vs 6%) SAEs (27% vs 23%)	[57]
Owonikoko et al. (ECOG-ACRIN 2511)	First-line ES-SCLC	Veliparib + cisplatin + etoposide Versus Cisplatin + etoposide + placebo	Phase II 64 versus 64	71.9% versus 65.6%	PFS—6.1 mo versus 5.5 mo OS—10.3 mo versus 8.9 mo	Lymphopenia G3 (8% vs 0%) Neutropenia G3/4 (49% vs 32%) 1 G5 FN in placebo	[61]
Byer et al.	First-line (Treatment-naïve) ES-SCLC	Veliparib + carboplatin + etoposide (EP) - > veliparib Versus Veliparib + EP - > placebo Versus Placebo + EP - > placebo	Phase II 61 versus 59 versus 61	77% versus 59.3% versus 63.9%	PFS—5.8 mo versus 5.7 mo versus 5.6 mo OS—10.1 mo versus 10.0 mo versus 12.4 mo	G3/4 AEs (82% vs 88% vs 68%) SAEs (55% vs 67% vs 45%)	[62]

(continued)

Table 9.1 (continued)

First author/study name	Cancer types	Treatments rendered (PARPi and chemotherapy)	Study phase/ number of patients	ORR	PFS (months) and OS (months)	Toxicities/ DLT	References
Pietanza et al.	Relapsed-sensitive or refractory ES-SCLC	Veliparib + temozolomide Versus Temozolomide + placebo	Phase II 55 versus 49	39% versus 14%	PFS—3.8 mo versus 2.0 mo OS—8.2 mo versus 7.0 mo	Thrombocytopenia G3/4 (50% vs 9%) Neutropenia G3/4 (31% vs 7%) FN (4% vs 0%)	[59]
Farago et al.	Relapsed ES-SCLC	Olaparib + temozolomide	Phase I/II 50	41.7%	PFS—4.2 mo OS—8.5 mo	Thrombocytopenia (68%), anemia (68%), neutropenia (54%) No DLT	[58]
Gastrointestinal malignancies including pancreatic cancer							
Pishvaian et al.	Metastatic pancreatic cancer	Veliparib + 5-Fluorouracil + Oxaliplatin	Phase I/II 64	26% (4 CR)	PFS—4.0 mo OS—7.8 mo	Neutropenia G3/4 (16%) Leukopenia G3/4 (5%) Nausea G3/4 (6%) Vomiting G3/4 (6%) 1 DLT	[65]
Chiorean et al. (SWOG S1513)	Metastatic pancreatic cancer	Veliparib + modified FOLFIRI Versus FOLFIRI	Phase II 59 versus 58	11% versus 10%	PFS—2.1 mo versus 2.9 mo OS—5.4 mo versus 6.5 mo	G3/4 AE (69% vs 58%) Neutropenia G3/4 (34% vs 22%)	[66]

(continued)

Table 9.1 (continued)

First author/study name	Cancer types	Treatments rendered (PARPi and chemotherapy)	Study phase/ number of patients	ORR	PFS (months) and OS (months)	Toxicities/ DLT	References
O'Reilly et al.	gBRCA/PALB2 mutant PDAC	Veliparib + cisplatin + gemcitabine Versus Cisplatin + gemcitabine	Phase II 27 versus 23	74% versus 65.2%	PFS—10.1 mo versus 9.7 mo OS—15.5 mo versus 16.4 mo	Anemia G3/4 (52% vs 35%) Neutropenia G3/4 (48% vs 30%) Thrombocytopenia G3/4 (55% vs 9%) FN G3/4 (4% vs 0%)	[64]
Gorbunova et al.	Metastatic colorectal cancer	Veliparib + FOLFIRI (± bevacizumab) Versus FOLFIRI (± bevacizumab)	Phase II 65 versus 65	57% versus 62%	PFS—12 mo versus 11 mo OS—25 mo versus 27 mo	Neutropenia G3/4 (59% vs 22%) Diarrhea G3/4 (17% vs 12%) Asthenia G3/4 (9% vs 3%) FN (5% vs 0%)	[63]
Bang et al.	Recurrent or metastatic gastric cancer	Olaparib + paclitaxel Versus Paclitaxel	Phase II 61 versus 62	26.4% versus 19.1%	PFS—3.91 mo versus 3.55 mo (HR 0.80, p = 0.131) OS—13.1 mo versus 8.3 mo (HR 0.56, p = 0.005)	Neutropenia G ≥ 3 (56% vs 39%) Anemia G ≥ 3 (11% vs 11%) Asthenia G ≥ 3 (3% vs 10%) SAE (27.9% vs 37.1%)	[67]

(continued)

Table 9.1 (continued)

First author/study name	Cancer types	Treatments rendered (PARPi and chemotherapy)	Study phase/ number of patients	ORR	PFS (months) and OS (months)	Toxicities/ DLT	References
Other cancers							
Sim et al. (VERTU study)	Unmethylated MGMT glioblastoma	Veliparib + radiation f/b veliparib + temozolomide Versus Temozoloide + radiation f/b temozolomide	Phase II 84 versus 41	NA	6-mo PFS—46% versus 31% (PFS—5.7 mo versus 4.2 mo) OS—12.7 mo versus 12.8 mo	Thrombocytopenia G3/4 (17% vs 8%) Neutropenia G3/4 (12% vs 3%) Seizures G3/4 (11% vs 5%) Fatigue G3/4 (7% vs 5%)	[76]
Jelinek et al. (Alliance A091101)	Locoregionally advanced head and neck squamous cell carcinoma	Veliparib + induction carboplatin/ paclitaxel	Phase I 18	55.6%	24-month PFS—66.7% 24-month OS—77.8%	Neutropenia G3/4 (33%) Thrombocytopenia G3/4 (33%) Anemia G3/4 (11%) Leucopenia G3/4 (11%) 1 DLT	[72]
Middleton et al.	Metastatic melanoma	Veliparib + temozolomide	Phase II 116/115 versus 115	10.3% and 8.7% 7%	PFS—3.7/3.6 mo versus 2.0 mo OS—10.8/13.6 mo versus 12.9 mo	Thrombocytopenia G3/4 (20%/28% vs 15%) Neutropenia G3/4 (16%/17% vs 5%) Fatigue G3/4 (7%/ 5% vs 5%) Anemia G3/4 (6%/ 4% vs 3%)	[71]

(continued)

Table 9.1 (continued)

First author/study name	Cancer types	Treatments rendered (PARPi and chemotherapy)	Study phase/ number of patients	ORR	PFS (months) and OS (months)	Toxicities/ DLT	References
Grignani et al. (TOMAS)	Advanced and non-resectable bone and soft tissue sarcomas	Olaparib + trabectedin	Phase Ib 54	14%	6-mo PFS—33% (PFS—8 mo in high PARP1 vs 2 mo in low PARP1) OS—11 mo	Lymphopenia G3/4 (64%) Neutropenia G3/4 (62%) Thrombocytopenia G3/4 (28%) Anemia G3/4 (28%) 3 DLTs	[70]
Tumors in Pediatric and Adolescents							
Schafer et al. (A COG Phase 1 Consortium study/ ADVL1411)	Refractory/ recurrent solid tumors including Ewing sarcoma	Talazoparib + temozolomide	Phase I/II 40 (15 Ewing Sarcoma)	1 PR (malignant glioma)	NA	Neutropenia $G \geq 3$ (26%) Lymphopenia $G \geq 3$ (14%) Thrombocytopenia $G \geq 3$ (13%) Anemia $G \geq 3$ (12%) 5 DLTs	[74]
Chugh, R. et al (SARC025)	Advanced Ewing sarcoma	Niraparib + temozolomide (Arm 1) Niraparib + irinotecan (Arm 2)	Phase I 17/12	8.3% (Arm 2)	PFS—9 weeks/ 16.3 weeks	Neutropenia $G \geq 3$ (18%/ 17%) Thrombocytopenia $G \geq 3$ (35%/8%) Leucopenia $G \geq 3$ (18%/ 8%) 5 DLTs/3 DLTs	[69]

(continued)

Table 9.1 (continued)

First author/study name	Cancer types	Treatments rendered (PARPi and chemotherapy)	Study phase/ number of patients	ORR	PFS (months) and OS (months)	Toxicities/ DLT	References
Federico et al	Recurrent/ refractory solid malignancies	Talazoparib + irinotecan (+ temozolomide in Arm B)	Phase I 41 (53% ES) Arm A—29 Arm B—12	1 CR, 5 PR (5 ES) 10.3% (Arm A) 25% (Arm B)	NA	Neutropenia $G \geq 3$ (78%/ 31%) Thrombocytopenia $G \geq 3$ (42%/31%) FN $G \geq 3$ (24%/ 14) Diarrhea $G \geq 3$ (21%/ 7%)	[73]
Baxter et al. (A Pediatric Brain Tumor Consortium study)	Newly diagnosed diffuse pontine glioma	Veliparib + radiation (RT) f/b veliparib + temozolomide maintenance	Phase I/II 65	14%	NA	Lymphopenia $G \geq 3$ (32.8%/ 50%) Neutropenia $G \geq 3$ (4.7%/32.7%) Leucopenia $G \geq 3$ (3.1%/30.8%) Thrombocytopenia $G \geq 3$ (1.6%/ 23.1%) 4 DLTs during RT + veliparib	[75]

Abbreviations: PARPi, poly (ADP-ribose) polymerase (PARP) inhibitors; ORR, objective response rate; CR, complete response; PR, partial response; PFS, progression-free survival; OS, overall survival; mo, months; HR, hazard ratio; DLT, dose-limiting toxicities; NA, not available; G2, grade 2; G4, grade 4; G3/ 4, grade 3/4; $G \geq 3$, grade 3 and above; OC, ovarian cancer; BC, breast cancer; O/PC, ovarian/ peritoneal cancers; gBRCAm, germline BReast CAncer genes (BRCA) mutation; SAEs, serious adverse events; FN, febrile neutropenia; LC, lung cancer; HGSOC, high grade serous ovarian cancer; BRCA + , BRCA mutation positive; BRCA w/uk, without BRCA mutation or BRCA mutation status unknown; IV, intravenous; TRAE, treatment-related adverse events; vs, versus; TNBC, triple-negative breast cancer; NSCLC, non-small cell lung cancer; ES-SCLC, extensive stage small cell lung cancer; ES, Ewing sarcoma; f/b, followed by; COG, children oncology group; FOLFIRI, irinotecan with fluorouracil and folinic acid; PDAC, pancreatic ductal adenocarcinoma was the most common adverse event reported. Veliparib was also studied in combination with irinotecan in advanced solid tumors in a phase 1 safety study [39]. Grade 3 febrile neutropenia, grade 4 neutropenia, grade 3 diarrhea and grade 3 fatigue were the four observed dose limiting toxicities (DLTs). The most prevalent adverse events were diarrhea, fatigue, nausea, neutropenia and leukopenia. Six out of 31 evaluable patients had PR, conferring objective response rate (ORR) of 19%. Appleman et al. [40] reported results of a phase 1 study employing veliparib with carboplatin and paclitaxel, one of the most commonly used chemotherapy regimens. Of 67 evaluable patients, 5 obtained complete response (CR), 22 had PR while 32 achieved SD, resulting in an ORR of 40%, with 9 of 13 breast cancer, and 7 of 16 lung cancer patients deriving clinical benefit. Neutropenia and febrile neutropenia were the most common DLTs observed.

In a study from Italian and Switzerland groups, Del Conte and colleagues studied oral olaparib with liposomal doxorubicin in 44 patients with advanced solid malignancies [41]. Sixty-one percent had grade 3 and above toxicities whereas 27% had serious adverse events. ORR was 33% and noteworthily, 13 of 14 responders were patients with ovarian cancer while 11 patients had gBRCA mutation. Olaparib was also studied in combination with carboplatin and/or paclitaxel in a phase 1 study: continuous and intermittent schedules [42, 43]. Bone marrow suppression was frequent in continuous schedules, and hence finding the optimal dosing regimen was onerous. In intermittent schedule (n = 132), ORR was 46% while 47% experienced neutropenia of any grade (39% experienced grade ≥ 3) and 39% had thrombocytopenia of any grade (13% experienced grade ≥ 3). Bone marrow toxicities frequently led to dose modifications despite using intermittent schedule. In another phase 1 study, olaparib and dacarbazine was studied in patients with advanced solid tumors where majority of patients had melanoma (82.5%) [44]. Of 40, two patients with melanoma (5%) achieved PR. As there was no response in melanoma patients who were chemo naïve, the study concluded that there was no added clinical advantage from the addition of PARP inhibitor compared to dacarbazine alone in this patient population.

Wilson and colleagues studied different chemotherapy combinations using intravenous and oral rucaparib in 85 patients with advanced solid tumors [45]. In the remaining arm with oral rucaparib after the intravenous arms were discontinued, 3 DLTs (grade 4 neutropenia and grade 4 thrombocytopenia) were observed while 75.3% had high grade adverse events. Grade 3 and above neutropenia, thrombocytopenia, fatigue and anemia, the most prevalent high grade adverse events, were 27.1%%, 18.8%, 12.9% and 11.8%, respectively.

9.5 Breast Cancer

Early phase study of veliparib in combination with cisplatin plus vinorelbine was conducted in patients with triple-negative and BRCAm-associated advanced breast cancers [46]. Thirty-five percent achieved ORR and median progression-free survival (PFS) was 5.5 months in the overall population. Detailed analysis revealed that patients with gBRCA mutation had higher median PFS and overall survival (OS); 9.2/22.6 months versus 4.2/8.7 months in gBRCA wild type. Fatigue and nausea were the most common adverse events whereas hematological toxicities were the most prevalent grade 3 and 4 (G3/4) adverse events. Another phase 1 study evaluated olaparib plus paclitaxel in 2 cohorts of patients with TNBC where cohort 2 was allowed to receive growth factor support [47]. Although 68% had grade 3 and above adverse events where the commonest high grade adverse event was neutropenia, 20% of patients in cohort 2 experienced high-grade neutropenia compared to 44% in cohort 1. Notably, 37% achieved partial responses.

Results of the combination of PARP inhibitor with chemotherapy were reported for the randomized BROCADE and BROCADE3 studies in patients with BRCA-mutated advanced breast cancer [48, 49]. In phase 2 BROCADE trial, 290 patients were randomized into 3 arms; Veliparib with temozolomide (VT) or carboplatin plus paclitaxel (VCP) versus placebo with carboplatin plus paclitaxel (CP). ORR were 61.3% in CP, 77.8% in VCP, and 28.6% in VT while median PFS and OS reported were 12.3/25.9 months in CP arm, 14.1/28.3 months in VCP arm, and 7.4/19.1 months in VT arm. Despite notable increase in ORR and numerical increasein survival from the addition of veliparib to carboplatin and paclitaxel without additional notable toxicities, there was no statistically significant difference in PFS and OS in patients receiving VCP versus CP, and VT was shown to be inferior to PCP. Given this intriguing result, VCP and CP was further studied in patients with HER2-negative gBRCA-mutated advanced breast cancer in the BROCADE3 trial. One difference between the two studies was that veliparib was continued as monotherapy if the chemotherapy was discontinued before progression in BRO-CADE3 trial. Although ORR was similar 75.8% versus 74.1%, median PFS was statistically significant at 14.5 months in VCP arm compared to 12.6 months in CP (HR 0.71, p = 0.0016). The study demonstrated that the addition of veliparib to carboplatin and paclitaxel was feasible and well tolerated with no additional discernable safety concerns and treatment discontinuation due to treatment-related adverse events was modest at less than 10%.

In the neoadjuvant setting, phase 3 BrighTNess trial was conducted utilizing veliparib plus carboplatin or carboplatin alone to standard neoadjuvant chemotherapy (VCP vs CP vs paclitaxel) in clinical stage II-III triple-negative breast cancer (Table 9.2) [50]. The reported rates of breast-conservation surgery after neoadjuvant chemotherapy were 62%, 44%, and 44% while pathological CR (pCR) was reported in 53%, 58%, and 31% respectively. Although VCP and CP increased the proportion of patients achieving pCR compared to paclitaxel arm, the addition of veliparib to CP failed to characterize extra benefit while similar safety profile with no increased toxicities were noted among VCP and CP arms.

Table 9.2 Randomized phase 3 clinical trials utilizing the combination PARP inhibitors and chemotherapy

First author/ study name	Study type/phase	Line of treatment	Number of Patients		Treatments Rendered		Median PFS and OS			Grade ≥ 3 toxicities	
			Combination	Control	Combination	Control	Combination	Control	Hazard ratio (HR) and p value	Combination	Control
Dieras et al. (BROCADE3)	Randomised, double- blind, placebo controlled	gBRCAm advanced HER2-negative BC	336	171	Veliparib + carboplatin + paclitaxel	Carboplatin + paclitaxel	14.5 mo 33.5 mo	12.6 mo 28.2 mo	HR 0.71; p = 0.0016 HR 0.95; p = 0.67	Neutropenia 81% Thrombocytopenia 40% Anemia 42%	Neutropenia 84% Thrombocytopenia 28% Anemia 40%
Ramalingam. et al.	Randomised, double- blind	Advanced metastatic squamous NSCLC	486	484	Veliparib + carboplatin + paclitaxel	Carboplatin + paclitaxel	5.6 mo 11.9 mo* 12.2 mo	5.6 mo 11.1 mo* 11.2 mo	HR 0.897; p = 0.107 HR 0.905; p = 0.266* HR 0.853; p = 0.032	Neutropenia 24% Thrombocytopenia 6% Anemia 10%	Neutropenia 20% Thrombocytopenia 7% Anemia 11%

(continued)

Table 9.2 (continued)

First author/ study name	Study type/phase	Line of treatment	Number of Patients		Treatments Rendered		Median PFS and OS			Grade ≥ 3 toxicities	
			Combination	Control	Combination	Control	Combination	Control	Hazard ratio (HR) and p value	Combination	Control
Bang et al. (GOLD)	Double-blind, randomised, placebo-controlled	Advanced gastric cancer	263	262	Olaparib + paclitaxel	Paclitaxel	3.7 mo 8.8 mo	3.2 mo 6.9 mo	HR 0.84; p = 0.065 HR 0.79; p = 0.026*	Neutropenia 30% Leucopenia 16% Anemia 14% FN 3%	Neutropenia 23% Leucopenia 11% Anemia 8% FN 2%
Loibl et al. (BrighTNess)	Randomised, double- blind, placebo controlled, multicenter, international	Stage II-III TNBC	313	158 157	Veliparib + carboplatin + paclitaxel (VCP)	Carboplatin + paclitaxel (CP) Paclitaxel (P)	Pathological complete response VCP versus P – 53% versus 31% (p < 0.0001) VCP versus CP – 53% versus 58% (p = 0.36)			Neutropenia 57% Anemia 25% Thrombocytopenia 11% FN 2%	Neutropenia 53% (CP), 3% (P) Anemia 17% (CP), 0% (P) Thrombocytopenia 6% (CP), 0% (P) FN 1% versus 0%

* Denotes no statistically significant difference

Abbreviations: PARPi, poly (ADP-ribose) polymerase (PARP) inhibitors; ORR, objective response rate; CR, complete response; PR, partial response; PFS, progression-free survival; OS, overall survival; mo, months; HR, hazard ratio; DLT, dose-limiting toxicities; NA, not available; G2, grade 2; G4, grade 4; G3/4, grade 3/4; G ≥ 3, grade 3 and above; OC, ovarian cancer; BC, breast cancer; gBRCAm, germline BReast CAncer genes (BRCA) mutation; SAEs, serious adverse events; FN, febrile neutropenia; LC, lung cancer; HGSOC, high grade serous ovarian cancer; BRCA + , BRCA mutation positive; BRCA w/uk, without BRCA mutation or BRCA mutation status unknown; TRAE, treatment-related adverse events; vs, versus; TNBC, triple-negative breast cancer; NSCLC, non-small cell lung cancer; ES-SCLC, extensive stage small cell lung cancer; ES, Ewing sarcoma; f/b, followed by; COG, children oncology group; FOLFIRI, irinotecan with fluorouracil and folinic acid; PDAC, pancreatic ductal adenocarcinoma

9.6   Gynecological Malignancies

Gray et al. [51] studied veliparib in combination with carboplatin and gemcitabine in 75 patients with advanced solid tumors, with majority of patients with ovarian and breast cancer (88%). Although 89% had any grade 3/4 adverse event while neutropenia and thrombocytopenia were the two DLTs observed, 69% of patients with BRCA-deficient ovarian cancer achieved ORR with a quarter achieving CR. Recently, ROLANDO study evaluated the efficacy of olaparib in combination with liposomal doxorubicin in 31 patients with platinum-resistant ovarian cancer with or without BRCA mutation (84% were BRCA wild-type), where 29% achieved PR and 48% had SD [52].

Olaparib in combination with chemotherapy, followed by maintenance monotherapy was compared to standard chemotherapy in patients with recurrent high-grade serous ovarian cancer who were platinum sensitive [53]. In the overall population, median PFS was statistically significant at 12.2 months in the experimental group versus 9.6 months in control group (HR 0.51, p = 0.0012). The difference in PFS was more pronounced in the patient subset carrying BRCA mutation (HR 0.21, p = 0.0015). Sixty-five percent experienced $\geq$ G3 adverse events in the combination group compared to 57% $\geq$ G3 adverse events in the control group, majority of these were hematological adverse events.

Coleman and colleagues subsequently reported the phase III VELIA study which randomized veliparib with first-line induction chemotherapy with carboplatin and paclitaxel and as single agent maintenance therapy compared to first-line chemotherapy in previously untreated high-grade serous ovarian cancer (Table 9.2) [54]. 1140 patients with previously untreated high-grade serous ovarian cancer were randomized, 26% harbored BRCA-mutation and 55% of tumors were HR deficient (HRD). HRD status was defined by patients who had tumors that were *BRCA*-mutated or had HRD according to the myChoice assay (score $\geq$ 33). Median PFS was statistically significant at 34.7 months in the veliparib-throughout arm compared to 22.0 months in the control arm (HR 0.44, P < 0.001), of the patients included in the BRCA-mutation group. In the HRD group, median PFS was 31.9 months versus 20.5 months, respectively (HR 0.57, P < 0.001). Fatigue, nausea, neutropenia and anemia were the most reported adverse events while hematological toxicities were the most prevalent G 3/4 adverse events in patients receiving veliparib in addition to chemotherapy.

The combination of veliparib with cisplatin and paclitaxel was shown safe and feasible in a phase 1 NRG Oncology study which enrolled 34 patients with recurrent cervical cancer [55]. ORR was reported at 34% and DLTs observed were grade 4 dyspnea, grade 3 neutropenia lasting $\geq$ 3 weeks, and febrile neutropenia.

9.7   Lung Cancers

In patients with metastatic non-small cell lung cancer (NSCLC), a randomized phase 2 study was conducted to determine the survival benefit of the addition of veliparib to standard carboplatin and paclitaxel [56]. Although there was a favorable trend in survival for patient with squamous histology, there was no statistical significance observed in median PFS (5.8 months versus 4.2 months, respectively; p = 0.17) and median OS (11.7 months versus 9.1 months, respectively; p = 0.27). No increased toxicities were observed, and high-grade hematological toxicities were comparable. Hence, Ramalingam and colleagues conducted the phase 3 study of carboplatin and paclitaxel with or without veliparib in patients with untreated metastatic squamous NSCLC [57]. However, the survival benefit was not confirmed in this phase 3 study from the addition of veliparib to conventional chemotherapy in patients with advanced squamous NSCLC who are current smokers.

In relapsed small cell lung cancer (SCLC), an early phase I/II study utilizing olaparib and temozolomide was performed [58]. Although increased hematological toxicities were observed with higher dose levels none met DLT criteria, and the recommended phase 2 dose was established at temozolomide 75 mg/m2 daily and olaparib 200 mg twice daily, both days 1 to 7 of a 21-day cycle. ORR was notable at 41.7% and median PFS and OS were 4.2 months and 8.5 months, respectively. Pietanza and colleagues reported the randomized phase 2 trial of temozolomide in combination with either veliparib or placebo in recurrent (relapsed-sensitive or refractory) SCLC [59]. The study did not meet the primary endpoint of improvement in 4-month PFS (36% vs 27%; p = 0.19) although there was significant increase in ORR (39% vs 14%; p = 0.016). However, statistically significant improvement in PFS (5.7 months vs 3.6 months; p = 0.009) and OS (12.2 months vs 7.5 months; p = 0.014) was noted in patients with SCLC harboring SLFN11 expression who had received temozolomide (TMZ) in combination with veliparib. SLFN11 regulates response to DNA damage and replication stress and hence, is a predictive marker of sensitivity to DNA-damaging chemotherapies [60]. TMZ by itself leads to cytotoxicity and apoptosis, but PARP-dependent base excision repair pathway is a known resistance mechanism for TMZ. Combination of these two agents has been shown to lead to greater tumor growth delay or regression. High grade hematological toxicities were observed more in the combination group compared to temozolomide alone.

ECOG-ACRIN 2511 study randomized either veliparib or placebo in combination with cisplatin and etoposide in patients with untreated extensive-stage small cell lung cancer [61]. Median PFS was 6.1 months versus 5.5 months (p = 0.06), and median OS was 10.3 months versus 8.9 months (p = 0.17) for the veliparib arm. ORR was 71.9% versus 65.6%, respectively. Grade 3 lymphopenia and grade 3/4 neutropenia were more common in the PARP containing regimen while other adverse events were comparable between the two groups. Recently, Byers and colleagues reported results of a randomized phase 2 study in treatment-naïve ES-SCLC where three arms were conducted; veliparib plus carboplatin and etoposide

(EP) followed by veliparib maintenance (veliparib throughout), veliparib plus EP followed by placebo (veliparib combination only), or EP (control) [62]. Improvement in PFS was observed in veliparib throughout group compared to control arm (HR, 0.67; 80% CI, 0.50–0.88; p = 0.059), yet this did not translate into an overall survival benefit as median OS was reported at 10.1 months in veliparib throughout group compared to 12.4 months in control arm (HR, 1.43; 80% CI, 1.09–1.88).

9.8 Gastrointestinal Malignancies

The addition of veliparib to first line FOLFIRI (with or without bevacizumab) in patients with metastatic colorectal cancer was evaluated in a phase 2 randomized study [63]. This study failed to demonstrate survival benefit, median PFS and OS were 12 months/25 months in veliparib group compared to 11 months/27 months in the control arm, respectively. Moreover, there was a significant increase in hematological adverse events observed in the veliparib containing regimen.

O'Reilly and group conducted a phase 2 randomized trial of the addition of veliparib to cisplatin and gemcitabine in patients with metastatic pancreatic cancer carrying gBRCA or PALB2 mutation, after a phase 1 trial demonstrated substantial antitumor activity in gBRCA-mutant metastatic pancreatic cancer [64]. ORR was 74.1% in the study arm versus 65.2% in control arm (p = 0.55). Median PFS and OS were 10.1 months/15.5 months in veliparib arm compared to 9.7 months/ 16.4 months in control group. Grade 3/4 hematological toxicities were doubled in the veliparib group compared to standard cisplatin plus gemcitabine arm. Pishvaian et al. [65] showed the safety and tolerability of veliparib in combination with 5-fluorouracil plus oxaliplatin (FOLFOX) in metastatic pancreatic cancer patients in a phase 1/2 study. The recommended phase 2 dose (RP2D) was veliparib 200 mg twice daily, days 1 to 7 of 14-day cycle. Although overall ORR was 26%, ORR was further heightened in HR-DDR mutated, platinum-naïve metastatic pancreatic cancer patients (57%). However, the randomized phase II SWOG S51513 study failed to demonstrate survival benefit of veliparib with modified FOLFIRI over FOLFIRI alone as second-line treatment of metastatic pancreatic cancer. In addition, grade 3/4 toxicities were more common in veliparib arm (69 vs 58%) [66].

A randomized phase 2 study was conducted to determine the efficacy of olaparib and paclitaxel in Asian patients with recurrent metastatic gastric cancer who had progressed following first-line therapy and had low levels of ATM [67]. Although there was no improvement in PFS, the addition of olaparib to paclitaxel demonstrated increment in OS in both the overall population (HR, 0.56; p = 0.005) as well as in metastatic gastric cancer patients with low or undetectable levels of ATM by immunohistochemistry (HR, 0.35; p = 0.002). Hence, the randomized phase 3 GOLD study was launched [68]. However, GOLD study failed to meet the primary endpoint of improvement in OS. In overall population, median OS was 8.8 months in olaparib/paclitaxel group versus 6.9 months in placebo arm. Median OS was 12 months versus 10 months, respectively, in ATM-negative population.

9.9   Other Cancers Including Cancers Affecting the Pediatric and Adolescent Population

Two arms in SARC025 trial evaluated the combination of niraparib with irinotecan or temozolomide in pretreated Ewing sarcoma [69]. Five of 29 patients had DLTs (hematological toxicities) in temozolomide arm and 3 patients in irinotecan arm experienced DLTs (gastrointestinal adverse events). One patient experiences a PR with ORR of 8.3% although two patients with SD remained on study for ~ 1.5 year. The phase 1b TOMAS trial from Italian sarcoma group also demonstrated the encouraging preliminary activity of olaparib in combination with trabectedin in 54 patients with advanced bone and soft tissue sarcomas [70]. While 14% attained PR, grade 3/4 hematological toxicities were frequently observed; 64, 62, 28 and 26% experienced grade 3/4 lymphopenia, neutropenia, thrombocytopenia and anemia, respectively.

In patients with unresectable stage III or IV metastatic melanoma, 346 patients were randomized to 3 groups (temozolomide plus veliparib 20 mg or 40 mg, or placebo) in a phase 2 study [71]. Median PFS/OS reported were similar among 3 arms: 3.7/10.8 months, 3.6/13.6 months, and 2/13.6 months, respectively. ORR was 10.3% versus 8.7% versuss 7.0%, and high-grade adverse events were 55%, 63%, and 41%, respectively. Hematological toxicities were the most commonly reported high-grade adverse events (42, 49 and 23%).

Recently, Alliance A091101 reported the early phase study of addition of veliparib to induction regimen (carboplatin and paclitaxel) in patients with locore-gionally advanced head and neck squamous cell carcinoma where ORR was 55.6%, 24-month OS was 77.8%, and 24-month PFS was 66.7% [72]. The study demonstrated the feasibility of the addition of veliparib to induction regimen while hematological toxicities were the most common G 3/4 adverse events.

A study led by St Jude Children's research hospital in 41 pediatric and young adults with refractory solid tumors (53% Ewing sarcoma) showed that talazoparib and irinotecan (± temozolomide) was feasible with hematological toxicities such as neutropenia and thrombocytopenia being the most reported G 3/4 adverse events [73]. In terms of efficacy, 10% obtained ORR from the doublet and 25% had ORR in the triplet group, where the correlation between SLFN11 positivity and effi-cacy was observed. Another phase 1 consortium study (ADVL1411) from COG demonstrated that talazoparib with low dose temozolomide was plausible with thrombocytopenia and neutropenia being the two DLT [74]. However modest activ-ity was reported while no to little efficacy was noted in Ewing sarcoma and CNS tumors. The feasibility of the combination of veliparib, temozolomide and radi-ation therapy was studied in a Pediatric Brain Tumor Consortium study [75]. However, the trial was stopped for futility following a planned interim analysis due to inability to show survival benefit despite the combination being clinically tolerable.

Recently, the VERTU study reported the results of randomized phase 2 study using veliparib and temozolomide plus radiation therapy (RT) versus standard of care concurrent temozolomide plus RT, in 125 patients with unmethylated O-6-methylguanine-DNA methyltransferase (MGMT) glioblastoma [76]. Although the addition of veliparib was well tolerated (similar grade 3/4 adverse events in both arms with 55%), and 6 months PFS in study group was higher at 46% compared to 31% in standard group, median OS was similar; 12.7 months in experimental arm versus 12.8 months in standard arm.

9.10   Challenges, Remaining Questions, and Future Directions

Although preclinical or early phase studies showed promise for the concept of chemopotentiation using the combination of PARP DNA repair pathway inhibitors and cytotoxic chemotherapeutic agents, the clinical value has been debatable with increased toxicities and marginal, if any, PFS/OS benefit despite higher response rates in some studies. The clinical experience to date underscores the need to pursue alternate, intermittent schedules to improve tolerability, and better defining patient selection to improve efficacy. Biomarkers beyond BRCA status, such as SLFN11, need to be studied, preclinically and in clinical trials, to identify patients likely to benefit. Development of more selective PARP1 targeting agents may lead to better tolerability. Initial single agent data was reported at AACR 2022 for AZ5305, a selective PARP1 inhibitor [77]. Further clinical evaluation is needed to establish whether selective targeting of PARP1 will result in better efficacy and ability to safely combine with chemotherapeutic agents.

PARP inhibitors are now widely available and approved in some tumor types, however optimal combination regimens with cytotoxic chemotherapies that have enhanced efficacy, while being well tolerated, are yet to be identified. Newer combination strategies for PARP inhibitors are focusing on immunotherapy or targeted agents such as the KEYLYNK or MEDIOLA studies. However, there remains a strong rationale to evaluate PARP inhibitors in combination with chemotherapy to broaden the population of patients who can derive benefit from this class of drugs. This will require carefully thought out trials with current and next generation PARP inhibitors that include patient selection based on novel biomarkers and evaluation of alternate schedules to optimize efficacy and tolerability.

Disclosures KZT No conflicts of interest.

RT No conflicts of interest.

SK Advisory board/consultant for Boehringer Ingelheim, Springworks Therapeutics, Gilead, EcoR1, Seagen, Mundibiopharma, Bayer, Genome & Company, Mirati, OxfordBiotherapeutics, and Harbour Biomed; co-founder and equity holder for PathomIQ, spouse is a scientific advisor for Cadila Pharmaceuticals ltd and founder of Arxeon Inc.

Acknowledgements None

Authorship Contributions All the authors have significantly contributed to the preparation of this manuscript and approved the final version.

References

1. Lu Y et al (2018) Double-barreled gun: combination of PARP inhibitor with conventional chemotherapy. Pharmacol Ther 188:168–175
2. Dias MP et al (2021) Understanding and overcoming resistance to PARP inhibitors in cancer therapy. Nat Rev Clin Oncol 18(12):773–791
3. Li H et al (2020) PARP inhibitor resistance: the underlying mechanisms and clinical implications. Mol Cancer 19(1):107
4. Howard SM, Yanez DA, Stark JM (2015) DNA damage response factors from diverse pathways, including DNA crosslink repair, mediate alternative end joining. PLoS Genet 11(1):e1004943
5. Cerrato A, Morra F, Celetti A (2016) Use of poly ADP-ribose polymerase [PARP] inhibitors in cancer cells bearing DDR defects: the rationale for their inclusion in the clinic. J Exp Clin Cancer Res 35(1):179
6. Satoh MS, Lindahl T (1992) Role of poly(ADP-ribose) formation in DNA repair. Nature 356(6367):356–358
7. Yap TA et al (2019) The DNA damaging revolution: PARP inhibitors and beyond. Am Soc Clin Oncol Educ Book 39:185–195
8. Nielsen FC, van Overeem Hansen T, Sørensen CS (2016) Hereditary breast and ovarian cancer: new genes in confined pathways. Nat Rev Cancer 16(9):599–612
9. (2011) Integrated genomic analyses of ovarian carcinoma. Nature 474(7353):609–15
10. Barkauskaite E, Jankevicius G, Ahel I (2015) Structures and mechanisms of enzymes employed in the synthesis and degradation of PARP-dependent protein ADP-ribosylation. Mol Cell 58(6):935–946
11. Lord CJ, Ashworth A (2017) PARP inhibitors: synthetic lethality in the clinic. Science 355(6330):1152–1158
12. Litton JK et al (2018) Talazoparib in patients with advanced breast cancer and a germline BRCA mutation. N Engl J Med 379(8):753–763
13. Moore K et al (2018) Maintenance olaparib in patients with newly diagnosed advanced ovarian cancer. N Engl J Med 379(26):2495–2505
14. Pujade-Lauraine E et al (2017) Olaparib tablets as maintenance therapy in patients with platinum-sensitive, relapsed ovarian cancer and a BRCA1/2 mutation (SOLO2/ENGOT-Ov21): a double-blind, randomised, placebo-controlled, phase 3 trial. Lancet Oncol 18(9):1274–1284
15. Penson RT et al (2020) Olaparib versus nonplatinum chemotherapy in patients with platinum-sensitive relapsed ovarian cancer and a germline BRCA1/2 Mutation (SOLO3): a randomized phase III trial. J Clin Oncol 38(11):1164–1174
16. Ray-Coquard I et al (2019) Olaparib plus bevacizumab as first-line maintenance in ovarian cancer. N Engl J Med 381(25):2416–2428
17. Golan T et al (2019) Maintenance olaparib for germline BRCA-mutated metastatic pancreatic cancer. N Engl J Med 381(4):317–327
18. Anscher MS et al (2021) FDA approval summary: rucaparib for the treatment of patients with deleterious BRCA-mutated metastatic castrate-resistant prostate cancer. Oncologist 26(2):139–146
19. Coleman RL et al (2017) Rucaparib maintenance treatment for recurrent ovarian carcinoma after response to platinum therapy (ARIEL3): a randomised, double-blind, placebo-controlled, phase 3 trial. Lancet 390(10106):1949–1961
20. González-Martín A et al (2019) Niraparib in patients with newly diagnosed advanced ovarian cancer. N Engl J Med 381(25):2391–2402

21. Mirza MR et al (2016) Niraparib maintenance therapy in platinum-sensitive, recurrent ovarian cancer. N Engl J Med 375(22):2154–2164
22. Farmer H et al (2005) Targeting the DNA repair defect in BRCA mutant cells as a therapeutic strategy. Nature 434(7035):917–921
23. Ekblad T et al (2013) PARP inhibitors: polypharmacology versus selective inhibition. Febs J 280(15):3563–3575
24. Donawho CK et al (2007) ABT-888, an orally active poly(ADP-ribose) polymerase inhibitor that potentiates DNA-damaging agents in preclinical tumor models. Clin Cancer Res 13(9):2728–2737
25. Wagner LM (2015) Profile of veliparib and its potential in the treatment of solid tumors. Onco Targets Ther 8:1931–1939
26. Su JM et al (2014) A phase I trial of veliparib (ABT-888) and temozolomide in children with recurrent CNS tumors: a pediatric brain tumor consortium report. Neuro Oncol 16(12):1661–1668
27. Murai J et al (2014) Stereospecific PARP trapping by BMN 673 and comparison with olaparib and rucaparib. Mol Cancer Ther 13(2):433–443
28. Murai J et al (2012) Trapping of PARP1 and PARP2 by clinical PARP inhibitors. Cancer Res 72(21):5588–5599
29. Litton JK et al (2020) Talazoparib versus chemotherapy in patients with germline BRCA1/2-mutated HER2-negative advanced breast cancer: final overall survival results from the EMBRACA trial. Ann Oncol 31(11):1526–1535
30. Golan T et al. (2021) Overall survival from the phase 3 POLO trial: Maintenance olaparib for germline BRCA-mutated metastatic pancreatic cancer. J Clinical Oncol 39(3_suppl):378–378
31. Michels J et al (2013) Cisplatin resistance associated with PARP hyperactivation. Cancer Res 73(7):2271–2280
32. Jacob DA et al (2007) Combination therapy of poly (ADP-ribose) polymerase inhibitor 3-aminobenzamide and gemcitabine shows strong antitumor activity in pancreatic cancer cells. J Gastroenterol Hepatol 22(5):738–748
33. Balmaña J et al (2014) Phase I trial of olaparib in combination with cisplatin for the treatment of patients with advanced breast, ovarian and other solid tumors. Ann Oncol 25(8):1656–1663
34. Kummar S et al (2015) Randomized trial of oral cyclophosphamide and Veliparib in high-grade serous ovarian, primary peritoneal, or fallopian tube cancers, or brca-mutant ovarian cancer. Clin Cancer Res 21(7):1574–1582
35. Lee JM et al. (2014) Phase I/Ib study of olaparib and carboplatin in BRCA1 or BRCA2 mutation-associated breast or ovarian cancer with biomarker analyses. J Natl Cancer Inst 106(6):dju089
36. Kummar S et al (2016) Randomized phase II trial of cyclophosphamide and the oral poly (ADP-ribose) polymerase inhibitor veliparib in patients with recurrent, advanced triple-negative breast cancer. Invest New Drugs 34(3):355–363
37. Xu J et al (2021) Phase II trial of veliparib and temozolomide in metastatic breast cancer patients with and without BRCA1/2 mutations. Breast Cancer Res Treat 189(3):641–651
38. Kummar S et al (2012) A phase I study of veliparib in combination with metronomic cyclophosphamide in adults with refractory solid tumors and lymphomas. Clin Cancer Res 18(6):1726–1734
39. LoRusso PM et al (2016) Phase I safety, pharmacokinetic, and pharmacodynamic study of the poly(ADP-ribose) polymerase (PARP) inhibitor Veliparib (ABT-888) in combination with irinotecan in patients with advanced solid tumors. Clin Cancer Res 22(13):3227–3237
40. Appleman LJ et al (2019) Phase 1 study of veliparib (ABT-888), a poly (ADP-ribose) polymerase inhibitor, with carboplatin and paclitaxel in advanced solid malignancies. Cancer Chemother Pharmacol 84(6):1289–1301
41. Del Conte G et al (2014) Phase I study of olaparib in combination with liposomal doxorubicin in patients with advanced solid tumours. Br J Cancer 111(4):651–659
42. van der Noll R et al (2020) Phase I study of continuous olaparib capsule dosing in combination with carboplatin and/or paclitaxel (Part 1). Invest New Drugs 38(4):1117–1128

43. van der Noll R et al (2020) Phase I study of intermittent olaparib capsule or tablet dosing in combination with carboplatin and paclitaxel (part 2). Invest New Drugs 38(4):1096–1107

44. Khan OA et al (2011) A phase I study of the safety and tolerability of olaparib (AZD2281, KU0059436) and dacarbazine in patients with advanced solid tumours. Br J Cancer 104(5):750–755

45. Wilson RH et al (2017) A phase I study of intravenous and oral rucaparib in combination with chemotherapy in patients with advanced solid tumours. Br J Cancer 116(7):884–892

46. Rodler ET et al (2016) Phase I study of Veliparib (ABT-888) combined with cisplatin and vinorelbine in advanced triple-negative breast cancer and/or BRCA mutation-associated breast cancer. Clin Cancer Res 22(12):2855–2864

47. Dent RA et al (2013) Phase I trial of the oral PARP inhibitor olaparib in combination with paclitaxel for first- or second-line treatment of patients with metastatic triple-negative breast cancer. Breast Cancer Res 15(5):R88

48. Diéras V et al (2020) Veliparib with carboplatin and paclitaxel in BRCA-mutated advanced breast cancer (BROCADE3): a randomised, double-blind, placebo-controlled, phase 3 trial. Lancet Oncol 21(10):1269–1282

49. Han HS et al (2018) Veliparib with temozolomide or carboplatin/paclitaxel versus placebo with carboplatin/paclitaxel in patients with BRCA1/2 locally recurrent/metastatic breast cancer: randomized phase II study. Ann Oncol 29(1):154–161

50. Loibl S et al (2018) Addition of the PARP inhibitor veliparib plus carboplatin or carboplatin alone to standard neoadjuvant chemotherapy in triple-negative breast cancer (BrighTNess): a randomised, phase 3 trial. Lancet Oncol 19(4):497–509

51. Gray HJ et al (2018) Phase I combination study of the PARP inhibitor veliparib plus carboplatin and gemcitabine in patients with advanced ovarian cancer and other solid malignancies. Gynecol Oncol 148(3):507–514

52. Perez-Fidalgo JA et al (2021) Olaparib in combination with pegylated liposomal doxorubicin for platinum-resistant ovarian cancer regardless of BRCA status: a GEICO phase II trial (ROLANDO study). ESMO Open 6(4):100212

53. Oza AM et al (2015) Olaparib combined with chemotherapy for recurrent platinum-sensitive ovarian cancer: a randomised phase 2 trial. Lancet Oncol 16(1):87–97

54. Coleman RL et al (2019) Veliparib with first-line chemotherapy and as maintenance therapy in ovarian cancer. N Engl J Med 381(25):2403–2415

55. Thaker PH et al (2017) A phase I trial of paclitaxel, cisplatin, and veliparib in the treatment of persistent or recurrent carcinoma of the cervix: an NRG oncology study (NCT#01281852). Ann Oncol 28(3):505–511

56. Ramalingam SS et al (2017) Randomized, placebo-controlled, phase II study of Veliparib in combination with carboplatin and paclitaxel for advanced/metastatic non-small cell lung cancer. Clin Cancer Res 23(8):1937–1944

57. Ramalingam SS et al (2021) Veliparib in combination with platinum-based chemotherapy for first-line treatment of advanced squamous cell lung cancer: a randomized, multicenter phase III study. J Clin Oncol 39(32):3633–3644

58. Farago AF et al (2019) Combination olaparib and temozolomide in relapsed small-cell lung cancer. Cancer Discov 9(10):1372–1387

59. Pietanza MC et al (2018) Randomized, double-blind, phase II study of Temozolomide in combination with either veliparib or placebo in patients with relapsed-sensitive or refractory small-cell lung cancer. J Clin Oncol 36(23):2386–2394

60. Murai J et al (2019) Schlafen 11 (SLFN11), a restriction factor for replicative stress induced by DNA-targeting anti-cancer therapies. Pharmacol Ther 201:94–102

61. Owonikoko TK et al (2019) Randomized phase II trial of cisplatin and etoposide in combination with veliparib or placebo for extensive-stage small-cell lung cancer: ECOG-ACRIN 2511 study. J Clin Oncol 37(3):222–229

62. Byers LA et al (2021) Veliparib in combination with carboplatin and etoposide in patients with treatment-naïve extensive-stage small cell lung cancer: a phase 2 randomized study. Clin Cancer Res 27(14):3884–3895

63. Gorbunova V et al (2019) A phase 2 randomised study of veliparib plus FOLFIRI±bevacizumab versus placebo plus FOLFIRI±bevacizumab in metastatic colorectal cancer. Br J Cancer 120(2):183–189
64. O'Reilly EM et al (2020) Randomized, multicenter, phase II trial of gemcitabine and cisplatin with or without veliparib in patients with pancreas adenocarcinoma and a germline BRCA/PALB2 mutation. J Clin Oncol 38(13):1378–1388
65. Pishvaian MJ et al (2020) A phase I/II study of Veliparib (ABT-888) in combination with 5-Fluorouracil and oxaliplatin in patients with metastatic pancreatic cancer. Clin Cancer Res 26(19):5092–5101
66. Chiorean EG et al (2021) Randomized phase II study of PARP inhibitor ABT-888 (Veliparib) with modified FOLFIRI versus FOLFIRI as second-line treatment of metastatic pancreatic Cancer: SWOG S1513. Clin Cancer Res 27(23):6314–6322
67. Bang YJ et al (2015) Randomized, double-blind phase II trial with prospective classification by ATM protein level to evaluate the efficacy and tolerability of olaparib plus paclitaxel in patients with recurrent or metastatic gastric cancer. J Clin Oncol 33(33):3858–3865
68. Bang YJ et al (2017) Olaparib in combination with paclitaxel in patients with advanced gastric cancer who have progressed following first-line therapy (GOLD): a double-blind, randomised, placebo-controlled, phase 3 trial. Lancet Oncol 18(12):1637–1651
69. Chugh R et al (2021) SARC025 arms 1 and 2: a phase 1 study of the poly(ADP-ribose) polymerase inhibitor niraparib with temozolomide or irinotecan in patients with advanced Ewing sarcoma. Cancer 127(8):1301–1310
70. Grignani G et al (2018) Trabectedin and olaparib in patients with advanced and non-resectable bone and soft-tissue sarcomas (TOMAS): an open-label, phase 1b study from the Italian Sarcoma Group. Lancet Oncol 19(10):1360–1371
71. Middleton MR et al (2015) Randomized phase II study evaluating veliparib (ABT-888) with temozolomide in patients with metastatic melanoma. Ann Oncol 26(10):2173–2179
72. Jelinek MJ et al (2021) A phase I trial adding poly(ADP-ribose) polymerase inhibitor veliparib to induction carboplatin-paclitaxel in patients with head and neck squamous cell carcinoma: alliance A091101. Oral Oncol 114:105171
73. Federico SM et al (2020) A phase I trial of talazoparib and irinotecan with and without temozolomide in children and young adults with recurrent or refractory solid malignancies. Eur J Cancer 137:204–213
74. Schafer ES et al (2020) Phase 1/2 trial of talazoparib in combination with temozolomide in children and adolescents with refractory/recurrent solid tumors including Ewing sarcoma: a children's oncology group phase 1 consortium study (ADVL1411). Pediatr Blood Cancer 67(2):e28073
75. Baxter PA et al (2020) A phase I/II study of veliparib (ABT-888) with radiation and temozolomide in newly diagnosed diffuse pontine glioma: a pediatric brain tumor consortium study. Neuro Oncol 22(6):875–885
76. Sim HW et al (2021) A randomized phase II trial of veliparib, radiotherapy, and temozolomide in patients with unmethylated MGMT glioblastoma: the VERTU study. Neuro Oncol 23(10):1736–1749
77. Yap TA et al. (2022) CT007—PETRA: first in class, first in human trial of the next generation PARP1-selective inhibitor AZD5305 in patients (pts) with BRCA1/2, PALB2 or RAD51C/D mutations. In: American Association for Cancer Research Annual Meeting 2022. New Orleans, LA

Rational Combinations of PARP Inhibitors with HRD-Inducing Molecularly Targeted Agents

10

Elizabeth K. Lee and Joyce F. Liu

10.1 Introduction

PARP inhibitors have a clear role in treating cancers with BRCA mutations and homologous recombination deficiency (HRD). However, preclinical and early clinical data suggest that PARP inhibitor combinations could expand the activity of PARP inhibitors across a range of tumor types and molecular backgrounds. In particular, homologous recombination (HR) proficient and BRCA-wildtype tumors, which represent a substantial proportion of cancers, may benefit from PARP inhibitor combination strategies. Additionally, acquired resistance to PARP inhibition is common, often due to restoration of homologous recombination repair (HRR), and represents an emergent area of unmet clinical need. Targeted agents which induce HRD or restore "BRCA-ness" are a promising strategy to re-sensitize cancers to PARP inhibition. In this chapter, we review molecularly-based targeted therapies associated with induction of HRD and evidence for effective combination with PARP inhibitors, summarized in Table 10.1. General principles and mechanisms are reviewed; however, as molecular features, genetic alterations, and pathway dependencies differ between various tumor and histologic subtypes, specific combinatorial strategies may not be active across all tumor types and will require validation in any tumor type of particular interest.

E. K. Lee · J. F. Liu (✉)
Dana-Farber Cancer Institute, Boston, USA
e-mail: joyce_liu@dfci.harvard.edu

E. K. Lee
e-mail: elizabethk_lee@dfci.harvard.edu

T. A. Yap and G. I. Shapiro (eds.), *Targeting the DNA Damage Response for Cancer Therapy*, Cancer Treatment and Research 186,
https://doi.org/10.1007/978-3-031-30065-3_10

Table 10.1 Mechanisms of HRD induction

Target	Mechanism of HRD induction by target inhibition	Combinations in clinical trials
VEGF/VEGFR (angiogenesis)	• BRCA1/2 downregulation • RAD51 downregulation	Cediranib/olaparib • Phase 2: cediranib/olaparib PFS 17.7 months versus olaparib PFS 9.0 months [1] • Phase 3 NRG-GY004: cediranib/olaparib PFS 10.4 months and ORR 69.4% versus chemotherapy PFS 10.3 months and ORR 71.3% [2] • Phase 2 EVOLVE: cediranib/olaparib ORR 3/34 patients [3] Bevacizumab/niraparib • Phase 2 AVANOVA: niraparib/bevacizumab PFS 11.9 months versus niraparib PFS 5.5 months [4] Bevacizumab/olaparib • Phase 3 PAOLA-1: olaparib/bevacizumab PFS 22.21 months versus bevacizumab 16.6 months [5]
PI3K pathway	• BRCA1/2 downregulation • Impaired non-oxidative pentose phosphate pathway, depleting the nucleotide pool • Depletion of MCL-1 • Suppression of SUV39H1 methyltransferase	Buparlisib/olaparib • Phase 1: ORR 29% ovarian cancer, ORR 28% breast cancer [6] Alpelisib/olaparib • Phase 1b: ORR 35% BRCA-wildtype ovarian cancer, ORR 30% BRCA-mutant ovarian cancer [7] • Phase 1b: ORR 18% breast cancer [8] Vistusertib/olaparib • Phase 1: ORR 27% endometrial cancer, ORR 20% ovarian cancer, ORR 6% breast cancer [9] Capivasertib/olaparib • Phase 1: ORR 25% advanced solid tumors [10] • Phase 1b: ORR 19% endometrial, ovarian, and breast cancer [11]

(continued)

Table 10.1 (continued)

Target	Mechanism of HRD induction by target inhibition	Combinations in clinical trials
MAPK pathway	• BRCA1/2, RAD50, RAD51,MRE11, NBN downregulation • Altered PARP1 expression	Selumetinib/olaparib • Phase 1 SOLAR: ORR 17% advanced solid tumors [12] • Phase 1 SOLAR dose expansion ongoing in ovarian and endometrial cancers (NCT03162627)
BET/BRD4	• BRCA1 downregulation • RAD51 downregulation • CtIP downregulation	AZD5153/olaparib • Phase 1: advanced solid tumors and lymphoma, ongoing NCT03205176 [13] NUV-868/olaparib • Phase 1: advanced solid tumors, ongoing NCT05252390 ZEN003694/talazoparib • Phase 1: ovarian cancer, ongoing NCT05071937 [14]
EZH2	• BRCA1/2 downregulation • REV7 upregulation	Tazemetostat/talazoparib • Phase 1: prostate cancer, ongoing NCT04846478 SHR2554/ SHR3162 • Phase 1: breast cancer, ongoing NCT04355858
HDAC	• BRCA1 depletion and downregulation • RAD51 downregulation • RAD50 downregulation • MRE11 downregulation	Vorinostat/olaparib • Phase 1: breast cancer, ongoing NCT03742245 Belinostat/talazoparib • Phase 1: breast, prostate, and ovarian cancers NCT04703920
Hsp90	• BRCA1 degradation • BRCA1/2 downregulation • RAD51 downregulation • MRE11 downregulation	Onalespib/olaparib – Phase 1: ORR 0% advanced solid tumors [15]
AXL	• Replication fork collapse • RAD51 downregulation • MRE11 downregulation	None

10.2 Anti-angiogenic Inhibition

Anti-angiogenic agents induce HRD through several mechanisms and pairing these with PARP inhibition is a compelling strategy. One mechanism of HRD induction through VEGF signaling blockade is via subsequent abrogation of VEGF-induced AKT-mediated non-homologous end-joining (NHEJ) and HRR, with increased levels of unresolved yH2AX foci and delayed resolution of DSBs [16]. Intratumoral hypoxia, whether chronic from tumor architecture or induced by VEGF/VEGFR inhibition and vascular pruning, is associated with down-regulation of BRCA1/2 and RAD51 expression, leading to defective HRR and increased susceptibility to DNA damage agents [17–22]. A second mechanism of HRD induction is via suppressed *BRCA1/2* expression; in preclinical studies in ovarian cancer cells, selective inhibition of VEGFR3 downregulated BRCA1 and BRCA2 mRNA levels by up to ninefold, effectively mimicking BRCA deficiency in *BRCA*-wildtype cells [23]. VEGFR3 inhibition re-sensitized platinum-resistant ovarian cancer cells and BRCA-reverted cells to platinum and inhibited tumor [23]. The combination of olaparib and cediranib, a small molecular oral VEGFR1/2/3 inhibitor, inhibited growth of ovarian cancer patient-derived xenografts (PDXs), with additive benefit in tumors resistant to platinum and to olaparib monotherapy, supporting the evidence of VEGF inhibitor-mediated induction of HRD and re-sensitization to PARP inhibition [24]. Enhancement of tumor cell apoptosis may be due to cediranib-induced AKT inhibition and subsequently increased FOX01-mediated apoptosis and cell cycle arrest [25].

Several clinical trials evaluating PARP and VEGFR inhibitor combinations provide promising evidence of clinical activity. In a Phase 2 trial, adding cediranib to olaparib resulted in an improved median PFS of 17.7 months compared to the control arm of 9.0 months with olaparib alone [1]. In post-hoc analyses, patients without a known germline *BRCA* mutation experienced a longer median progression-free survival (PFS, 23.7 months) and median overall survival (OS, 37.8 months) compared to those receiving olaparib alone (PFS 5.7 months; OS 23.0 months), suggesting potential synergism in the HR-proficient setting [1]. In a subsequent phase 3 trial, combination olaparib/cediranib was compared to platinum-based chemotherapy in patients with platinum-sensitive ovarian cancer; while the trial did not meet the primary endpoint of improved PFS compared to standard platinum-based chemotherapy, substantial activity of the combination was observed, with median PFS of 10.4 months and ORR 69.4% compared to 10.3 months and 71.3% for chemotherapy. In contrast, while formal statistical comparison was not performed, olaparib monotherapy in this population resulted in a PFS of 8.2 months and an ORR of 52.4% [2]. Similarly, in the phase 2 AVANOVA trial randomizing patients with recurrent platinum-sensitive ovarian cancer to niraparib or combined niraparib and bevacizumab, combination therapy demonstrated a PFS benefit of 11.9 months compared to 5.5 months with PARP inhibition alone [4]. PFS prolongation was seen even in patients with HR proficiency or BRCA wild-type disease, again reflecting the potential PARP inhibitor-sensitizing effects of VEGFR blockade. In the PAOLA-1 trial randomizing ovarian cancer patients to maintenance bevacizumab or olaparib/bevacizumab following response to first-line chemotherapy, the combination of olaparib/bevacizumab was superior to bevacizumab monotherapy across the study population (PFS of 22.1 months vs. 16.6 months) [5]. A direct comparison of combined PARP inhibitor and anti-angiogenic to PARP inhibitor monotherapy as first-line maintenance therapy in ovarian cancer has not been performed; a population-adjusted indirect treatment comparison of olaparib/bevacizumab to ola-parib as first-line maintenance in patients with *BRCA*-mutated suggested a slight numerical but not statistically significant improvement in PFS [26]. Whether other populations might benefit from the combination and whether benefit would be seen in a direct head-to-head comparison remains unknown.

As more patients with ovarian and other cancers receive PARP inhibitors as monotherapy, an emerging question is whether combined PARP and VEGFR inhi-bition can overcome resistance to prior PARP inhibitor monotherapy. Combined olaparib/cediranib after progression on prior PARP inhibitor was evaluated fur-ther in the phase 2 EVOLVE trial in women with recurrent ovarian cancer [3]. In this trial, only 3 of 34 patients achieved a partial response to treatment with ola-parib/cediranib [3]. Evaluation of tumor specimens obtained after progression on prior PARP inhibitor sheds light on mechanisms of acquired PARP inhibitor resis-tance, including *RAD51B* reversion mutation, *BRCA1/2* reversion mutations, and *BRCA1/2* amplification or overexpression, overall suggesting restoration of HRR and were associated with worse outcomes. Interestingly, one patient with amplifi-cation of *BRCA1*, *RAD51C*, *BRIP1*, and *NBN* after progression on PARP inhibitor was able to achieve a response with olaparib/cediranib [3]. However, the overall low response rate in this study suggests that mechanisms of resistance to PARP inhibitors are likely to affect response to combined VEGF/PARP inhibition and indicates a need to incorporate molecular characteristics in determining the most appropriate patient population to receive this treatment. The ongoing KGOG 3056 trial evaluating bevacizumab and niraparib in ovarian cancer patients previously treated with a PARP inhibitor will provide further insight into this combinatorial strategy in PARP inhibitor-exposed patients [27].

10.3   PI3K Pathway Inhibition

The phosphatidylinositol 3-kinase (PI3K) pathway has broad oncogenic roles in cell metabolism, proliferation, and survival and can aberrantly mediate chemore-sistance [28]. Inhibition of the PI3K pathway suppresses *BRCA1/2* transcription via ERK-regulated phosphorylation of the ETS1 transcription factor, establishing an HRD phenotype [29]. PI3K inhibition reduces flux through the non-oxidative pen-tose phosphate pathway, depleting the nucleotide pool available for DNA repair [30]. Additionally, glycolytic activity is reduced with PI3K inhibition, affecting amino acid synthesis; this impairs synthesis of bases and further inhibits DNA repair [30]. Upregulation of PARylation in the setting of PI3K inhibition provides further rationale for synthetic lethality from paired PARP and PI3K inhibition. In fact, combined PI3K/PARP inhibition impairs the pentose phosphate pathway more than either alone [30]. Interestingly, inhibition of PI3K but not AKT, a signal-ing partner downstream of PI3K, was associated with reduced pentose phosphate pathway flux and a DNA damage phenotype, demonstrating that signaling partners within a pathway may have disparate downstream effects [30].

In support of combining PI3K and PARP inhibition, *in vitro* and *in vivo* models demonstrated greater DNA damage and tumor growth inhibition with combined PI3K pathway and PARP blockade in HR proficient or *BRCA*-wildtype settings, including in breast, ovarian, endometrial, and cervical cancers [31–38]. A phase 1 trial combining buparlisib, an inhibitor of all PI3K isoforms, and olaparib, yielded an ORR of 29% in ovarian cancer and ORR 28% in breast cancer, including in patients without germline *BRCA* mutations [6]. A phase 1b trial of olaparib with alpelisib, a PI3Kα isoform-specific inhibitor, yielded similar results in ovarian cancer with an ORR of 35% (6/17) in those without germline *BRCA* mutations and an ORR of 30% (3/10) in those with germline *BRCA* mutations, in a trial population that was almost fully comprised of platinum resistant or refractory disease as a surrogate marker of HR proficiency [7]. In patients with triple-negative breast cancer, including many with *BRCA* wild-type tumors, activity was also seen, with an ORR of 18% (3/17) and disease control of 59% (10/17) [8]. Although the numbers are limited, these results suggest that PI3K inhibition can effectively induce HRD and sensitize tumors to PARP inhibition in these settings. An international phase 3 trial randomizing patients with germline *BRCA*-wildtype platinum resistant ovarian cancer to combined olaparib/alpelisib or chemotherapy is underway (NCT04729387).

Studies evaluating inhibition of mTOR, a downstream signaling partner within the PI3K pathway, shed further light on additional mechanisms of HRD induction. This may occur by depleting MCL-1, an anti-apoptotic BCL-2 protein [39]. Depleting MCL-1 switches the preferential DNA repair pathway from HRR to error-prone NHEJ and inhibits resolution of stalled replication forks [40]. mTOR inhibition, possibly reflecting overall PI3K pathway inhibition, also suppresses the expression of the epigenetic regulator SUV39H1 histone methyltransferase [41], which regulates heterochromatin stability and has been implicated in double-strand DNA break repair [42, 43]. Loss of SUV39H1 suppresses HRR [44]. mTOR inhibition, utilizing everolimus and KU, sensitized BRCA-proficient triple-negative breast cancer cells *in vitro* and *in vivo* to olaparib and talazoparib, increasing apoptosis, reducing cell viability, and inhibiting xenograft tumor growth more than mTOR inhibition or PARP inhibition alone [41]. Combining mTOR inhibition with PARP inhibition has also been shown to synergistically suppress tumor growth in other xenograft models of colorectal cancer, glioblastoma multiforme, and breast cancer [39, 45]. In a phase 1 trial of patients with of predominantly BRCA-wildtype endometrial, ovarian, and breast cancer, the combination of olaparib and vistusertib, an mTOR inhibitor, yielded ORRs of 27%, 20%, and 6% respectively [9]. These preliminary efficacy results may speak to different effects of mTOR/PARP inhibition in different cancer types.

The AKT serine/threonine kinases are downstream PI3K pathway mediators which are also implicated as oncogenic drivers. In xenograft models of glioblastoma, AKT inhibition using the small molecule inhibitor MK-2206 had more pronounced effects increasing γH2AX, delaying double-strand break repair, and sensitizing to radiotherapy than VEGF inhibition [16], an intriguing finding considering the evidence for paired VEGF/PARP inhibition. *In vitro, BRCA*-deficient, but not -proficient, ovarian cancer cells are sensitive to combined MK-2206 and olaparib [46]. This may reflect *BRCA* deficiency-associated upregulation of AKT activity as a primary survival mechanism, and renders AKT inhibition an attractive strategy to further impair cancer cell survival [46]. Results from early phase clinical trials support utilizing combined AKT/PARP inhibition. In a phase 1 trial of olaparib and capivasertib, a pan-AKT inhibitor, in advanced/recurrent solid tumors, 25% of evaluable patients (14/56) achieved partial responses and an additional 20% (11/56) achieved stable disease (SD) for at least 4 months [10]. The majority of the enrolled patients harbored germline *BRCA* mutations, other pathogenic DNA repair mutations, or PI3K pathway alterations. Fourteen of the 25 patients (56%) achieving clinical benefit (CR + PR + SD ≥ 4 months) had germline *BRCA* mutations. Interestingly, 4 patients who were previously resistant to PARP inhibition experienced clinical benefit with combined olaparib/capivasertib, with 2 of these patients achieving prolonged stable disease of 56 and 115 weeks respectively, supporting the hypothesis of re-sensitization to PARP inhibition [10]. On-treatment tumor biopsies showed an increase in phosphorylated ERK, supporting the pre-clinical rationale of ERK-mediated suppression of *BRCA* expression and induction of HRD [10]. The combination of olaparib/capivasertib was further studied in a phase 1b trial in endometrial, ovarian, and breast cancer patients, yielding a 19% response rate with an additional 22% experiencing stable disease for 4 months or greater [11]. High receptor tyrosine kinase and RAS/MAPK pathway activation in baseline tumor samples was associated with poor outcome to olaparib/capivasertib, suggesting upregulation of bypass survival pathways and a potential biomarker of resistance [11]. Preclinical evidence supports this translational finding, in which combined PI3K/PARP inhibition did not show synergistic activity in RAS-mutated cells [47].

10.4 MAPK Pathway Inhibition

Upregulation of the mitogen-activated protein kinase (MAPK) pathway has been demonstrated in the setting of PARP inhibitor resistance, and RAS mutations confer resistance to PARP inhibitors *in vitro* [47, 48]. Expression of *BRCA1/2*, *RAD50*, *RAD51*, *MRE11*, and *NBN* are reduced in the setting of MEK inhibition, at least partly through regulation of the E2F transcription factor, thereby inducing HRD [23, 47, 49]. DNA damage checkpoint proteins CHK1, CHK2, and Wee1 are also reduced in response to MEK inhibition, further exacerbating replication stress [47]. Through induction of FOXO3a, a forkhead family transcription factor, MEK inhibition also alters PARP1 expression and decreases sensing of DNA damage [11]. As VEGF production is mediated by mutant RAS and FOXO3a, MEK inhibition may decrease vascularity and indirectly promote HRD through increased intratumoral hypoxia [47, 50, 51].

In vitro synergy between the PARP inhibitors olaparib and talazoparib and two MEK inhibitors, including selumetinib, was demonstrated in ovarian cancer cell lines with and without *BRCA* mutations, suggesting that these combinations may increase the efficacy and spectrum of PARP inhibitor activity even in HR proficient settings [47]. The presence of *KRAS* mutations were found to be the most significant predictor of MEK/PARP inhibitor synergy, possibly by blocking adaptive responses induced by each drug on its own and inducing a synthetic lethal interaction [47]. RAS mutation may therefore be a biomarker of response to combined MEK/PARP inhibition. A phase 1 trial of olaparib and selumetinib in solid tumors with RAS pathway alterations reported an ORR of 17% and clinical benefit rate of 33% in 12 evaluable patients [12]. Enrollment to dose expansion cohorts, including ovarian and endometrial cancers with RAS pathway alterations and PARP inhibitor-resistant ovarian cancer, is ongoing (NCT03162627). Modulation of anti-tumor immunity may be an additional mechanism of synergy between MEK and PARP inhibition; MEK inhibition amplifies the DNA damage, cGAS/STING pathway activation, and immune microenvironment changes associated with PARP inhibition [48], providing rationale for adding PD-1/PD-L1 blockade to MEK/PARP inhibition.

10.5 BET Inhibition

The bromodomain and extraterminal (BET) protein family controls the transcription of many genes involved in inflammation, immunity, and pattern recognition receptors [52]. PARP inhibition increases expression of BRD4, a BET family member; upregulated BRD4 expression is associated with increased expression of aldehyde dehydrogenase, which promotes the NHEJ DNA repair pathway and drives PARP inhibitor resistance [53]. Therefore, targeting BET family proteins represents a rational strategy for reversing PARP inhibitor resistance. Drug-combination screens identified BET inhibitors as potential synergistic partners to olaparib, confirmed on siRNA knockdown of the BET proteins BRD2, BRD3, and BRD4 [54].

Specific inhibition of BRD4 presents an opportunity for PARP inhibition in HR proficient settings. BRD4 inhibition reduces transcription of and depletes C-terminal binding protein interacting protein (CtIP), which is crucial for HRR by interacting with the MRN complex at double-strand DNA breaks, promoting the nuclease activity of MRN, and facilitating DNA end-resection to generate single-stranded DNA and RAD51 loading. HRR is further impaired by BRD4-associated downregulation of *BRCA1* and *RAD51* [54–56]. BRD4 inhibition generates an HRD gene signature, confirming the overall effect and opportunity for synthetic lethality with PARP inhibition [57].

Combined BRD4/PARP inhibition demonstrated anti-cancer synergy broadly across multiple ovarian, endometrial, and breast cancer cell lines [57], regardless of BRCA status. Acquired resistance to PARP inhibition *in vitro* was reversed with BRD4 inhibition, specifically circumventing PARP inhibitor resistance mechanisms of 53BP1 or PARP1 loss [57]. Marked anti-tumor synergy of combined BRD4/PARP inhibition was seen in HR-proficient xenograft models of ovarian, breast, and pancreatic cancer which were resistant to PARP inhibitor monotherapy

[57]. Dual BET/PARP inhibitor synergy has also been demonstrated in pancreatic and cholangiocarcinoma models [56, 58]. This is a compelling treatment strategy under active clinical study. Early phase trials are ongoing, evaluating the combination of olaparib and BET inhibitor AZD5153 (NCT03205176) [13], olaparib and BET inhibitor NUV-868 (NCT05252390), and talazoparib and BET inhibitor ZEN003694 (NCT05071937) [14].

10.6 EZH2 Inhibitors

EZH2 is the catalytic subunit of the polycomb repressive complex 2 (PRC2), which trimethylates histone H3 at lysine 27 to epigenetically silence target genes [59]. EZH2 is recruited to sites of DNA damage, implying a role in modulating the DNA damage response [60]. Significant changes in DNA damage response-related genes by gene enrichment analysis in response to EZH2 inhibition, including reduced BRCA1/2 expression, provides further support for the combinatorial strategy of paired EZH2 and PARP inhibition [61]. EZH2 inhibition or knockdown also sensitized lung adenocarcinoma cells to platinum-based chemotherapy, further bolstering the hypothesis that EZH2 inhibition causes functional HRD that sensitizes cells to agents such as platinum and PARP inhibitors [62].

One mechanism of EZH2 inhibition-induced HRD is through altering the shieldin complex, which typically promotes HRR by localizing to double-strand DNA breaks in a 53BP1-dependent manner. Inhibiting EZH2 upregulates the REV7 component of the shieldin complex and decreases DNA end-resection, thereby suppressing HRR, promoting error-prone NHEJ, and sensitizing HR-proficient ovarian cancer cells to PARP inhibition [63]. Of note, this effect was seen only in *CARM1*-amplified ovarian cancer cells and xenografts [63]. CARM1, also known as PRMT4, is an arginine methyltransferase epigenetic regulator, and amplification of *CARM1* is typically mutually exclusive with *BRCA1*/2 mutations [63]. CARM1 drives a switch from SWI/SNF complex-mediated gene silencing to that of EZH2, with subsequent effects on NHEJ-associated genes, such as *REV7* [63]. Therefore, *CARM1* amplification is necessary for effective HRR suppression in the setting of EZH2 inhibition. CARM1 may therefore serve as a predictive biomarker of response to dual EZH2/PARP inhibition in ovarian cancer, although whether the same molecular context is necessary in other cancer types must be investigated.

This combinatorial strategy is under active clinical investigation, with early phase trials evaluating the combination of SHR2554 (EZH2 inhibitor) and SHR3162 (PARP inhibitor) in breast cancer (NCT04355858) and the combination of talazoparib and tazemetostat in prostate cancer (NCT04846478). Additionally, novel dual EZH2/PARP inhibitors are also in development as a separate strategy to effect combined simultaneous EZH2 and PARP inhibition. A first-in-class dual EZH2/PARP inhibitor was effective *in vitro* in reducing cell growth of

BRCA-wildtype triple-negative breast cancer cells, with improved activity compared to olaparib monotherapy, tazemetostat (an EZH2 inhibitor) monotherapy, or combined olaparib/tazemetostat [64].

10.7 HDAC Inhibition

Histone deacetylases (HDACs) regulate gene expression by acetylating histones and have multiple effects on base excision repair, nucleotide excision repair, double-strand DNA damage signaling and repair, and NHEJ [65–67]. The repair of double-strand DNA breaks relies on HDAC modulation of chromatin accessibility and interaction with ATM [67]. Pan-HDAC inhibition downregulates *RAD50* and *MRE11* [68], altering DNA end-resection and impairing HRR [67]. In prostate cancer and lung adenocarcinoma cells, vorinostat, a pan-HDAC inhibitor, induced double-strand DNA breaks, suppressed RAD50 and MRE11 protein expression, and induced cell death [68]. These effects were not seen in normal cells, suggesting selectivity of effect, likely due to normal cells' retained ability to repair DNA damage.

In prostate cancer cells *in vitro*, HDAC inhibition concomitantly depleted the ubiquitin ligase UHRF1 and BRCA1 protein, likely acting on the UHRF1-BRCA complex, thus sensitizing to cells to PARP inhibition [69]. Combined HDAC and PARP inhibition also reduced levels of BRCA1 and RAD51 [70] and synergistically inhibited tumor growth in prostate xenograft models [69]. Similarly, HDAC inhibition in pancreatic cancer cells decreased RAD51 and CHK1 via proteasomal degradation, thereby enhancing anti-tumor effect with PARP inhibition [71]. In glioblastoma cells treated with vorinostat (HDAC inhibitor) and olaparib, BRCA1 and RAD51 protein expression were reduced, double-strand DNA breaks significantly increased, and apoptosis markedly increased [72]. Oxidative damage to DNA bases from vorinostat-induced reactive oxygen species may have further contributed to increased DNA damage, replication stress, and the synergy of dual HDAC/PARP inhibition [72]. Similar synergy has been demonstrated *in vitro* in anaplastic thyroid cancer [73] and breast cancer [74]. Notably, there were differing levels of sensitivity to HDAC inhibition and PARP inhibition across cell lines in preclinical studies, underscoring the importance of validation in cancer- and histology-specific contexts. Dual PARP/HDAC inhibitors are under development and demonstrate preclinical anti-tumor activity [75, 76]. Compound P1, a dual PARP/HDAC inhibitor, effectively reduced cell viability and increased apoptosis across a number of vorinostat-resistant cancer types, including in breast cancer and Burkitt lymphoma cell lines, underscoring the efficacy of the combination [75]. The clinical effectiveness of combined HDAC/PARP inhibition is being explored in trials of olaparib/vorinostat in breast cancer (NCT03742245) and talazoparib/belinostat in breast, prostate, and ovarian cancer (NCT04703920).

10.8   Hsp90 Inhibition

Heat shock protein 90 (Hsp90) is a molecular chaperone that facilitates the appropriate folding, conformational stability, and function of numerous client proteins, thereby regulating cell cycle, survival, and intracellular signaling pathways; it is now understood to also have a role in DNA damage repair [77].

In *BRCA*-mutated breast cancer cells with acquired PARP inhibitor resistance due to an abnormal BRCA C-terminal domain, Hsp90 promoted protein folding and conformational stability, preventing degradation of the mutant BRCA protein and preserving HRR [78]. This finding suggests that inhibiting Hsp90 could re-sensitize a subset of PARP inhibitor-resistant, *BRCA*-mutant cells to DNA-damaging treatment. Additionally, Hsp90 inhibition induces BRCA1 ubiquitination, proteasomal degradation of BRCA1, and inhibition of both HRR and NHEJ, thereby sensitizing cancer cells to radiation and platinum-based therapy [79, 80]. Mitotic catastrophe was most pronounced in BRCA-mutant cells; however, inhibiting Hsp90 with the small molecule ganetespib was able to synergistically sensitize BRCA-wildtype ovarian cancer cells to talazoparib [81]. In these BRCA-wildtype ovarian cancer cells, ganetespib treatment was associated with reduced BRCA1 and BRCA2 levels, as well as reduced levels of RAD51, MRE11 (a member of the MRN complex), ATM, and CHK1, providing evidence of a broad range of Hsp90-associated client proteins involved in DNA repair [81]. Preclinically, even sub-lethal levels of Hsp90 inhibitors are sufficient to synergize HR-proficient ovarian cancer cells to platinum therapy [82].

In high grade glioma cells and xenograft models, inhibiting Hsp90 with brain-penetrant onalespib depleted RAD51 and CHK1, reduced expression of *BRCA1/2* and *XRCC2*, attenuated HRR, and sensitized glioma cells to treatment with radiation and the alkylating chemotherapy temozolomide [83]. Addition of onalespib to chemoradiation extended survival of murine glioblastoma models compared to chemoradiation alone, providing support for this approach in this and other tumor types. In p53-mutated squamous cell carcinoma of the head and neck, Hsp90 inhibition induced chromosomal fragmentation and sensitized to platinum-based chemoradiation as well [84].

In clinical studies, a phase 1 trial of olaparib and onalespib in advanced solid tumors did not report any objective responses, although 32% of patients (7/22) experienced stable disease lasting 24 weeks or more [15]. Two of these 7 patients had previously progressed through PARP inhibitor therapy. One of the patients had *CCNE1* amplification; Cyclin E is also an Hsp90 client protein, and in this patient, may have been an additional effect by onalespib to promote disease stability. While no responses were seen in this study, the significant portion of patients that had disease stability with dual Hsp90 and PARP inhibition despite being heavily pretreated supports that this treatment strategy may still have merit, but additional work will be required to identify the optimal patient population.

10.9 GAS6/AXL Inhibition

Growth arrest-specific 6 (GAS6) is a ligand of the receptor tyrosine kinase AXL, as well as Mer and Tyro3. Axl is expressed on endothelial and cancer cell surfaces and is implicated in epithelial to mesenchymal transition, invasion, and cancer metastasis [85]. High GAS6 serum levels are associated with a poor prognosis in ovarian cancer patients, with poor response to neoadjuvant chemotherapy, and shorter PFS and OS [86]. Evidence suggests a role for AXL in modulating HRR potentially through activation of DNA-PK [87], altered MAPK and PI3K signaling [88], and changes in replication fork dynamics via DNA damage response-associated proteins CHK1 and CHK2 [89].

AVB-S6-500, a high-affinity AXL decoy receptor which disrupts GAS6/AXL signaling, increased responses in ovarian cancer cells *in vitro* and in murine xenograft models when given in combination with carboplatin [86, 90]. Mechanistically, this was due to increased DNA damage as evidenced by significantly more γH2AX foci in comparison to carboplatin monotherapy, altered replication fork dynamics, and reduced RAD51 foci. These changes were seen in HRD as well as HR proficient settings, providing evidence that GAS6/AXL inhibition induces HRR [86]. AVB-S6-500 sensitized ovarian cancer cells to olaparib, reducing cell viability and impairing xenograft tumor growth more than olaparib alone. Similar findings with AXL inhibition were seen in models of lung, breast, and head and neck cancers, in which combined AXL/PARP inhibition also diminished protein levels of RAD51 and MRE11 [85, 91]. Thus, combined GAS6/AXL and PARP inhibition may represent a novel approach to improve response to or re-sensitize cancer cells to PARP inhibitors in ovarian and other solid tumors.

10.10 Conclusion

PARP inhibitors have transformed the treatment paradigm for *BRCA*-mutated cancers and have become an FDA-approved therapy across a number of disease types, including ovarian, breast, prostate, and pancreatic cancers. However, challenges remain in the clinical development of PARP inhibitors, including whether PARP inhibitor sensitivity can be induced in cancer cells that are homologous recombination proficient or otherwise intrinsically not susceptible to PARP inhibitor monotherapy. An additional unmet need includes a rapidly growing number of patients who have received a PARP inhibitor and developed resistance to monotherapy; how PARP inhibitor resistance can be reversed, and if PARP inhibitors can be used effectively again, remain questions of significant clinical interest. Multiple lines of preclinical evidence suggest that certain combinatorial strategies can leverage agents that induce HR deficiency and thereby increase PARP inhibitor sensitivity. Whether these combinatorial strategies can be successfully deployed in the clinical arena, and if they can overcome acquired or *de novo* PARP inhibitor resistance, are areas of active investigation. Overall, these combinatorial strategies guide our understanding of HRR as a whole and hold potential to broaden the population of patients who may benefit from treatment with PARP inhibitors.

References

1. Liu JF, Barry WT, Birrer M et al (2019) Overall survival and updated progression-free survival outcomes in a randomized phase II study of combination cediranib and olaparib versus olaparib in relapsed platinum-sensitive ovarian cancer. Ann Oncol 30:551–557
2. Liu JF, Brady MF, Matulonis UA et al (2020) A phase III study comparing single-agent olaparib or the combination of cediranib and olaparib to standard platinum-based chemotherapy in recurrent platinum-sensitive ovarian cancer. J Clin Oncol 38:6003
3. Lheureux S, Oaknin A, Garg S et al (2020) EVOLVE: a multicenter open-label single-arm clinical and translational phase II trial of cediranib plus olaparib for ovarian cancer after PARP inhibition progression. Clin Cancer Res 26:4206–4215
4. Mirza MR, Åvall Lundqvist E, Birrer MJ et al (2019) Niraparib plus bevacizumab versus niraparib alone for platinum-sensitive recurrent ovarian cancer (NSGO-AVANOVA2/ENGOT-ov24): a randomised, phase 2, superiority trial. Lancet Oncol 20:1409–1419
5. Ray-Coquard I, Pautier P, Pignata S et al (2019) Olaparib plus bevacizumab as first-line maintenance in ovarian cancer. N Engl J Med 381:2416–2428
6. Matulonis UA, Wulf GM, Barry WT et al (2017) Phase I dose escalation study of the PI3kinase pathway inhibitor BKM120 and the oral poly (ADP ribose) polymerase (PARP) inhibitor olaparib for the treatment of high-grade serous ovarian and breast cancer. Ann Oncol 28:512–518
7. Konstantinopoulos PA, Barry WT, Birrer M et al (2019) Olaparib and α-specific PI3K inhibitor alpelisib for patients with epithelial ovarian cancer: a dose-escalation and dose-expansion phase 1b trial. Lancet Oncol 20:570–580
8. Batalini F, Xiong N, Tayob N et al (2022) Phase 1b clinical trial with alpelisib plus olaparib for patients with advanced triple-negative breast canceralpelisib plus olaparib for triple-negative breast cancer. Clin Cancer Res 28:1493–1499
9. Westin SN, Litton JK, Williams RA et al (2018) Phase I trial of olaparib (PARP inhibitor) and vistusertib (mTORC1/2 inhibitor) in recurrent endometrial, ovarian and triple negative breast cancer. J Clin Oncol 36:5504
10. Yap TA, Kristeleit R, Michalarea V et al (2020) Phase i trial of the parp inhibitor olaparib and akt inhibitor capivasertib in patients with brca1/2-and non–brca1/2-mutant cancers. Cancer Discov 10:1528–1543
11. Westin SN, Labrie M, Litton JK et al (2021) Phase Ib dose expansion and translational analyses of olaparib in combination with capivasertib in recurrent endometrial, triple-negative breast, and ovarian cancer. Clin Cancer Res 27:6354–6365
12. Kurnit KC, Meric-Bernstam F, Hess K, et al (2019) Abstract CT020: Phase I dose escalation of olaparib (PARP inhibitor) and selumetinib (MEK Inhibitor) combination in solid tumors with Ras pathway alterations. Cancer Research 79:CT020–CT020
13. Wang JS-Z, de Vita S, Karlix JL et al (2019) First-in-human study of AZD5153, a small molecule inhibitor of bromodomain protein 4 (BRD4), in patients (pts) with relapsed/refractory (RR) malignant solid tumor and lymphoma: Preliminary data. J Clin Oncol 37:3085
14. Kharenko OA, Patel R, Calosing C (2021) Abstract 1129: combination of ZEN-3694 with talazoparib is a novel therapeutic approach in ER positive breast cancer resistant to CDK4/6 inhibitors, independent of BRCA status. Can Res 81:1129
15. Konstantinopoulos PA, Cheng SC, Supko JG et al (2022) Combined PARP and HSP90 inhibition: preclinical and phase 1 evaluation in patients with advanced solid tumours. Br J Cancer 126:1027–1036

16. Gomez-Roman N, Chong MY, Chahal SK, Caragher SP, Jackson MR, Stevenson KH, Dongre SA, Chalmers AJ (2020) Radiation responses of 2D and 3D glioblastoma cells: a novel, 3D-specific radioprotective role of VEGF/Akt signaling through functional activation of NHEJ. Mol Cancer Ther 19:575–589

17. Bindra RS, Schaffer PJ, Meng A, Woo J, Maseide K, Roth ME, Lizardi P, Hedley DW, Bristow RG, Glazer PM (2004) Down-regulation of Rad51 and decreased homologous recombination in hypoxic cancer cells. Mol Cell Biol 24:8504–8518

18. Bindra RS, Gibson SL, Meng A, Westermark U, Jasin M, Pierce AJ, Bristow RG, Classon MK, Glazer PM (2005) Hypoxia-induced down-regulation of BRCA1 expression by E2Fs. Can Res 65:11597–11604

19. Chan N, Koritzinsky M, Zhao H, Bindra R, Glazer PM, Powell S, Belmaaza A, Wouters B, Bristow RG (2008) Chronic hypoxia decreases synthesis of homologous recombination proteins to offset chemoresistance and radioresistance. Can Res 68:605–614

20. Kumareswaran R, Ludkovski O, Meng A, Sykes J, Pintilie M, Bristow RG (2012) Chronic hypoxia compromises repair of DNA double-strand breaks to drive genetic instability. J Cell Sci 125:189–199

21. Bristow RG, Hill RP (2008) Hypoxia and metabolism: hypoxia, DNA repair and genetic instability. Nat Rev Cancer 8:180–192

22. Kaplan AR, Gueble SE, Liu Y, Oeck S, Kim H, Yun Z, Glazer PM (2019) Cediranib suppresses homology-directed DNA repair through down-regulation of BRCA1/2 and RAD51. Science Translational Medicine 11:4508

23. Lim J, Yang K, Taylor-Harding B, Ruprecht Wiedemeyer W, Buckanovich RJ (2014) VEGFR3 inhibition chemosensitizes ovarian cancer stemlike cells through down-regulation of BRCA1 and BRCA2. Neoplasia (United States) 16:343-353.e2

24. Bizzaro F, Fuso Nerini I, Taylor MA et al (2021) VEGF pathway inhibition potentiates PARP inhibitor efficacy in ovarian cancer independent of BRCA status. J Hematol Oncol 14:186

25. Ping Lin Z, Zhu YL, Lo YC, Moscarelli J, Xiong A, Korayem Y, Huang PH, Giri S, LoRusso P, Ratner ES (2018) Combination of triapine, olaparib, and cediranib suppresses progression of BRCA-wild type and PARP inhibitor-resistant epithelial ovarian cancer. PLoS ONE. https://doi.org/10.1371/journal.pone.0207399

26. Vergote I, Ray-Coquard I, Anderson DM et al (2021) Population-adjusted indirect treatment comparison of the SOLO1 and PAOLA-1/ENGOT-ov25 trials evaluating maintenance olaparib or bevacizumab or the combination of both in newly diagnosed, advanced BRCA-mutated ovarian cancer. Eur J Cancer 157:415–423

27. Park J, Lim MC, Lee J-K, Jeong DH, Kim SI, Choi MC, Kim B-G, Lee J-Y (2022) A single-arm, phase II study of niraparib and bevacizumab maintenance therapy in platinum-sensitive, recurrent ovarian cancer patients previously treated with a PARP inhibitor: Korean Gynecologic Oncology Group (KGOG 3056)/NIRVANA-R trial. J Gynecol Oncol. https://doi.org/10.3802/jgo.2022.33.e12

28. Thorpe LM, Yuzugullu H, Zhao JJ (2015) PI3K in cancer: divergent roles of isoforms, modes of activation and therapeutic targeting. Nat Rev Cancer 15:7–24

29. Ibrahim YH, García-García C, Serra V et al (2012) PI3K inhibition impairs BRCA1/2 expression and sensitizes BRCA-proficient triple-negative breast cancer to PARP inhibition. Cancer Discov 2:1036–1047

30. Juvekar A, Hu H, Yadegarynia S et al (2016) Phosphoinositide 3-kinase inhibitors induce DNA damage through nucleoside depletion. Proc Natl Acad Sci U S A 113:E4338–E4347

31. Juvekar A, Burga LN, Hu H et al (2012) Combining a PI3K inhibitor with a PARP inhibitor provides an effective therapy for BRCA1-related breast cancer. Cancer Discov 2:1048–1063

32. De P, Sun Y, Carlson JH, Friedman LS, Leyland-Jones BR, Dey N (2014) Doubling down on the PI3k-AKT-mTOR pathway enhances the antitumor efficacy of PARP inhibitor in triple negative breast cancer model beyond BRCA-ness. Neoplasia (United States) 16:43–72

33. Wang J, He G, Li H, Ge Y, Wang S, Xu Y, Zhu Q (2021) Discovery of novel PARP/PI3K dual inhibitors with high efficiency against BRCA-proficient triple negative breast cancer. Eur J Med Chem. https://doi.org/10.1016/j.ejmech.2020.113054

34. Wang D, Wang M, Jiang N, Zhang Y, Bian X, Wang X, Roberts TM, Zhao JJ, Liu P, Cheng H (2016) Effective use of PI3K inhibitor BKM120 and PARP inhibitor olaparib to treat PIK3CA mutant ovarian cancer. Oncotarget 7:13153–13166
35. Wang D, Li C, Zhang Y et al (2016) Combined inhibition of PI3K and PARP is effective in the treatment of ovarian cancer cells with wild-type PIK3CA genes. Gynecol Oncol 142:548–556
36. Cao P, Wang Y, Lv Y et al (2019) PI3K p110α inhibition sensitizes cervical cancer cells with aberrant PI3K signaling activation to PARP inhibitor BMN673. Oncol Rep 42:2097–2107
37. Philip CA, Laskov I, Beauchamp MC et al (2017) Inhibition of PI3K-AKT-mTOR pathway sensitizes endometrial cancer cell lines to PARP inhibitors. BMC Cancer. https://doi.org/10.1186/s12885-017-3639-0
38. Guney Eskiler G, Ozturk Sezgin M (2022) Therapeutic potential of the PI3K inhibitor LY294002 and PARP inhibitor talazoparib combination in BRCA-deficient triple negative breast cancer cells. Cell Signal. https://doi.org/10.1016/j.cellsig.2021.110229
39. Mattoo AR, Joun A, Milburn Jessup J (2019) Repurposing of mTOR complex inhibitors attenuates Mcl-1 and sensitizes to PARP inhibition. Mol Cancer Res 17:42–53
40. Mattoo AR, Pandita RK, Chakraborty S, Charaka V, Mujoo K, Hunt CR, Pandita TK (2017) MCL-1 depletion impairs DNA double-strand break repair and reinitiation of stalled DNA replication forks. Mol Cell Biol. https://doi.org/10.1128/mcb.00535-16
41. Mo W, Liu Q, Lin CCJ et al (2016) mTOR inhibitors suppress homologous recombination repair and synergize with PARP inhibitors via regulating SUV39H1 in BRCA-proficient triple-negative breast cancer. Clin Cancer Res 22:1699–1712
42. Peters AHFM, O'Carroll D, Scherthan H et al (2001) Loss of the Suv39h histone methyltransferases impairs mammalian heterochromatin and genome stability. Cell 107:323–337
43. Peng JC, Karpen GH (2009) Heterochromatic genome stability requires regulators of histone H3 K9 methylation. PLoS Genet 5:1000435
44. Ayrapetov MK, Gursoy-Yuzugullu O, Xu C, Xu Y, Price BD (2014) DNA double-strand breaks promote methylation of histone H3 on lysine 9 and transient formation of repressive chromatin. Proc Natl Acad Sci U S A 111:9169–9174
45. el Botty R, Coussy F, Hatem R et al (2018) Inhibition of mTOR downregulates expression of DNA repair proteins and is highly efficient against BRCA2-mutated breast cancer in combination to PARP inhibition. Oncotarget 9:29587–29600
46. Whicker ME, Lin ZP, Hanna R, Sartorelli AC, Ratner ES (2016) MK-2206 sensitizes BRCA-deficient epithelial ovarian adenocarcinoma to cisplatin and olaparib. BMC Cancer 16:550
47. Sun C, Fang Y, Yin J et al (2017) Rational combination therapy with PARP and MEK inhibitors capitalizes on therapeutic liabilities in RAS mutant cancers. Sci Transl Med. https://doi.org/10.1126/scitranslmed.aal5148
48. Yang B, Li X, Fu Y et al (2021) MEK inhibition remodels the immune landscape of mutant KRAS tumors to overcome resistance to PARP and immune checkpoint inhibitors. Can Res 81:2714–2729
49. Vena F, Jia R, Esfandiari A et al (2018) MEK inhibition leads to BRCA2 downregulation and sensitization to DNA damaging agents in pancreas and ovarian cancer models. Oncotarget 9:11592–11603
50. Karadedou CT, Gomes AR, Chen J et al (2012) FOXO3a represses VEGF expression through FOXM1-dependent and -independent mechanisms in breast cancer. Oncogene 31:1845–1858
51. Okada F, Rak JW, St. Croix B, Lieubeau B, Kaya M, Roncari L, Shirasawa S, Sasazuki T, Kerbel RS (1998) Impact of oncogenes in tumor angiogenesis: Mutant K-ras up-regulation of vascular endothelial growth factor/vascular permeability factor is necessary, but not sufficient for tumorigenicity of human colorectal carcinoma cells. Proc Natl Acad Sci U S A 95:3609–3614
52. Wang N, Wu R, Tang D, Kang R (2021) The BET family in immunity and disease. Signal Transduct Target Ther. https://doi.org/10.1038/s41392-020-00384-4
53. Liu L, Cai S, Han C et al (2020) ALDH1A1 contributes to PARP inhibitor resistance via enhancing DNA repair in BRCA2-/- ovarian cancer cells. Mol Cancer Ther 19:199–210

54. Yang L, Zhang Y, Shan W et al (2017) Repression of BET activity sensitizes homologous recombination-proficient cancers to PARP inhibition. Sci Transl Med. https://doi.org/10.1126/scitranslmed.aal1645

55. Wilson AJ, Stubbs M, Liu P, Ruggeri B, Khabele D (2018) The BET inhibitor INCB054329 reduces homologous recombination efficiency and augments PARP inhibitor activity in ovarian cancer. Gynecol Oncol 149:575–584

56. Miller AL, Fehling SC, Garcia PL, Gamblin TL, Council LN, van Waardenburg RCAM, Yang ES, Bradner JE, Yoon KJ (2019) The BET inhibitor JQ1 attenuates double-strand break repair and sensitizes models of pancreatic ductal adenocarcinoma to PARP inhibitors. EBioMedicine 44:419–430

57. Sun C, Yin J, Fang Y et al (2018) BRD4 inhibition is synthetic lethal with PARP inhibitors through the induction of homologous recombination deficiency. Cancer Cell 33:401-416.e8

58. Fehling SC, Miller AL, Garcia PL, Vance RB, Yoon KJ (2020) The combination of BET and PARP inhibitors is synergistic in models of cholangiocarcinoma. Cancer Lett 468:48–58

59. Kim KH, Roberts CWM (2016) Targeting EZH2 in cancer. Nat Med 22:128–134

60. Campbell S, Ismail IH, Young LC, Poirier GG, Hendzel MJ (2013) Polycomb repressive complex 2 contributes to DNA double-strand break repair. Cell Cycle 12:2675–2683

61. Garner IM, Su Z, Hu S, Wu Y, McNeish IA, Fuchter MJ, Brown R (2021) Abstract 2066: Modulation of homologous recombination repair pathway gene expression by a dual EZH2 and EHMT2 histone methyltransferase inhibitor and synergy with PARP inhibitors in ovarian cancer. Can Res 81:2066

62. Riquelme E, Suraokar M, Behrens C et al (2014) VEGF/VEGFR-2 upregulates EZH2 expression in lung adenocarcinoma cells and EZH2 depletion enhances the response to platinum-based and VEGFR-2-targeted therapy. Clin Cancer Res 20:3849–3861

63. Karakashev S, Fukumoto T, Zhao B et al (2020) EZH2 inhibition sensitizes CARM1-high, homologous recombination proficient ovarian cancers to PARP inhibition. Cancer Cell 37:157-167.e6

64. Wang C, Qu L, Li S et al (2021) Discovery of first-in-class dual PARP and EZH2 inhibitors for triple-negative breast cancer with wild-type BRCA. J Med Chem 64:12630–12650

65. Bhaskara S, Jacques V, Rusche JR, Olson EN, Cairns BR, Chandrasekharan MB (2013) Histone deacetylases 1 and 2 maintain S-phase chromatin and DNA replication fork progression. Epigenetics Chromatin. https://doi.org/10.1186/1756-8935-6-27

66. Bhaskara S (2015) Cell Cycle Histone deacetylases 1 and 2 regulate DNA replication and DNA repair: potential targets for genome stability-mechanism-based therapeutics for a subset of cancers Histone deacetylases 1 and 2 regulate DNA replication and DNA repair: potential targets for genome stability-mechanism-based therapeutics for a subset of cancers. Cell Cycle 14:1779–1785

67. Roos P, Krumm A (2016) The multifaceted influence of histone deacetylases on DNA damage signalling and DNA repair. Nucleic Acids Res 44:10017–10030

68. Lee JH, Choy ML, Ngo L, Foster SS, Marks PA (2010) Histone deacetylase inhibitor induces DNA damage, which normal but not transformed cells can repair. Proc Natl Acad Sci U S A 107:14639–14644

69. Yin L, Liu Y, Peng Y et al (2018) PARP inhibitor veliparib and HDAC inhibitor SAHA synergistically co-target the UHRF1/BRCA1 DNA damage repair complex in prostate cancer cells. J Exp Clin Cancer Res. https://doi.org/10.1186/s13046-018-0810-7

70. Chao OS, Goodman OB DNA damage and repair synergistic loss of prostate cancer cell viability by coinhibition of HDAC and PARP. https://doi.org/10.1158/1541-7786.MCR-14-0173

71. Romeo MA, Saveria M, Montani G, Benedetti R, Arena A, D'orazi G, Cirone M (2022) VPA and TSA interrupt the interplay between mutp53 and HSP70, leading to CHK1 and RAD51 down-regulation and sensitizing pancreatic cancer cells to AZD2461 PARP inhibitor. J Mol Sci 2022:2268

72. Rasmussen RD, Gajjar MK, Jensen KE, Hamerlik P (2016) Enhanced efficacy of combined HDAC and PARP targeting in glioblastoma. Mol Oncol 10:751–763

73. Baldan F, Mio C, Allegri L, Puppin C, Russo D, Filetti S, Damante G (2015) Synergy between HDAC and PARP inhibitors on proliferation of a human anaplastic thyroid cancer-derived cell line. Int J Endocrinol. https://doi.org/10.1155/2015/978371

74. Min A, Im SA, Kim DK et al (2015) Histone deacetylase inhibitor, suberoylanilide hydroxamic acid (SAHA), enhances anti-tumor effects of the poly (ADP-ribose) polymerase (PARP) inhibitor olaparib in triple-negative breast cancer cells. Breast Cancer Res. https://doi.org/10.1186/s13058-015-0534-y

75. Yuan Z, Chen S, Sun Q, Wang N, Li D, Miao S, Gao C, Chen Y, Tan C, Jiang Y (2017) Olaparib hydroxamic acid derivatives as dual PARP and HDAC inhibitors for cancer therapy. Bioorg Med Chem 25:4100–4109

76. Truong S, Ghaidi F, Ramos L, Joshi J, Brown D, Sankar N, Langlands J, Bacha J, Shen W, Daugaard M (2021) Abstract P081: In vitro activity and efficacy of novel dual PARP-HDAC inhibitors. Mol Cancer Ther 20:P081–P081

77. Schopf FH, Biebl MM, Buchner J (2017) The HSP90 chaperone machinery. Nat Rev Mol Cell Biol 18:345–360

78. Johnson N, Johnson SF, Yao W et al (2013) Stabilization of mutant BRCA1 protein confers PARP inhibitor and platinum resistance. Proc Natl Acad Sci U S A 110:17041–17046

79. Stecklein SR, Kumaraswamy E, Behbod F, Wang W, Chaguturu V, Harlan-Williams LM, Jensen RA (2012) BRCA1 and HSP90 cooperate in homologous and non-homologous DNA double-strand-break repair and G2/M checkpoint activation. Proc Natl Acad Sci U S A 109:13650–13655

80. Lee Y, Li HK, Masaoka A, Sunada S, Hirakawa H, Fujimori A, Nickoloff JA, Okayasu R (2016) The purine scaffold Hsp90 inhibitor PU-H71 sensitizes cancer cells to heavy ion radiation by inhibiting DNA repair by homologous recombination and non-homologous end joining. Radiother Oncol 121:162–168

81. Gabbasov R, Benrubi ID, O'Brien SW, Krais JJ, Johnson N, Litwin S, Connolly DC (2019) Targeted blockade of HSP90 impairs DNA-damage response proteins and increases the sensitivity of ovarian carcinoma cells to PARP inhibition. Cancer Biol Ther 20:1035–1045

82. Choi YE, Battelli C, Watson J, Liu J, Curtis J, Morse AN, Matulonis UA, Chowdhury D, Konstantinopoulos PA (2014) Sublethal concentrations of 17-AAG suppress homologous recombination DNA repair and enhance sensitivity to carboplatin and olaparib in HR proficient ovarian cancer cells. Oncotarget 5:2678–2687

83. Xu J, Wu P-J, Lai T-H et al (2022) Disruption of DNA repair and survival pathways through heat shock protein inhibition by onalespib to sensitize malignant gliomas to chemoradiation therapy. Clin Cancer Res. clincanres.0468.2020

84. McLaughlin M, Barker HE, Khan AA et al (2017) HSP90 inhibition sensitizes head and neck cancer to platin-based chemoradiotherapy by modulation of the DNA damage response resulting in chromosomal fragmentation. BMC Cancer. https://doi.org/10.1186/s12885-017-3084-0

85. Balaji K, Vijayaraghavan S, Diao L et al (2017) AXL inhibition suppresses the DNA damage response and sensitizes cells to PARP inhibition in multiple cancers. Mol Cancer Res 15:45–58

86. Mullen MM, Lomonosova E, Toboni MD et al (2022) GAS6/AXL inhibition enhances ovarian cancer sensitivity to chemotherapy and PARP inhibition through increased DNA damage and enhanced replication stress. Mol Cancer Res 20:265–279

87. Brand TM, Iida M, Stein AP et al (2015) AXL is a logical molecular target in head and neck squamous cell carcinoma. Clin Cancer Res 21:2601–2612

88. Flem-Karlsen K, McFadden E, Omar N, Haugen MH, Oy GF, Ryder T, Gullestad HP, Hermann R, Mælandsmo GM, Flørenes VA (2020) Targeting AXL and the DNA damage response pathway as a novel therapeutic strategy in melanoma. Mol Cancer Ther 19:895–905

89. Kariolis MS, Miao YR, Diep A et al (2017) Inhibition of the GAS6/AXL pathway augments the efficacy of chemotherapies. J Clin Investig 127:183–198
90. Quinn JM, Greenwade MM, Palisoul ML et al (2019) Therapeutic inhibition of the receptor tyrosine kinase AXL improves sensitivity to platinum and taxane in ovarian cancer. Mol Cancer Ther 18:389–398
91. Ramkumar K, Stewart CA, Cargill KR et al (2021) AXL inhibition induces DNA damage and replication stress in non-small cell lung cancer cells and promotes sensitivity to ATR inhibitors. Mol Cancer Res 19:485–497

Combination DNA Damage Response (DDR) Inhibitors to Overcome Drug Resistance in Ovarian Cancer

Dimitrios Nasioudis, Erin M. George, Haineng Xu, Hyoung Kim, and Fiona Simpkins

11.1 Introduction

The DNA damage response (DDR) results in the activation of a series of key target kinases such as ATM, ATR, CHK1/2, DNA-PK and WEE1 that response to different DNA damage insults (Yap et al. 2015; Khanna et al. 2001). DNA double strand breaks (DSB) activate ATM and DNA-dependent protein kinases while accumulation of single stranded DNA breaks will active ATR and the downstream CHK1 and WEE1 (Caldecott et al. 2014; Bakkenist et al. 2003; Bartek et al. 2007). DNA damage response coordinates cell-cycle progression and permits DNA repair [1]. Tumor cells rely on these pathways to trigger cell cycle arrest cell, stall replication forks and permit DNA repair thus maintaining genomic stability. Inhibition of these pathways permits cell cycle progression, stalled replication forks leading to DNA replication stress and accumulation of DNA damage, ultimately triggering

D. Nasioudis · E. M. George · H. Xu · H. Kim · F. Simpkins (✉)
Division of Gynecologic Oncology, Department of Obstetrics and Gynecology, Perelman School of Medicine, Ovarian Cancer Research Center, University of Pennsylvania, Philadelphia, PA 19104, USA
e-mail: fiona.simpkins@pennmedicine.upenn.edu

D. Nasioudis
e-mail: dimitrios.nasioudis@pennmedicine.upenn.edu

E. M. George
e-mail: erin.george@pennmedicine.upenn.edu

H. Xu
e-mail: haineng@pennmedicine.upenn.edu

H. Kim
e-mail: hyoungk@pennmedicine.upenn.edu

© The Author(s), under exclusive license to Springer Nature Switzerland AG 2023
T. A. Yap and G. I. Shapiro (eds.), *Targeting the DNA Damage Response for Cancer Therapy*, Cancer Treatment and Research 186,
https://doi.org/10.1007/978-3-031-30065-3_11

apoptosis if DNA damage is irreparable [2]. Certain tumors have higher levels of DNA replication stress such as those with oncogene activation (e.g. *CCNE1* amplification, *KRAS* mutations) or *BRCA1/2* mutations, which sensitize cancer cells to agents targeting DNA damage response (Primo et al. 2019).

Monotherapy activity of DDR targeting agents such as PARP inhibitors (PARPi), ATR/CHK1/WEE1 inhibitors, usually correlate with the underlying tumor mutational profile (e.g. PARPi in HRD deficient tumors, WEE1 inhibitors [WEE1i] in *CCNE1* amplified tumors, and ATR inhibitors [ATRi] in ATM deficient tumors) but responses are often not durable even for biomarker-selected populations [3–5]. In addition, emergence of resistance to monotherapy for oncogene-addicted tumors is almost universal [6]. Identification of patients with tumors harboring specific DNA alterations that increase DNA replication stress (referred to any condition that compromises the fidelity of genome replication) may allow lower dose strategies making combinations tolerable without jeopardizing antitumor activity. For example, homologous recombination deficient (HRD) tumors as well as *CCNE1* amplified tumors are characterized by high levels of replication stress and represent a population that could benefit from DDR inhibitor combinations (DDR-DDR). *CCNE1* amplified ovarian tumors are typically platinum-resistant and carry an extremely poor prognosis. Moreover, with the widespread adoption of PARPi for HRD tumors, overcoming resistance is another clinically unmet need. In the present chapter we discuss rationale of DDR-DDR strategies that capitalize on genomic alterations found in ovarian cancer and may provide in the near future, new treatment options for these patients.

11.2   Mechanisms of Resistance to PARPi

Resistance to PARPi can be classified into HR-dependent and HR-independent mechanisms [3]. HR-independent mechanisms include upregulation of drug efflux pumps, alteration of PARP activity and activation of alterative pathways such as RAS/RAF/MEK, and PI3K/AKT pathways. Although, preclinical work has identified, overexpression of drug-efflux transporter genes (e.g. *ABCB1*, *ABCD1*, and *ABCG2*) and subsequent decreased cellular availability of PARPi as a resistance mechanism, the clinical significance of this resistance of this mechanism has yet to be elucidated. For HR-proficient cells (or cells with residual BRCA1 activity secondary to hypomorphic *BRCA1* mutations) emergence of *PARP1* mutations can decrease protein binding to DNA (PARP trapping) or preserve the endogenous functions of the enzyme when bound to a PARPi leading to the emergence of PARPi resistance [7]. PARG is responsible for degradation of PAR chains from target proteins. PARG loss can restore PARylation, diminish PARP1 trapping and lead to PARPi resistance [8]. Again, the clinical significance of this resistance mechanism is not well established.

HR-dependent mechanisms of resistance to PAPRi are clinically relevant given the widespread adoption of PARPi for HRD tumors and include: (i) reversion of HR gene mutations, (ii) HR pathway rewiring facilitating BRCA1 independent end resection, and (iii) stabilization of the DNA replication forks [3]. Reversion of HR gene mutations and restoration of DNA repair function has been observed in the clinic as a major PARP resistance mechanism (Domchek et al. 2017), [9]. Since most mutations in the *BRCA1/2* genes are single-nucleotide mutations or short insertions/deletions leading to frameshifts, under selection pressure, tumors can acquire secondary reversion mutations leading to frame-restoration and restored protein function. Reversion mutations in other HRD genes such as *RAD51C, RAD51D,* and *PALB2* have also been described (Noordermeer et al. 2019). Demethylation of the hypermethylated *BRCA1* gene promoter has also been described [10]. Another HR-dependent resistance mechanism is reactivation of the HR pathway by rewiring facilitating BRCA1-independent end resection; loss of proteins involved in non-homologous end joining (NHEJ; TP53BP1, RIF1 and REV7) suppress the HR-counteracting pathway leading to PARPi resistance [11]. Another important resistance mechanism in HRD tumors is stabilization of the stalled DNA replication forks [12, 13]. Cell cycle arrest triggered by DNA damage permits tumor cells to repair DNA by recruiting BRCA1/2 that stabilizes and protects the stalled replication fork. For *BRCA1/2* mutant tumors, EZH2 and PTIP recruit the nucleases MRE11 and MUS81 that degrade the replication forks leading to chromosomal aberrations [13], (Lemacon et al. 2018). Fork collapse is potentiated by PARPi. Resistance to PARPi can occur following fork reversal by chromatin remodelers (e.g. SMARCAL1, ZRANB3, HLTF), by EZH2-mediated methylation of H3K27, by methylation of H3K4 or by loss of SLFN11, a replication stress effector (Noordermeer et al. 2019). It should be underlined that clinically, PARPi resistance can be multifactorial since multiple resistance mechanisms can be observed following PARPi progression. Restoration of HR and replication fork protection can simultaneously occur during the process of PARPi resistance [11].

11.2.1 Strategies to Overcome PARP-Resistance with DDR-DDR Combinations

PARPi have revolutionized the treatment landscape of ovarian cancer. Following success in the recurrent setting, over the past few years PARPi has moved to frontline maintenance treatment. It is currently standard of care for patients with HRD tumors to receive PARPi maintenance with remarkable prolongation of progression-free interval (Washington et al. 2021), [14]; however, resistance ultimately emerges. Although there is less clinical benefit in HR proficient tumors [15] it is anticipated that most ovarian cancer patients will receive a PARPi either as maintenance or in the recurrent setting. Understanding and battling PARPi resistance is a clinically unmet need. A recent phase III blind randomized trial (OReO/ ENGOT Ov-38) examined the role of PARPi maintenance in platinum-sensitive recurrent ovarian cancer who had previously received PARPi [16]. Among patients with *BRCA1/2* mutations, only a modest increase in PFS was observed after platinum doublet followed by PARPi maintenance treatment compared to placebo (median PFS 4.3 vs. 2.8 months, HR 0.57 (95% CI: 0.37, 0.87) suggesting that novel strategies to overcome PARPi resistance are needed [16]. DDR-DDR combinations is a rationale strategy to overcome multiple resistance mechanisms and could provide a therapeutic avenue for these patients.

ATR is activated by replication stress, stabilizes replication forks and causes cell cycle arrest at the S and G2-M checkpoints that permit DNA repair (Fig. 11.1). ATR inhibition (ATRi) can result in replication fork collapse and generation of DSB (Dunwala et al. 2015). ATRi also results in the loss of the G2/M checkpoint that allows tumor cells with damaged DNA to progress prematurely into M phase leasing to mitotic catastrophe and apoptosis [17]. Treatment with PARPi results in generation of DSB that are repaired by HR requiring BRCA1/2 proteins. PARPi resistant cells regain the ability of RAD51 loading to DNA double strand breaks and stalled replication forks and become heavily dependent on the ATR pathway to maintain genomic integrity (Kim et al. 2020), [11]. For these tumors, ATRi further disrupts HR repair and fork protection leading to replication fork collapse and bypass PARPi resistance (Kim et al. 2020), [11]. Interestingly, among PARPi resistant tumor cells lines, ATR pathway activation was more pronounced in cell lines with acquired PARPi resistance (Kim et al. 2020). The combination of PARPi-ATRi (PARPi, olaparib and ATRi, ceralasertib) demonstrated strong in vitro synergy across multiple PARPi resistant cell lines and various genetic contexts (e.g. *BRCA1/2* reversions, *CCNE1* amplification). ATRi re-sensitizes PARPi/platinum-resistant cells by impairing HR (Kim et al. 2020). In addition, in PDX models, the combination of PARPi-ATRi led to durable tumor regression in PARPi-resistant models as well as platinum-resistant PDX models derived from *BRCA1/2* mutant patients (Kim et al. 2020).

The strong preclinical evidence supported the further exploration of PARP–ATR inhibitor combinations in clinical trials targeting PARPi resistance in the HRD ovarian cancer. In the ceralasertib-olaparib arm of the exploratory OLAPCO basket trial that enrolled patients with tumor mutations in HR and other DDR genes included 7 patients with high-grade serous ovarian cancer and *BRCA1/2* mutations who had received prior PARPi and had progressed during their most recent PARPi treatment. In that group the ORR was 14% (n = 1) while the clinical benefit rate was 85.7% (n = 6). A multicohort non-randomized trial (CAPRI, NCT03462342) examines the safety and efficacy of dual PARPi-ATRi (olaparib-ceralasertib) in recurrent HGSOC. A total of 13 patients with *BRCA1/2* mutations or tumors with evidence of HRD (Cohort C) and platinum-sensitive disease who benefited but then progressed on PARPi at their last therapy, received a median of 8 cycles. Based on 12 patients, the ORR was 50% (6 partial responses) with a median PFS of 7.5 months. Overall, the toxicity profile of the combination was acceptable (31% grade 3 toxicity; 23% grade 3 thrombocytopenia, 8% anemia and 8% neutropenia) with no patient discontinuing treatment secondary to toxicity [18]. The cohort had received a median of 3 prior lines of therapy and had been on PARPi for a median of 13 months (range 4–60 months) while the majority (84.6%) had progressed while on PARPi. Multiple other early clinical trials are currently open to enrollment and if preclinical evidence is confirmed in phase II/III trials, in

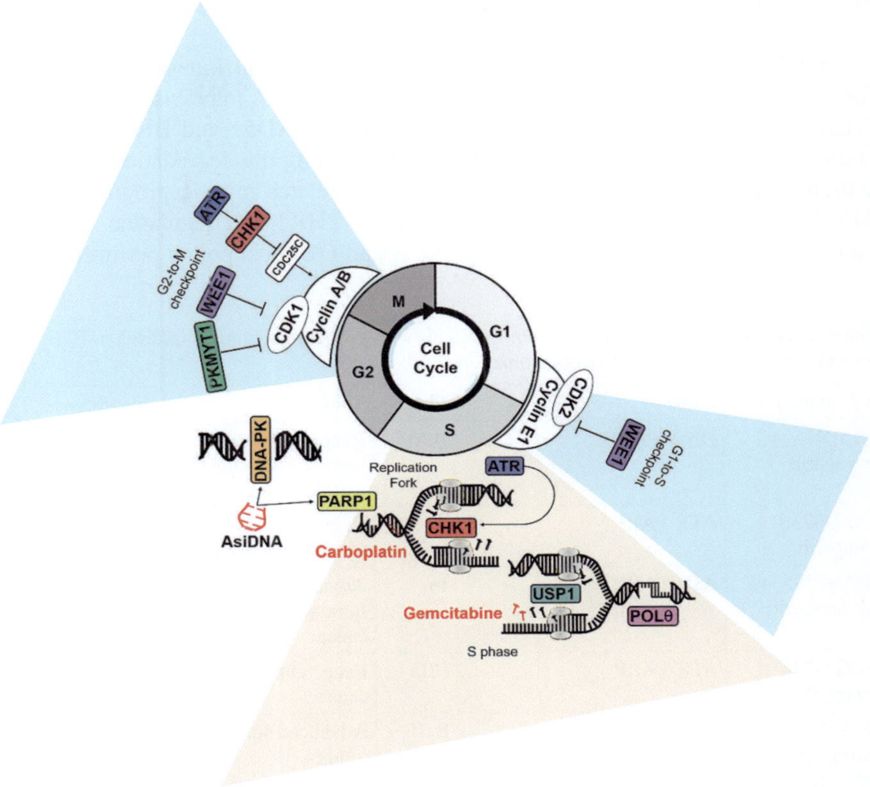

Fig. 11.1 DDR targets for combination strategies. Available DDR inhibitors have different roles in affecting the cell cycle and DNA damage repair. WEE1 acts at both G1/S and G2/M checkpoints by phosphorylation of CDK1 and CDK2. Inhibition of WEE1 leads to hyper-activation of the Cyclin E1—CDK2 complex leading to dysregulation at the G1/S checkpoint and also premature entry into M-phase because of its role in regulating the Cyclin A/B—CDK1 complex. ATR/CHK1, while also playing a role to halt DNA progression at the G2/M checkpoint to allow time for DNA repair, also helps stabilize replication forks in S phase. PKMYT1, similar to WEE1, phosphorylates CDK1 at the G2/M checkpoint to regulate cell cycle entry into M phase. DNA-PK can act through all phases of the cell cycle to help promote double strand break (DSB) repair through NHEJ. PARP1 is involved in single strand break (SSB) repair. When inhibited during S phase, there is an accumulation of SSBs, which will lead to DSBs, which then need to be repaired by homologous recombination. In BRCA1 deficient tumor cells, Ubiquitin Specific Protease—1 (USP1) is localized at the replication fork and is pivotal for its protection and stabilization. USP1 inhibition is synthetically lethal with BRCA1 deficiency. POLθ is a DNA repair enzyme required for double strand break (DSB) repair through MMEJ. DNA-PK can act through all phases of the cell cycle to help promote DSB repair through NHEJ. AsiDNA is a double-helix DNA molecule that mimics DSBs and leads to hyperactivation of PARP1 and DNA-PK, which prevents detection of DNA breaks and recruitment of proteins involved in HR and NHEJ. Chemotherapies can also interfere with DDR. Gemcitabine exacerbates replication stress by incorporation into DNA and also inhibits ribonucleotide reductase leading to depletion of deoxyribonucleotide pools. Carboplatin causes intra- and inter-strand crosslinks in DNA, which interferes with DNA damage and repair

the near future, PARPi-ATRi may become a treatment option to overcome PARPi resistance (Table 11.1).

CHK1, downstream of ATR, is a cell cycle checkpoint kinase that is critical for HR repair (Fig. 11.1; Sorensen et al. 2005). CHK1 interacts and phosphorylates RAD51 facilitating the interaction between RAD51 and BRCA2 [19]. In addition, CHK1 induces cell cycle arrest by facilitating the degradation or sequestration of CDC25 phosphatases, while it also regulates mitotic progression [20, 21]. Following DNA damage and activation of CHK1 and regulation of CDK2 and CDK1, cell cycle arrests occurs at the S and G2 checkpoints permitting time

Table 11.1 Active clinical trials enrolling patients with gynecologic tumors (phase I or II) or solid tumors (phase I) exploring DDRi combinations

Combination	Class	Phase	Tumors	Identifier
AsiDNA + niraparib	Dbait-PARP	Ib/II	Recurrent platinum-sensitive ovarian cancer	NCT04826198
AZD6738 + olaparib	ATR-PARP	II	Relapsed gynecological tumors	NCT04065269
BAY1895344 + niraparib	ATR-PARP	Ib	Advanced solid tumors and ovarian cancer	NCT04267939
AZD6738 + olaparib	ATR-PARP	I/IIa	Recurrent ovarian cancer	NCT03462342
RP-3500 + niraparib or olaparib	ATR-PARP	Ib/II	Advanced solid tumors	NCT04972110
M1774 + niraparib	ATR-PARP	I	Metastatic or locally advanced unresectable solid tumors	NCT04170153
Adavosertib + olaparib	WEE1-PARP	II	Recurrent ovarian cancer progressed on PARPi	NCT03579316
ZN-c3 + niraparib	WEE1-PARP	I/II	Platinum-resistant ovarian cancer	NCT05198804
RP-6306 + Gemcitabine	PKMYT1—chemotherapy	I	Advanced solid tumors	NCT05147272
RP-6306 + RP-3500	PKYT1—ATR	I	Advanced solid tumors	NCT04855656
KSQ-4279 + PARPi	USP1—PARP	I	Advanced solid tumors	NCT05240898
ART4215 + talazoparib or niraparib	Pol theta—PARP	I/IIa	Advanced or metastatic solid tumors	NCT04991480

for DNA repair (Dai et al. 2010). To maintain genome integrity, HR-deficient high-grade serous ovarian cancer cells, heavily rely on an intact ATR/CHK1 pathway to allow adequate time for DNA repair [22]. In patient-derived xenograft models established from PARPi resistant *BRCA1* mutant tumors that demonstrated HR restoration, CHK1/CHK2 inhibition (CHKi) with prexasertib exhibited monotherapy activity (Parmar et al. 2019). In addition, in *BRCA1*-mutant PARPi resistant high-grade serous ovarian cancer tumor cells, prexasertib was able reverse stabilization of replication forks likely by preventing RAD51 accumulation at sites of stalling and also compromise HR repair (Parmar et al. 2019). Combination of olaparib with CHK1i was also in vitro markedly synergistic in a *BRCA1* mutant ovarian cancer cell line rendered resistant to olaparib following long-term exposure [23]. Given the strong preclinical evidence demonstrating that CHK1 can target HR restoration and replication fork protection, two major PARP resistance mechanisms in HR-deficient cells, a recent phase I trial explored the combination of olaparib (PARPi) and prexasertib (CHK1i) in high-grade serous ovarian cancer and other solid tumors, using an attenuated course of olaparib to avoid overlapping hematologic toxicities [24]. A patient expansion cohort included HGSOC patients with *BRCA1/2* mutations who had received at least 6 months of prior PARPi and derived clinical benefit. A total of 29 patients were enrolled and the most common dose-limiting toxicities were grade 3 neutropenia and febrile neutropenia. The recommended phase 2 dose was 70 mg/m^2 IV for prexasertib and olaparib 100 mg twice daily [24]. Paired tumor biopsies further elucidated the mechanism of action. Following combination treatment, CHK1 mediated modulation of HR repair was observed by reduction of RAD51 foci formation and induction of replicative stress leading to increased replication stress. In the cohort of patients with *BRCA1/2*-mutant, PARP-resistant HGSOC (n = 18) encouraging antitumor activity was observed with 4 (22%) patients achieving a partial response while 10 (56%) patients remained on the study for at least 4 cycles [24]. These patients were heavily pretreated with the majority progressing within 6 months on first-line platinum-based chemotherapy while tumor biopsies demonstrated HR restoration as the mechanism of resistance to PARPi. By preventing RAD51 foci formation and RAD51 transnuclear localization, CHK1i can enhance the anti-tumor activity of PAPRi in *BRCA1/2* wild-type high-grade serous ovarian cancer models [25], (Parmar et al. 2019). For *BRCA1/2* proficient HGSOC cells, inhibition of CHK1/CHK2 by prexasertib can lead to an impaired G2/M checkpoint and a mitotic catastrophe in the presence of a PARPi [26]. It should be noted that heavily pretreated tumors may be less responsive to CHK1i, secondary to downregulation of cyclin B [27]. In addition, FAM122A expression level can serve as a biomarker predicting CHK1i sensitivity, since loss of FAM122A expression is associated with resistance to ATR-CHK1 inhibition secondary to WEE1 stabilization [27, 28].

As previously discussed, PARPi induce DNA damage and cell dependency on S-phase and G2/M checkpoint regulation. WEE1, down stream of ATR and CHK1 through phosphorylation of CDK2 and CDK1 prevents cell cycle progression from G1 to S and from S/G2 to M (Fig. 11.1). Inhibition of WEE1 can lead cancer cells with unrepaired DNA alterations to enter mitosis prematurely resulting in a mitotic catastrophe [29]. Also, WEE1 inhibition increases replication stress through uncontrolled firing of replication origins and nucleotide starvation leads to genomic instability [30]. While PARPi induces two key mitotic gatekeepers (CDC2Y15 and FOXM1), a decrease in expression is observed when combined with WEE1i [31]. PARPi induces G2 cell cycle arrest, however WEE1i is able to promote entry into M phase and override the effects of PARPi [31]. While the combination of WEE1i-PARPi has demonstrated synergy across multiple tumors models [32–34] dual WEEi-PARPi is also a rational strategy to overcome PARPi resistance. As previously discussed, overlapping toxicity profiles is a major limitation of DDR-DDR combinations. A phase I dose escalation clinical trial examining the combination of adavosertib with olaparib in 119 patients with refractory solid tumors reported a high incidence of grade 3+ hematologic toxicity (anemia 23.5%, neutropenia 21.8% and thrombocytopenia 16.8%). However, antitumor activity was observed (ORR 11.1% in the total population) while activity was noted in both *BRCA1/2* mutant and wild-type tumors. A recently presented phase II non-comparative study (EFFORT trial) enrolled patients with recurrent PARPi-resistant ovarian cancer and randomized to adavosertib with (n = 35) or without olaparib (n = 35) [35]. It should be noted that benefit from prior PARPi was not required while intervening chemotherapy following PARPi was permitted and eligibility was agnostic to HRD status. ORR in the monotherapy and combination arms was 23% and 29% with a clinical benefit rate of 63% and 89% respectively. Median duration of response was 5.5 months in the adavosertib arm and 6.4 months in the combination arm. A high incidence of grade 3/4 toxicity was observed (76%) in the combination arm compared to monotherapy (51%); most commonly involving thrombocytopenia (20%) and neutropenia (15%). A total of 36 (88%) of patients required at least one dose interruption, while 29 (71%) required dose reduction, and 4 (10%) did not restart due to toxicity [35].

Preclinical work using ovarian cancer PDX models has demonstrated that following cessation of monotherapy treatment with PARPi or WEE1i, the effects of the inhibitors persist, as such sequential treatment can be as efficacious as concurrent treatment while ameliorating the toxicity of the combination [31]. Presence of high levels of endogenous replication stress only in tumor cells but not normal cells is key for the efficacy of the combination [31]. The sequential combination of olaparib followed by adavosertib is being currently evaluated in a phase I trial (STAR study, NCT04197713) that is enrolling patients with advanced solid tumors with PARPi resistance. Patients are eligible if they have germline or somatic mutations in *BRCA1/2* genes and evidence of progression at their 1st restaging while on PARPi (intrinsic resistance) as well as patients with germline or somatic mutation in any of the DDR genes (*BRCA1, BRCA2, BRIP1, FANCA, PALB2*) or *CCNE1* amplification who had prior complete or partial response to PARPi (acquired resistance). Patients are receiving olaparib twice daily on days 1–5 and 15–19 of each cycle and adavosertib once daily on days 8–12 and 22–26 of each cycle.

AsiDNA is a double-helix DNA molecule that mimics a double-strand break and is part of a new class of DNA damage repair pathway inhibitors, Dbait [36]. AsiDNA acting as an agonist, hyper-activates PARP1 and DNA-PK, prevents the detection of DNA breaks and recruitment of other proteins involved in HR and NHEJ, thus disorganizing the DNA damage response. In vitro AsiDNA increases the efficacy of PARP inhibition across multiple cancer cell lines irrespective of their *BRCA1/2* or HRD status without exerting additive toxic effect on normal cells [37]. The combination of AsiDNA and olaparib induced a transient HRD status and prevented the recruitment of XRCC1 and RAD51/53BP1 enzymes at areas of DNA damage [37, 38]. Interestingly, AsiDNA potentiated the effect of PARPi irrespective of their mechanism of action suggesting that trapping of PARP on DNA is not required. Moreover, *in vitro* treatment with AsiDNA abrogated PARPi resistance emerged following repeated exposure to PARPi [38]. Since acquired resistance to AsiDNA is less likely to occur, the combination of PARPi-AsiDNA is an attractive option for patients who have previously received PARPi. A phase IB/II (NCT04826198) is currently evaluating the safety of the combination of AsiDNA and niraparib (PARPi) in patients with relapsed platinum-sensitive ovarian cancer that have already received a prior line of PARP for at least 6 months (Table 11.1).

Although DDR-DDR combinations demonstrate encouraging activity to overcome multiple PARPi resistance mechanisms further studies are required to define the optimal biomarker that will drive their use in the clinic. In addition, overlapping toxicity profiles require non-conventional dosing regimens and limit their clinical application. However, with the introduction of the next generation PARP1 selective inhibitors (such as AZD5305 that recently demonstrated acceptable safety and efficacy in the phase I/II PETRA trial), DDR combinations using PARPi may be more tolerable [39].

11.2.2 DDR Inhibitor Combinations in the Setting of Platinum-Resistance

Patients with high-grade serous ovarian cancer initially respond to platinum-based chemotherapy. However, after multiple lines of treatment, platinum-resistance ultimately emerges. Prognosis of patients with platinum-resistant ovarian cancer is poor and novel treatment options are urgently needed [40]. DDR combinations are a strategy to exploit the unique genomic alterations of high-grade serous ovarian cancer that are characterized by a high incidence of Cyclin E overexpression and increased replication stress (Karst et al. 2014). CCNE1 complexes with CDK2 to promote cell-cycle progression from G1 to S phase and its overexpression promotes premature entry into S phase resulting in increased stress at the replication forks and double-strand DNA breaks (Fig. 11.1; Jones et al. 2013). Along the DDR pathway, WEE1 is an attractive target for *TP53* mutant tumors such as high-grade serous ovarian cancer cells given that loss of p53 regulation of the G1 checkpoint results in increased reliance on the G2 checkpoint controlled by WEE1 (Kawabe et al. 2004). WEE1 through phosphorylation of CDK2 and CDK1, prevents cell cycle progression from G1 to S and from S/G2 to M and protects the stability of stalled DNA replication forks (Heald et al. 1992; Elbaek). Inhibition of WEE1 can lead cancer cells with unrepaired DNA alterations to enter mitosis prematurely resulting in a mitotic catastrophe [41]. Also, WEE1 inhibition increases replication stress through uncontrolled firing of replication origins and nucleotide starvation leads to genomic instability [30].

Given that WEE1i leads to premature mitotic entrance of tumor cells with unrepaired DNA alterations, combination of WEE1i with DNA-damaging chemotherapy agents such as carboplatin (causes intra and inter-stand DNA cross-links) is a rational approach to potentiate the effects of chemotherapy and overcome resistance to platinum. Combinations of WEE1i with chemotherapy have already been explored in the setting of recurrent platinum resistant disease demonstrating encouraging results. The majority of trials examine the safety and efficacy of adavosertib in combination of chemotherapy. In a proof-of-principle phase II trial enrolling 24 patients with recurrent platinum-resistant or refractory *TP53* mutated ovarian cancer that evaluated the combination of carboplatin (AUC5) with adavosertib (225 mg twice daily over 2.5 days every 21-day cycle), based on 21 patients the ORR was 43% with a median PFS and OS of 5.3 and 12.6 months respectively, though hematologic toxicity was significant with 48% having grade 4 thrombocytopenia and 39% grade ≥ 3 neutropenia [42]. An open label four arm multicenter phase II study enrolled 94 patients with primary platinum-resistant ovarian cancer and evaluated the addition of adavosertib to gemcitabine, carboplatin, pactitaxel and gemcitabine (Moore et al. 2021). A signal of efficacy was observed in the combination of adavosertib with carboplatin with a ORR of 66.7% and a median PFS of 12 months among patients in the C2 arm (n = 12) who received adavosertib 225 mg twice daily on days 1–3,, 8–10, 15–17 and carboplatin AUC5 on day 1 of a 21 day cycle. Another phase II randomized trial enrolling 99 patients with platinum-resistant or refractory high-grade serous ovarian cancer evaluated the addition of adavosertib administered as 175 mg/po on D1-2, D8-9 and D15-16 of a 28 cycle to gemcitabine (1000 mg/m^2) and demonstrated improved PFS (median 4.6 vs. 3.0 months, HR 0.56, 95% CI: 0.35–0.90), partial response rate (21% vs. 3%, $p = 0.02$) and OS (median 11.5 vs. 7.2 months, HR 0.56, 95% CI: 0.34, 0.92) compared to placebo [43]. Grade 3 or worse hematological toxicities were more common in the combination arm and included neutropenia (62% vs. 30%), and thrombocytopenia (31% vs. 6%). In all aforementioned trials, incidence of grade ≥ 3 hematologic toxicity was high. In a dose escalation phase I trial, a novel WEE1 inhibitor (ZN-c3) demonstrated improved bone marrow toxicity with less than 10% of patients experiencing hematologic toxicities [44]. A phase IB dose escalation trial evaluating the safety and preliminary clinical acitivity of ZN-c3 in combination with chemotherapy for heavily pretreated patients with platinum-resistant or refractory ovarian cancer, encouraging responses were observed in combination with carboplatin (n = 11, ORR 45.5%), and paclitaxel (n = 8, 62.5%) but not with pegylated-doxorubicin (n = 24, 12.5%). Combination was well tolerated with the rate of grade ≥ 3 neutropenia (34.1%), thrombocytopenia (17.1%) and anemia (9.8%) being relatively low compared to other WEE1i agents [45]. A fourth cohort exploring the combination of ZN-c3 with gemcitabine in the same patient population is anticipated to open enrollment soon.

Gemcitabine is a chemotherapy agent that inhibits DNA repair by incorporation in DNA helix and inhibits ribonucleotide reductase leading to depletion of deoxyribonucleotide pool utilized for DNA repair (de Sousa Cavalcante et al. 2014). As such, gemcitabine can exacerbate replication stress in high-grade serous ovarian cancer and is a rationale combination partner for other DDRi agents such as ATRi and WEEi. In a recent phase II trial enrolling 70 patients with platinum-resistant ovarian cancer (including 18 who previously received PARPi) the addition of ATRi (berzosertib) to gemcitabine was superior to gemcitabine alone (median PFS 22.9 vs. 14.7 weeks, $p = 0.044$) with no increase in the rate of serious adverse events (26% vs. 28%) [3].

Using a CRISPR synthetically lethal screen, PKYT1 inhibition has been recently identified as a synthetically lethal combination with CCNE1 amplification [46]. For CCNE1 overexpressing tumors, elevated DNA replication stress and MMB-FOXM1 transcription increase cyclin B-CDK1 levels and activity in S phase. Since PKMYT1 is a negative regulator of CDK1, PKYT1i can promote early mitosis in cells that undergo DNA synthesis leading to catastrophic genomic instability (Fig. 11.1, [46]). For CCNE1 overexpressing ovarian cancer tumor models, enhancement of replication stress with gemcitabine was highly synergistic with PKYT1i in vivo [46]. A phase I trial (MAGNETIC is now exploring the combination of gemcitabine with PKYT1i (RP-6306 in patients with advanced solid tumor (NCT05147272. PKMYT1 (RP-6306 is also being evaluated in combination with ATRi (RP-3500) in a Phase I trial (MYTHIC, NCT04855656).

CCNE1 overexpression also activates the ATR/CHK1/WEE1 signaling. Dual WEE1i-ATRi is synergistic in *CCNE1* amplified tumors that are characterized by high levels of replication stress. In tumor cells with high CCNE1 expression, induction with a low-dose of WEE1i leads to defective DNA replication at S-phase entry and increasing tumor cell reliance on ATR signaling for replication fork stability [4]. Addition of an ATRi increased M-phase entry and replication fork instability, leading to fork collapse in early S phase. ATRi also blocked the WEE1-mediated induction of the feedback loop. More importantly, dual WEE1i-ATRi required low doses to elicit robust antitumor effect sparing normal cells from treatment toxicity which is critical for moving the combination to the clinic. In vitro and in vivo experiments identified increased CCNE1 expression as a biomarker predictive of response to the combination of WEE1i-ATRi in ovarian and uterine cancer models. Promising antitumor activity of the WEE1i-ATRi combination has also been demonstrated in other biomarker unselected tumors [47, 48] (Bukhari et al. 2020).

11.3 Other DDR-DDR Combinations

DNA-PK is a protein part of the PI3K-related kinase family that is pivotal in the classic non-homologous end joining (NHEJ) DNA repair process (Fig. 11.1) [49]. Following binding of the Ku70/Ku80 heterodimer complex in double-stranded

DNA break ends, DNA-Pks are recruited and activated following autophospory-lation that leads to recruitment of other complexes such as the endonuclease ARTEMIS, gH2AX and XRCC4 [50]. DNA-PKcs are also involved in DNA repli-cation stress response through phosphorylation of RPA32 [51]. Repair of DSB generated from topoisomerase inhibitors or ionizing radiation heavily relies on DNA-PKcs [52]. Several DNA-PKcs inhibitors have been previously developed but their clinical application has been limited secondary to a poor in vivo phar-macokinetic profile and lack of selectivity [53]. However, a new generation of DNA-PKcs are currently being explored AZD7648, nedisertib, CC-115, samo-tolisib, voxtalisib [54]. Inhibition of NHEJ may represent an important strategy for HR proficient tumors. Loss of *ATM* gene was associated with sensitivity to a DNA-PKc inhibitor (AZD7648) [52]. Combination of AZD7648 and olaparib was synergistic in ATM-deficient preclinical models, however the combination with doxorubicin was selected for further evaluation in a phase I trial (NCT03907969).

ATM is a key serine/threonine phosphoinositide 3-kinase-related protein kinase involved in DDR by orchestrating homologous recombination following activation by DSBs. Activation of ATM potentiates the DNA-damage signal and generates dockings sites for other proteins such as BRCA1 [55]. In addition, ATM can con-trol cell cycle following generation of DNA damage; activation of ATM results in an increase of p21 levels and G1 arrest as well as activation of CHK1/2 and G2 arrest. Sensitivity of ATM deficient tumors (such as prostate cancer) to ionizing radiation as well as PARPi has been previously demonstrated, however only a small fraction of tumors harbor ATM gene mutations. *In vitro* for ATM proficient tumor cells, combination of ATMi and PARPi was synergistic and resulted in G2-M cell cycle arrest, and cell growth inhibition [56, 57]. In preclinical tumor models, ATMi created a DDR-deficient phenotype and potentiated the anti-tumor effects of olaparib both *in vitro* across multiple cell lines and well as *in vivo* in two triple-negative breast cancer tumor models [57]. A phase I trial evaluating the safety and efficacy of escalating doses of ATMi (AZD0156) as monotherapy or in com-bination with chemotherapy (FOLFIRI) or olaparib has been recently concluded (NCT02588105) and results are awaited. As previously discussed, DNA-PKcs are involved in c-nNHEJ as such dual ATM and DNA-PKc inhibition could be syn-thetically lethal. For ATM-defective tumor cells DNA-PKcs inhibition results in accumulation of DSB and generation of ssDNA repair intermediates that trigger apoptotic pathways.

USP1 is also another emerging target involved in the DDR pathway that is overexpressed in *BRCA1* deficient tumors promoting the stabilization of repli-cation forks [58]. USP1 inhibition with KSQ-4279 had antitumor activity either as monotherapy or in combination with PARP inhibitors in ovarian cancer PDX models [59]. A phase I clinical trial explores KSQ-4279 as monotherapy or in combination with PARPi or platinum-based chemotherapy (NCT05240898). DNA polymerase theta (Polθ) is a multifunctional DNA repair enzyme with dual poly-merase and helicase activity required for the repair of dsDNA strand breaks through Microhomology-mediated End Joining [60, 61]. Polθ is overexpressed in tumors with homologous recombination deficiency serving as an alternative mechanism of DSB repair. Inhibition of Polθ is synthetic lethal with HR, in vitro and in vivo. In addition, Polθ inhibition can overcome or prevent acquired PARPi resistance [60, 61]. A phase I trial exploring ART4215 a Polθ inhibitor as monotherapy or in combination with PARPi are open to enrollment (NCT04991480).

References

1. Foster SS, De S, Johnson LK, Petrini JH, Stracker TH (2012) Cell cycle- and DNA repair pathway-specific effects of apoptosis on tumor suppression. Proc Natl Acad Sci U S A 109(25):9953–9958
2. Pearl LH, Schierz AC, Ward SE et al (2015) Therapeutic opportunities within the DNA damage response. Nat Rev Cancer 15:166–180
3. Konstantinopoulos PA, Cheng SC, Wahner Hendrickson AE et al (2020) Berzosertib plus gemcitabine versus gemcitabine alone in platinum-resistant high-grade serous ovarian cancer: a multicentre, open-label, randomised, phase 2 trial. Lancet Oncol 21(7):957–968. https://doi.org/10.1016/S1470-2045(20)30180-7. Epub 2020 Jun 15. PMID: 32553118; PMCID: PMC8023719
4. Xu H, George E, Kinose Y, Kim H, Shah JB, Peake JD, Ferman B, Medvedev S, Murtha T, Barger CJ, Devins KM, D'Andrea K, Wubbenhorst B, Schwartz LE, Hwang WT, Mills GB, Nathanson KL, Karpf AR, Drapkin R, Brown EJ, Simpkins F (2021) CCNE1 copy number is a biomarker for response to combination WEE1-ATR inhibition in ovarian and endometrial cancer models. Cell Rep Med. 2(9):100394
5. Rafiei S, Fitzpatrick K, Liu D, Cai MY, Elmarakeby HA, Park J, Ricker C, Kochupurakkal BS, Choudhury AD, Hahn WC, Balk SP, Hwang JH, Van Allen EM, Mouw KW (2020) ATM loss confers greater sensitivity to ATR inhibition than PARP inhibition in prostate cancer. Cancer Res 80(11):2094–2100
6. Lim SY, Menzies AM, Rizos H (2017) Mechanisms and strategies to overcome resistance to molecularly targeted therapy for melanoma. Cancer 123(S11):2118–2129
7. Pettitt SJ, Krastev DB, Brandsma I, Dréan A, Song F, Aleksandrov R, Harrell MI, Menon M, Brough R, Campbell J et al (2018) Genome-wide and high-density CRISPR-Cas9 screens identify point mutations in PARP1 causing PARP inhibitor resistance. Nat Commun 9:1849
8. Gogola E, Duarte AA, de Ruiter JR, Wiegant WW, Schmid JA, de Bruijn R, James DI, Guerrero Llobet S, Vis DJ, Annunziato S et al (2018) Selective loss of PARG restores PARylation and counteracts PARP inhibitor-mediated synthetic lethality. Cancer Cell 33(1078–93):e1012
9. Quigley D, Alumkal JJ, Wyatt AW, Kothari V, Foye A, Lloyd P, Aggarwal R, Kim W, Lu E, Schwartzman J, Beja K, Annala M, Das R, Diolaiti M, Pritchard C, Thomas G, Tomlins S, Knudsen K, Lord CJ, Ryan C, Youngren J, Beer TM, Ashworth A, Small EJ, Feng FY (2017) Analysis of circulating cell-free DNA identifies multiclonal heterogeneity of BRCA2 reversion mutations associated with resistance to PARP inhibitors. Cancer Discov 7(9):999–1005
10. Ter Brugge P et al (2016) Mechanisms of therapy resistance in patient-derived xenograft models of BRCA1-deficient breast cancer. J Natl Cancer Inst 108
11. Yazinski SA, Comaills V, Buisson R, Genois MM, Nguyen HD, Ho CK, Todorova Kwan T, Morris R, Lauffer S, Nussenzweig A, Ramaswamy S, Benes CH, Haber DA, Maheswaran S, Birrer MJ, Zou L (2017) ATR inhibition disrupts rewired homologous recombination and fork protection pathways in PARP inhibitor-resistant BRCA-deficient cancer cells. Genes Dev 31(3):318–332. https://doi.org/10.1101/gad.290957.116. Epub 2017 Feb 27. PMID: 28242626; PMCID: PMC5358727
12. Taglialatela A, Alvarez S, Leuzzi G, Sannino V, Ranjha L, Huang JW et al (2017) Restoration of replication fork stability in BRCA1- and BRCA2-deficient cells by inactivation of SNF2-family fork remodelers. Mol Cell 68:414-430.e8

13. Rondinelli B, Gogola E, Yücel H, Duarte AA, van de Ven M, van der Sluijs R et al (2017) EZH2 promotes degradation of stalled replication forks by recruiting MUS81 through histone H3 trimethylation. Nat Cell Biol 19:1371–1378

14. Moore K, Colombo N, Scambia G, Kim BG, Oaknin A, Friedlander M, Lisyanskaya A, Floquet A, Leary A, Sonke GS, Gourley C, Banerjee S, Oza A, González-Martín A, Aghajanian C, Bradley W, Mathews C, Liu J, Lowe ES, Bloomfield R, DiSilvestro P (2018) Maintenance olaparib in patients with newly diagnosed advanced ovarian cancer. N Engl J Med 379(26):2495–2505

15. González-Martín A, Pothuri B, Vergote I, DePont Christensen R, Graybill W, Mirza MR, McCormick C, Lorusso D, Hoskins P, Freyer G, Baumann K, Jardon K, Redondo A, Moore RG, Vulsteke C, O'Cearbhaill RE, Lund B, Backes F, Barretina-Ginesta P, Haggerty AF, Rubio-Pérez MJ, Shahin MS, Mangili G, Bradley WH, Bruchim I, Sun K, Malinowska IA, Li Y, Gupta D, Monk BJ (2019) PRIMA/ENGOT-OV26/GOG-3012 investigators. Niraparib in patients with newly diagnosed advanced ovarian cancer. N Engl J Med 381(25):2391–2402

16. Pujade-Lauraine E, Selle F, Scambia G et al (2021) Maintenance olaparib rechallenge in patients with ovarian carcinoma previously treated with a PARP inhibitor. Phase IIIb OReO/ENGOT OV-38 trial. In: ESMO congress 2021. Abstract LBA33. Presented September 18, 2021

17. Saldivar JC, Hamperl S, Bocek MJ, Chung M, Bass TE, Cisneros-Soberanis F, Samejima K, Xie L, Paulson JR, Earnshaw WC, Cortez D, Meyer T, Cimprich KA (2018) An intrinsic S/G2 checkpoint enforced by ATR. Science 361(6404):806–810. https://doi.org/10.1126/science.aap9346.PMID:30139873;PMCID:PMC6365305

18. Wethington SL, Shah PD, Martin LP, Tanyi JL, Latif NA, Morgan MA, Torigian DA, Pagan C, Rodriguez D, Domchek SM, Drapkin R, Shih Ie-M, Smith S, Dean E, Armstrong DK, Gaillard S, Simpkins F (2021) Combination of PARP and ATR inhibitors (olaparib and ceralasertib) shows clinical activity in acquired PARP inhibitor-resistant recurrent ovarian cancer. J Clin Oncol 39:(15_suppl):5516

19. Bahassi EM, Ovesen JL, Riesenberg AL, Bernstein WZ, Hasty PE, Stambrook PJ (2008) The checkpoint kinases Chk1 and Chk2 regulate the functional associations between hBRCA2 and Rad51 in response to DNA damage Oncogene 27(28):3977–3985

20. Wang JL, Wang X, Wang H, Iliakis G, Wang Y (2002) CHK1-regulated S-phase checkpoint response reduces camptothecin cytotoxicity. Cell Cycle 1(4):267–272

21. Tang J, Erikson RL, Liu X (2006) Checkpoint kinase 1 (Chk1) is required for mitotic progression through negative regulation of polo-like kinase 1 (Plk1). Proc Natl Acad Sci U S A 103(32):11964–11969

22. Gralewska P, Gajek A, Marczak A, Mikuła M, Ostrowski J, Śliwińska A, Rogalska A (2020) PARP inhibition increases the reliance on ATR/CHK1 checkpoint signaling leading to synthetic lethality-an alternative treatment strategy for epithelial ovarian cancer cells independent from HR effectiveness. Int J Mol Sci 21(24):9715. https://doi.org/10.3390/ijms21249715

23. Burgess BT, Anderson AM, McCorkle JR, Wu J, Ueland FR, Kolesar JM (2020) Olaparib combined with an ATR or Chk1 inhibitor as a treatment strategy for acquired olaparib-resistant BRCA1 mutant ovarian cells. Diagnostics (Basel) 10(2):121. https://doi.org/10.3390/diagnostics10020121.PMID:32098452;PMCID:PMC7168282

24. Do KT, Kochupurakkal B, Kelland S, de Jonge A, Hedglin J, Powers A, Quinn N, Gannon C, Vuong L, Parmar K, Lazaro JB, D'Andrea AD, Shapiro GI (2021) Phase 1 combination study of the CHK1 inhibitor prexasertib and the PARP inhibitor olaparib in high-grade serous ovarian cancer and other solid tumors. Clin Cancer Res 27(17):4710–4716

25. Brill E, Yokoyama T, Nair J, Yu M, Ahn YR, Lee JM (2017) Prexasertib, a cell cycle checkpoint kinases 1 and 2 inhibitor, increases in vitro toxicity of PARP inhibition by preventing Rad51 foci formation in BRCA wild type high-grade serous ovarian cancer. Oncotarget 8(67):111026–111040

26. Cho HY, Kim YB, Park WH, No JH (2021) Enhanced efficacy of combined therapy with checkpoint kinase 1 inhibitor and rucaparib via regulation of Rad51 expression in BRCA wild-type epithelial ovarian cancer cells. Cancer Res Treat 53(3):819–828

27. Nair BH, Huang TT, Lee JM (2018) Downregulation of cyclin B1 as a potential mechanism of resistance to the cell cycle checkpoint kinase 1 (CHK1) inhibitor, prexasertib (Prex). Eur J Cancer 103S1:e21–e148. Abstract 354 (PB-017)

28. Li F, Kozono D, Deraska P, Branigan T, Dunn C, Zheng XF, Parmar K, Nguyen H, DeCaprio J, Shapiro GI, Chowdhury D, D'Andrea AD (2020) CHK1 Inhibitor blocks phosphorylation of FAM122A and promotes replication stress. Mol Cell 80(3):410-422.e6

29. Aarts M, Sharpe R, Garcia-Murillas I, Gevensleben H, Hurd MS, Shumway SD, Toniatti C, Ashworth A, Turner NC (2012) Forced mitotic entry of S-phase cells as a therapeutic strategy induced by inhibition of WEE1. Cancer Discov 2:524–539

30. Beck H, Nahse-Kumpf V, Larsen MS, O'Hanlon KA, Patzke S, Holmberg C et al (2012) Cyclin-dependent kinase suppression by WEE1 kinase protects the genome through control of replication initiation and nucleotide consumption. Mol Cell Biol 32(20):4226–4236. https://doi.org/10.1128/MCB.00412-12

31. Fang Y, McGrail DJ, Sun C, Labrie M, Chen X, Zhang D, Ju Z, Vellano CP, Lu Y, Li Y, Jeong KJ, Ding Z, Liang J, Wang SW, Dai H, Lee S, Sahni N, Mercado-Uribe I, Kim TB, Chen K, Lin SY, Peng G, Westin SN, Liu J, O'Connor MJ, Yap TA, Mills GB (2019) Sequential therapy with PARP and WEE1 inhibitors minimizes toxicity while maintaining efficacy. Cancer Cell 35(6):851-867.e7. https://doi.org/10.1016/j.ccell.2019.05.001.PMID:31185210;PMCID:PMC6642675

32. Lin X, Chen D, Zhang C, Zhang X, Li Z, Dong B, Gao J, Shen L (2018) Augmented antitumor activity by olaparib plus AZD1775 in gastric cancer through disrupting DNA damage repair pathways and DNA damage checkpoint. J Exp Clin Cancer Res 37(1):129. https://doi.org/10.1186/s13046-018-0790-7.PMID:29954437;PMCID:PMC6027790

33. Meng X, Bi J, Li Y, Yang S, Zhang Y, Li M, Liu H, Li Y, Mcdonald ME, Thiel KW, Wen KK, Wang X, Wu M, Leslie KK (2018) AZD1775 increases sensitivity to olaparib and gemcitabine in cancer cells with p53 mutations. Cancers (Basel) 10(5):149. https://doi.org/10.3390/cancers10050149.PMID:29783721;PMCID:PMC5977122

34. Lallo A, Frese KK, Morrow CJ, Sloane R, Gulati S, Schenk MW, Trapani F, Simms N, Galvin M, Brown S, Hodgkinson CL, Priest L, Hughes A, Lai Z, Cadogan E, Khandelwal G, Simpson KL, Miller C, Blackhall F, O'Connor MJ, Dive C (2018) The combination of the PARP inhibitor olaparib and the WEE1 inhibitor AZD1775 as a new therapeutic option for small cell lung cancer. Clin Cancer Res 24(20):5153–5164

35. Westin SN, Coleman RL, Fellman BM, Yuan Y, Sood AK, Soliman PT, Wright AA, Horowitz NS, Campos SM, Konstantinopoulos PA, Levenback CF, Gershenson DM, Lu KH, Bayer V, Tukdi S, Rabbit A, Ottesen L, Godin R, Mills GB, Liu JF (2021) EFFORT: EFFicacy of adavosertib in parp ResisTance: a randomized two-arm non-comparative phase II study of adavosertib with or without olaparib in women with PARP-resistant ovarian cancer. J Clin Oncol 39:(15_suppl):5505

36. Le Tourneau C, Delord JP, Kotecki N, Borcoman E, Gomez-Roca C, Hescot S, Jungels C, Vincent-Salomon A, Cockenpot V, Eberst L, Molé A, Jdey W, Bono F, Trochon-Joseph V, Toussaint H, Zandanel C, Adamiec O, de Beaumont O, Cassier PA (2020) A Phase 1 dose-escalation study to evaluate safety, pharmacokinetics and pharmacodynamics of AsiDNA, a first-in-class DNA repair inhibitor, administered intravenously in patients with advanced solid tumours. Br J Cancer 123(10):1481–1489

37. Jdey W, Thierry S, Russo C, Devun F, Al Abo M, Noguiez-Hellin P, Sun JS, Barillot E, Zinovyev A, Kuperstein I, Pommier Y, Dutreix M (2017) Drug-driven synthetic lethality: bypassing tumor cell genetics with a combination of AsiDNA and PARP inhibitors. Clin Cancer Res 23(4):1001–1011

38. Jdey W, Lascaux P, Bono F (2019) Abstract 3797: AsiDNA abrogates acquired resistance to PARP inhibitors. Cancer Res 79(13_Supplement) 3797. https://doi.org/10.1158/1538-7445.AM2019-3797

39. Yap TA, Im SA, Schram AM et al (2022) PETRA: first in class, first in human trial of the next generation PARP1-selective inhibitor AZD5305 in patients with BRCA1/2, PALB2, or

RAD51C/D mutations. In: AACR Annual Meeting 2022. Abstract CT007. Presented April 10, 2022

40. Marchetti C, De Felice F, Romito A, Iacobelli V, Sassu CM, Corrado G, Ricci C, Scambia G, Fagotti A (2021) Chemotherapy resistance in epithelial ovarian cancer: mechanisms and emerging treatments. Semin Cancer Biol 77:144–166

41. Bukhari AB, Chan GK, Gamper AM (2022) Targeting the DNA damage response for cancer therapy by inhibiting the kinase Wee1. Front Oncol 17(12):828684

42. Leijen S, van Geel RM, Sonke GS, de Jong D, Rosenberg EH, Marchetti S, Pluim D, van Werkhoven E, Rose S, Lee MA, Freshwater T, Beijnen JH, Schellens JH (2016) Phase II study of WEE1 inhibitor AZD1775 plus carboplatin in patients with TP53-mutated ovarian cancer refractory or resistant to first-line therapy within 3 months. J Clin Oncol 34(36):4354–4361

43. Lheureux S, Cristea MC, Bruce JP, Garg S, Cabanero M, Mantia-Smaldone G, Olawaiye AB, Ellard SL, Weberpals JI, Wahner Hendrickson AE, Fleming GF, Welch S, Dhani NC, Stockley T, Rath P, Karakasis K, Jones GN, Jenkins S, Rodriguez-Canales J, Tracy M, Tan Q, Bowering V, Udagani S, Wang L, Kunos CA, Chen E, Pugh TJ, Oza AM (2021) Adavosertib plus gemcitabine for platinum-resistant or platinum-refractory recurrent ovarian cancer: a double-blind, randomised, placebo-controlled, phase 2 trial. Lancet 397(10271):281–292

44. Tolcher A, Mamdani H, Chalasani P, Meric-Bernstam F, Gazdoiu M, Makris L, Pultar P, Voliotis D (2021) Abstract CT016: clinical activity of single-agent ZN-c3, an oral WEE1 inhibitor, in a phase 1 dose-escalation trial in patients with advanced solid tumors. Cancer Res 81(13_Supplement):CT016. https://doi.org/10.1158/1538-7445.AM2021-CT016

45. Pasic et al (2022) CT148/15—a phase 1b dose-escalation study of ZN-c3, a WEE1 inhibitor, in combination with chemotherapy (CT) in subjects with platinum-resistant or refractory ovarian, peritoneal, or fallopian tube cancer AACR 2022 Conference New Orleans

46. Gallo D, Young JTF, Fourtounis J et al (2022) CCNE1 amplification is synthetic lethal with PKMYT1 kinase inhibition. Nature 604:749–756. https://doi.org/10.1038/s41586-022-04638-9

47. Young LA, O'Connor LO, de Renty C, Veldman-Jones MH, Dorval T, Wilson Z, Jones DR, Lawson D, Odedra R, Maya-Mendoza A, Reimer C, Bartek J, Lau A, O'Connor MJ (2019) Differential activity of ATR and WEE1 inhibitors in a highly sensitive subpopulation of DLBCL linked to replication stress. Cancer Res 79(14):3762–3775

48. Jin J, Fang H, Yang F, Ji W, Guan N, Sun Z, Shi Y, Zhou G, Guan X (2018) Combined inhibition of ATR and WEE1 as a novel therapeutic strategy in triple-negative breast cancer. Neoplasia 20(5):478–488

49. Shrivastav M, De Haro LP, Nickoloff JA (2008) Regulation of DNA double-strand break repair pathway choice. Cell Res 18:134–147

50. Drouet J, Frit P, Delteil C, de Villartay JP, Salles B, Calsou P (2006) Interplay between Ku, Artemis, and the DNA-dependent protein kinase catalytic subunit at DNA ends. J Biol Chem 281:27784–27793

51. Ashley AK, Shrivastav M, Nie J, Amerin C, Troksa K, Glanzer JG, Liu S, Opiyo SO, Dimitrova DD, Le P, Sishc B, Bailey SM, Oakley GG, Nickoloff JA (2014) DNA-PK phosphorylation of RPA32 Ser4/Ser8 regulates replication stress checkpoint activation, fork restart, homologous recombination and mitotic catastrophe. DNA Repair (Amst) 21:131–139

52. Fok JHL, Ramos-Montoya A, Vazquez-Chantada M, Wijnhoven PWG, Follia V, James N, Farrington PM, Karmokar A, Willis SE, Cairns J, Nikkilä J, Beattie D, Lamont GM, Finlay MRV, Wilson J, Smith A, O'Connor LO, Ling S, Fawell SE, O'Connor MJ, Hollingsworth SJ, Dean E, Goldberg FW, Davies BR, Cadogan EB (2019) AZD7648 is a potent and selective DNA-PK inhibitor that enhances radiation, chemotherapy and olaparib activity. Nat Commun 10(1):5065

53. Harnor SJ, Brennan A, Cano C (2017) Targeting DNA-dependent protein kinase for cancer therapy. ChemMedChem 12:895–900

54. Hu S, Hui Z, Lirussi F, Garrido C, Ye XY, Xie T (2021) Small molecule DNA-PK inhibitors as potential cancer therapy: a patent review (2010-present). Expert Opin Ther Pat 31(5):435–452

55. Lavin MF, Delia D, Chessa L (2006) ATM and the DNA damage response. Workshop on ataxia-telangiectasia and related syndromes. EMBO Rep 7(2):154–160. https://doi.org/10.1038/sj.embor.7400629. PMID: 16439996; PMCID: PMC1369257

56. Mak JPY, Ma HT, Poon RYC (2020) Synergism between ATM and PARP1 inhibition involves DNA damage and abrogating the G2 DNA damage checkpoint. Mol Cancer Ther 19(1):123–134

57. Riches LC, Trinidad AG, Hughes G, Jones GN, Hughes AM, Thomason AG, Gavine P, Cui A, Ling S, Stott J, Clark R, Peel S, Gill P, Goodwin LM, Smith A, Pike KG, Barlaam B, Pass M, O'Connor MJ, Smith G, Cadogan EB (2020) Pharmacology of the ATM Inhibitor AZD0156: potentiation of irradiation and olaparib responses preclinically. Mol Cancer Ther 19(1):13–25

58. Lim KS, Li H, Roberts EA, Gaudiano EF, Clairmont C, Sambel LA, Ponnienselvan K, Liu JC, Yang C, Kozono D, Parmar K, Yusufzai T, Zheng N, D'Andrea AD (2018) USP1 is required for replication fork protection in BRCA1-deficient tumors. Mol Cell 72(6):925-941.e4

59. Cadzow L et al (2020) Development of KSQ-4279 as a first-in-class USP1 inhibitor for the treatment of BRCA-deficient cancers. Eur J Cancer 138:S52

60. Zhou J, Gelot C, Pantelidou C, Li A, Yücel H, Davis RE, Färkkilä A, Kochupurakkal B, Syed A, Shapiro GI, Tainer JA, Blagg BSJ, Ceccaldi R, D'Andrea AD (2021) A first-in-class polymerase theta inhibitor selectively targets homologous-recombination-deficient tumors. Nat Cancer 2(6):598–610

61. Zatreanu D, Robinson HMR, Alkhatib O et al (2021) Polθ inhibitors elicit BRCA-gene synthetic lethality and target PARP inhibitor resistance. Nat Commun 12(1):3636

62. Yazinski SA, Comaills V, Buisson R, Genois MM, Nguyen HD, Ho CK, Todorova Kwan T, Morris R, Lauffer S, Nussenzweig A, Ramaswamy S, Benes CH, Haber DA, Maheswaran S, Birrer MJ, Zou L (2017) ATR inhibition disrupts rewired homologous recombination and fork protection pathways in PARP inhibitor-resistant BRCA-deficient cancer cells. Genes Dev 31(3):318–332. https://doi.org/10.1101/gad.290957.116

63. Sørensen CS, Hansen LT, Dziegielewski J, Syljuåsen RG, Lundin C, Bartek J, Helleday T (2005) The cell-cycle checkpoint kinase Chk1 is required for mammalian homologous recombination repair. Nat Cell Biol 7(2):195–201

64. Dai Y, Grant S (2010) New insights into checkpoint kinase 1 in the DNA damage response signaling network. Clin Cancer Res 16:376–383

65. Moore KN, Chambers SK, Hamilton EP, Chen LM, Oza AM, Ghamande SA, Konecny GE, Plaxe SC, Spitz DL, Geenen JJJ, Troso-Sandoval TA, Cragun JM, Rodrigo Imedio E, Kumar S, Mugundu GM, Lai Z, Chmielecki J, Jones SF, Spigel DR, Cadoo KA (2022) Adavosertib with chemotherapy in patients with primary platinum-resistant ovarian, fallopian tube, or peritoneal cancer: an open-label, four-arm, phase II study. Clin Cancer Res 28(1):36–44

66. Kawabe T (2004) G2 checkpoint abrogators as anticancer drugs. Mol Cancer Ther 3:513–519

67. Ghelli Luserna di Rorà A, Cerchione C, Martinelli G et al (2020) A WEE1 family business: regulation of mitosis, cancer progression, and therapeutic target. J Hematol Oncol 13:126. https://doi.org/10.1186/s13045-020-00959-2

68. Heald R, McLoughlin M, McKeon F (1993) Human Wee1 maintains mitotic timing by protecting the nucleus from cytoplasmically activated Cdc2 kinase. Cell 74(3):463–474

69. Elbæk CR, Petrosius V, Benada J, Erichsen L, Damgaard RB, Sørensen CS (2022) WEE1 kinase protects the stability of stalled DNA replication forks by limiting CDK2 activity. Cell Rep 38(3):110261

70. Bukhari AB, Lewis CW, Pearce JJ, Luong D, Chan GK, Gamper AM (2019) Inhibiting Wee1 and ATR kinases produces tumor-selective synthetic lethality and suppresses metastasis. J Clin Invest 129(3):1329–1344. https://doi.org/10.1172/JCI122622

71. Konstantinopoulos PA, Lheureux S, Moore KN (2020) PARP inhibitors for ovarian cancer: current indications, future combinations, and novel assets in development to target DNA damage repair. Am Soc Clin Oncol Educ Book 40:e116–e131

72. Washington CR, Moore KN (2021) PARP inhibitors in the treatment of ovarian cancer: a review. Curr Opin Obstet Gynecol 33(1):1–6

73. Yazinski SA et al (2017) ATR inhibition disrupts rewired homologous recombination and fork protection pathways in PARP inhibitor-resistant BRCA-deficient cancer cells. Genes Dev 31:318–332

74. Lemaçon D, Jackson J, Quinet A, Brickner JR, Li S, Yazinski S, You Z, Ira G, Zou L, Mosammaparast N, Vindigni A (2017) MRE11 and EXO1 nucleases degrade reversed forks and elicit MUS81-dependent fork rescue in BRCA2-deficient cells. Nat Commun 8(1):860. https://doi.org/10.1038/s41467-017-01180-5.PMID:29038425;PMCID:PMC5643552

75. Mahdi H, Hafez N, Doroshow D, Sohal D, Keedy V, Do KT, LoRusso P, Jürgensmeier J, Avedissian M, Sklar J, Glover C, Felicetti B, Dean E, Mortimer P, Shapiro GI, Eder JP (2021) Ceralasertib-mediated ATR inhibition combined with olaparib in advanced cancers harboring DNA damage response and repair alterations (olaparib combinations). JCO Precis Oncol 5:PO.20.00439. https://doi.org/10.1200/PO.20.00439. PMID: 34527850; PMCID: PMC8437220

76. Domchek SM (2017) Reversion mutations with clinical use of PARP inhibitors: many genes, many versions. Cancer Discov 7(9):937–939

77. Dungrawala H et al (2015) The replication checkpoint prevents two types of fork collapse without regulating replisome stability. Mol Cell 59:998–1010

78. Beck H, Nähse-Kumpf V, Larsen MS, O'Hanlon KA, Patzke S, Holmberg C, Mejlvang J, Groth A, Nielsen O, Syljuåsen RG, Sørensen CS (2012) Cyclin-dependent kinase suppression by WEE1 kinase protects the genome through control of replication initiation and nucleotide consumption. Mol Cell Biol 32(20):4226–4236. https://doi.org/10.1128/MCB.00412-12. Epub 2012 Aug 20. PMID: 22907750; PMCID: PMC3457333

79. de Sousa CL, Monteiro G (2014) Gemcitabine: metabolism and molecular mechanisms of action, sensitivity and chemoresistance in pancreatic cancer. Eur J Pharmacol 15(741):8–16

80. Primo LMF, Teixeira LK (2019) DNA replication stress: oncogenes in the spotlight. Genet Mol Biol 43(1 suppl 1):e20190138

81. Bakkenist CJ, Kastan MB (2003) DNA damage activates ATM through intermolecular autophosphorylation and dimer dissociation. Nature 421(6922):499–506

82. Bartek J, Lukas J (2007) DNA damage checkpoints: from initiation to recovery or adaptation. Curr Opin Cell Biol 19:238–245

83. Khanna KK, Jackson SP (2001) DNA double-strand breaks: signalling, repair and the cancer connection. Nature Genet 27:247–254

Combining PARP Inhibition and Immunotherapy in BRCA-Associated Cancers

Geoffrey I. Shapiro and Suzanne M. Barry

12.1 Cytotoxic T-Cell Recruitment and Activation in Response to PARP Inhibition in BRCA-Deficient Cancers

Effects of PARP inhibition on cytotoxic T-cell infiltration and activation have been extensively investigated in breast cancer models, including the immunocompetent *K14-Cre-Brca1^{f/f};Trp53^{f/f}* genetically engineered mouse model (GEMM) of BRCA1-deficient triple-negative breast cancer (TNBC) [1]. When individual tumors arising from this model were transplanted into syngeneic mice, olaparib significantly increased CD3+ and granzyme B-positive CD8+ T-cell infiltration as early as 3 days after exposure. Olaparib also increased infiltration of CD4+ T-cells, without affecting the proportion of T-regulatory FOXP3+ CD4+ T-cells (Tregs), suggesting an increase in CD4+ T-helper cells, further contributing to an effective immune response. Importantly, the critical role of activated cytotoxic T-cell infiltration in the response to PARP inhibition was demonstrated by the significantly reduced efficacy of olaparib with anti-CD8 antibody-mediated T-cell depletion and the more prolonged survival afforded by olaparib against tumors expanded in immunocompetent versus immunodeficient mice [1]. Similar findings have been described in a BRCA1-deficient TNBC MDA-MB-436 xenograft model expanded in humanized mice, where PARP inhibition was also associated with an increased T-cell infiltrate and activated interferon signaling demonstrated on transcriptomic analysis [2].

In the context of breast cancer preclinical models, modulation of the immune microenvironment has been largely restricted to a BRCA-deficient background.

G. I. Shapiro (✉) · S. M. Barry
Department of Medical Oncology and Center for DNA Damage and Repair, Dana-Farber Cancer Institute and Harvard Medical School, Boston, USA
e-mail: geoffrey_shapiro@dfci.harvard.edu

© The Author(s), under exclusive license to Springer Nature Switzerland AG 2023
T. A. Yap and G. I. Shapiro (eds.), *Targeting the DNA Damage Response for Cancer Therapy*, Cancer Treatment and Research 186,
https://doi.org/10.1007/978-3-031-30065-3_12

For example, when tumors were established using a cell line derived from the Brca1-deficient TNBC GEMM and a Brca1-reconstituted isogenic cell line, treatment with olaparib only caused accumulation of significantly higher CD3+, CD8+, and granzyme B-positive CD8+T-cell proportions in Brca1-deficient tumors [1]. Additionally, in the syngeneic Brca-proficient EMT6 model, PARP inhibition was shown to decrease T-cell infiltration and increase PD-L1 expression via GSK3β inactivation, contributing to immunosuppression, albeit reversed by the addition of an anti-PD-L1 antibody [3].

12.2   Mechanisms of PARP Inhibitor-Induced T-Cell Infiltration and Activation

cGAS-STING pathway activation. PARP inhibitor-mediated DNA damage in HR-deficient breast cancer has been associated with activation of the cGAS-STING pathway [1], a component of the innate immune system, activated primarily in response to micronucleation and the presence of cytosolic DNA (Fig. 12.1). Double-strand breaks that are inadequately repaired promote chromosomal misseg-regation and formation of micronuclei, a source of immunostimulatory cytosolic DNA. Detection of cytosolic DNA by cyclic GMP-AMP synthase (cGAS) leads to its activation and subsequent production of the second messenger 2′3′ cyclic GMP-AMP (cGAMP). cGAMP activates STING (Stimulator of Interferon Genes), which goes on to recruit TANK-binding kinase 1 (TBK1), promote TBK1 autophospho-rylation, and subsequent phosphorylation of interferon regulatory factor 3 (IRF3). Phosphorylated IRF3 then enters the nucleus and induces the expression of type 1 interferon genes, interferon stimulating genes, and other inflammatory mediators/chemokines, including CCL5 and CXCL10 [4], thereby triggering the immune system and mediating the infiltration of immune cells, including T-cells [5, 6].

Evidence for the importance of the cGAS/STING pathway in breast cancer was first recognized in a molecular subtype identified as DNA damage response-deficient (DDRD), characterized by a 44-gene assay that was validated as predicting benefit from DNA-damaging chemotherapy [7]. This gene signature was defined by upregulation of interferon-related genes and interferon signaling. Follow-up work in a group of 184 primary breast cancer patients demonstrated that the DDRD subtype was associated with CD4+ and CD8+ T lymphocyte infiltration [8].

In isogenic cell lines representing DDRD-positive and negative subtypes, there were significantly higher levels of the chemokines CCL5 and CXCL10 in DDRD cells compared to DNA damage response-proficient T-cells. Conditioned medium from DDRD cells attracted significantly more PBMCs when compared with medium from DNA damage response-proficient T-cells, which was dependent on CCL5 and CXCL10. Importantly, DDRD cells demonstrated increased cytosolic DNA and constitutive activation of the cGAS/STING pathway, related to endogenous S-phase DNA damage. DDRD cells also demonstrated expression of PD-L1 in a STING-dependent manner [8].

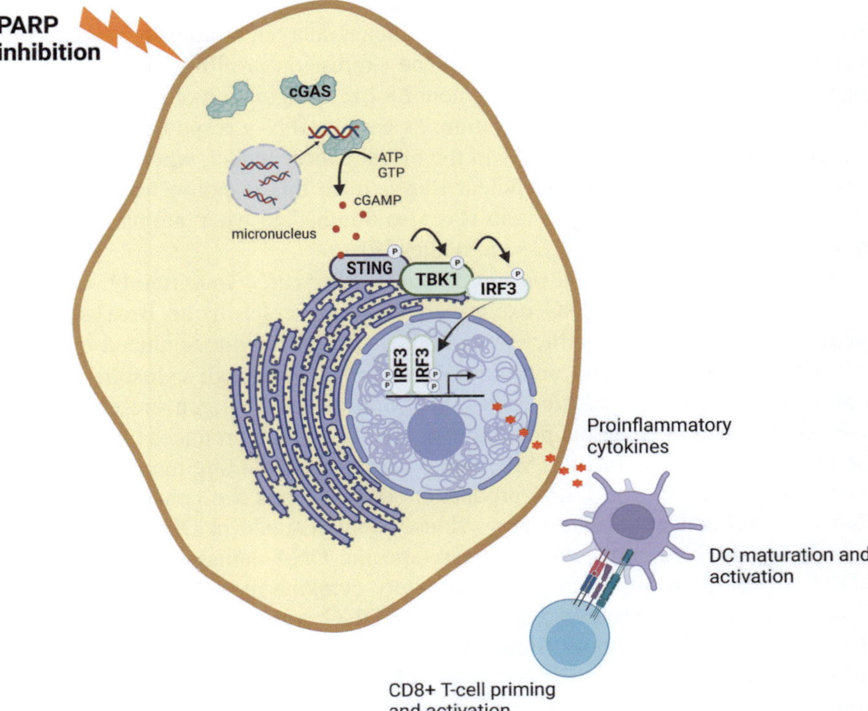

Fig. 12.1 cGAS/STING pathway. Sensing of cytosolic DNA by cGAS catalyzes the formation of cGAMP, leading to activation of STING. Activated STING recruits TBK1, resulting in the phosphorylation of IRF3. Phosphorylated IRF3 translocates to the nucleus and induces the expression of type 1 interferon genes, interferon stimulating genes, and inflammatory chemokines. Image generated with BioRender

These results suggested cGAS/STING activation as a potential mechanism by which tumor cells deficient in DNA repair processes mount an inflammatory response in response to endogenous DNA damage that may be further augmented by exposure to exogenous damage. Consistent with this hypothesis, it has been demonstrated that in response to olaparib, the cGAS/STING pathway is activated *in vivo* in Brca1-deficient tumor cells derived from the *K14-Cre-Brca1^{f/f};Trp53^{f/f}* model but not in Brca1-proficient tumor cells, which was correlated with the induction of DNA damage, as demonstrated by the convergence of immunofluorescence for pIRF3 and γ-H2AX in Brca1-deficient tumor cells after olaparib exposure [1].

Notably, similar results have been reported in models of high-grade serous ovarian cancer (HGSOC) [9]. Olaparib-induced effects on the immune system were dependent on HR status, with effects confined to the HR-deficient setting and not observed in HR-proficient models. In a pair of syngeneic Brca-deficient (*Trp53-/-; Brca1-/-; c-Myc*; PBM) or Brca-proficient (*Trp53-/-; Pten-/-; c-Myc*; PPM) HGSOC

GEMMs, olaparib treatment led to activation of the cGAS-STING pathway in PBM tumor-bearing mice, along with a significant delay in tumor progression compared to vehicle control-treated mice. Gene expression profiling after 18 days of olaparib treatment indicated an enrichment for the upregulation of genes associated with immune response, T-cell activation, as well as IFN-γ response, compared to vehicle control-treated animals. As in the breast cancer model, when PBM tumors were engrafted on to immunodeficient Rag-/- mice this response was attenuated; tumor growth inhibition by olaparib was also diminished when animals were also exposed to neutralizing anti-CD8 antibodies [9].

Effects of PARP inhibition on antigen presenting cells. Importantly, CRISPR-mediated knockout of STING exclusively in tumor cells in the Brca1-deficient breast cancer model was sufficient to abolish PARP inhibitor-induced cytotoxic CD8+T-cell infiltration and antitumor efficacy [1]. Although cytosolic DNA is a known activator of dendritic cells (DCs) into effector antigen presenting cells (APCs) [10], and DCs are the predominant T-cell type that produces type I IFNs in the tumor microenvironment (TME), other cell types, including tumor cells themselves, may also be type I IFN producers. These results are consistent with the cGAS/STING activation that was previously demonstrated in DDRD breast cancer cell lines, where endogenous S phase-specific DNA damage activated cGAS/STING signaling, resulting in proinflammatory cytokine production [8].

Although PARP inhibition activated the STING pathway with elevated levels of pTBK1 and pIRF3 in both Brca-deficient breast tumor cells and dendritic cells *in vivo*, olaparib did not directly induce TBK1/IRF3 signaling in DCs isolated from bone marrow and treated *ex vivo* [1]. This was also observed in the study of Brca-deficient ovarian cancer models, in which olaparib treatment led to DCs present in the TME expressing elevated levels of costimulatory markers CD80 and CD86 and antigen presentation molecules (MHC class II), although there was no activation of the cGAS/STING pathway when DCs alone were cultured with olaparib. In contrast, co-culture of olaparib-treated ovarian cancer cells with naïve DCs led to increased TBK1, IRF3, CXCL10, and IFNβ [9]. These results indicate that STING-mediated signaling exclusively within tumor cells is necessary and sufficient for the cytotoxic CD8+T-cell infiltration in olaparib-treated tumors and imply that olaparib- induced maturation of DCs is reliant upon paracrine signaling from neighboring cells rather than direct activation.

Effects of PARP inhibition on tumor mutational burden. Given the induction of DNA damage by PARP inhibition in an HR repair-deficient setting, it has been considered whether treatment could result in mutagenicity and increased mutational burden, thereby contributing to the induction of an anti-tumor immune response. Whole genome sequencing (WGS) following long term exposure to niraparib in several cell line models, including *BRCA1*-mutant SUM149PT TNBC cells, found no significant increase in the number of genomic alterations, including single nucleotide variations, short indels, deletions, and genomic rearrangements, compared to vehicle-treated cells [11]. Similar results were observed *in vivo*, where there was no contribution of niraparib to subclonal mutations arising in breast cancer-derived xenografts. However, it should be noted that SUM149PT-cells carry an exon 11 mutation that results in expression of a truncated BRCA1 Δ11b isoform that may retain residual HR function. Additionally, the patient-derived xenografts studied were both BRCA wild-type. Indeed, the *BRCA* wild-type xenografts were used to model the lack of mutagenesis expected in the heterozygous somatic tissue of patients with BRCA-deficient tumors.

Nonetheless, similar results were observed in both *BRCA* WT and *BRCA1–/–* DT40 cells exposed to PARP inhibition. However, there was an increase in microhomology-mediated deletions in *BRCA1–/–* DT40 cells. The large *BRCA1* deletion in these cells precluded reversion mutation, but recent reports indicate that reversion mutations in *BRCA1-* or *BRCA2*-mutated breast and ovarian cancers arising during PARP inhibitor treatment are mediated by microhomology-mediated end joining (MMEJ) [12]. These results present several testable implications. First, suppression of MMEJ via POLθ inhibition [13, 14] may prevent or delay the emergence of deletions associated with functional reversion and PARP inhibitor resistance. Conversely, it is possible that BRCA reversion mutants may create an increase in neoantigen load, capable of T-cell activation and ultimate sensitization to immune checkpoint blockade. One provocative clinical result that supports the latter hypothesis are the impressive responses to ipilimumab combined with nivolumab observed among patients with heavily pretreated pancreatic ductal adenocarcinoma (PDAC) harboring *BRCA1/2* or *RAD51C/D* mutations, suggesting an increased tumor mutational burden capable of conferring sensitivity to immune checkpoint blockade [15].

Mutational frequencies following veliparib have also been studied in *BRCA1*-mutant and BRCA1-complemented HCC1937 TNBC cells using WGS and whole exome sequencing (WES) [16]. TMB was found to be low in BRCA-deficient T-cells treated with veliparib. Surprisingly, in BRCA1-complemented cells, TMB was increased approximately twofold. Bioinformatic algorithms were used to model the MHC binding affinity for predicted neoantigens and indicated that in *BRCA1*-deficient T-cells there was limited effect compared to untreated controls. However, in BRCA1-complemented cells, some predicted neoantigens were identified and were modeled to have a significantly higher affinity compared to untreated controls, indicating that PARP inhibitors may potentially prime the immune system in some *BRCA1* wild-type cells. The underlying mechanism by which this occurs requires further elucidation.

12.3 PARP Inhibition and PD-L1 Expression

Based on the activation of interferon signaling in response to PARP inhibition in HR repair-deficient cancer cells, it is not surprising that PARP inhibition increases PD-L1 levels in various cancer models, including ovarian cancer [9, 17] breast cancer [2, 3] and pancreatic cancer [18]. Effects of PARP inhibition on PD-L1 expression have been observed both *in vitro* and *in vivo* and may be a direct consequence of cGAS/STING pathway activation. Although PD-L1 upregulation has been more strongly linked to type II interferons, it may also be upregulated by a type I response [19]. Beyond use of olaparib, similar findings have been observed in studies using other PARP inhibitors, as well as in gene silencing experiments; in ovarian cancer cell line and mouse models, both niraparib and siRNA-directed PARP1 knockdown resulted in increased PD-L1 expression [17]. While PARP inhibitor-mediated induction of PD-L1 expression may contribute to PARP inhibitor resistance, it also provides rationale for combining PARP inhibition with PD-1/PD-L1 blockade. In GEMM models of HGSOC, immune checkpoint blockade targeting PD-1 plus olaparib resulted in sustained inhibition of tumor growth with concurrent prolonged survival compared to olaparib alone, indicating that activation of the immune inhibitory activity of PD-1/PD-L1 by olaparib may limit its activity, but may be overcome by combining with PD-1 blockade [9]. In HGSOC models, PARP inhibition has also been successfully combined with CTLA-4 blockade [20]. Notably, however, in MDA-MB-436 *BRCA1*-mutant breast cancer xenografts established in humanized mice, the addition of PD-1 blockade to niraparib resulted in only modest combinatorial benefit [2].

12.4 Clinical Trials of Combination PARP Inhibitors and Immuno-Oncology Agents

Non-randomized studies in HGSOC and breast cancer. Preclinical results have stimulated numerous clinical trials combining PARP inhibition with immune checkpoint blockade in solid tumors. The KEYNOTE-162/TOPACIO trial (NCT02657889) was a phase 1/2 trial of the PARP inhibitor niraparib in combination with the anti-PD1 antibody pembrolizumab in PARP inhibitor-naïve patients with either platinum-resistant HGSOC [21] or TNBC [22] irrespective of *BRCA1/2* mutational status or PD-L1 expression. In the phase 1 part of this study, the recommended phase 2 dose (RP2D) was established as 200 mg niraparib once daily and 200 mg pembrolizumab on day 1 of each 21-day cycle.

In contrast, the MEDIOLA trial (NCT02734004) was a phase 1/2 basket study of olaparib and durvalumab in patients with PARP inhibitor-naïve solid tumors, focusing on germline *BRCA1/2*-mutated, metastatic ovarian cancer (without and with bevacizumab) [23] and germline *BRCA1/2*-mutated, metastatic breast cancer [24], as well as gastric cancer and small-cell lung cancer [25]. Patients received olaparib lead-in dosing of 300 mg orally, twice daily for 4 weeks, followed by olaparib (300 mg, twice daily) and durvalumab 1.5 g (IV, every four weeks). There were no new safety signals nor excess immune-mediated adverse events observed. The olaparib/durvalumab combination was also examined in a single-site study of patients with recurrent HGSOC.

A third program included two large trials evaluating the PARP inhibitor talazoparib combined with avelumab-mediated PD-L1 blockade in PARP inhibitor-naïve patients. In the JAVELIN PARP Medley phase 1b/2 basket trial (NCT03330405), the combination was studied in 223 patients assigned to 10 cohorts based on presence of *BRCA1/2* mutations, DDR defects (DDR+) defined using a 34-gene panel, or those with immune checkpoint blockade-sensitive advanced tumors. Among the 10 cohorts were those for recurrent, platinum-sensitive ovarian cancer, and recurrent, platinum-sensitive, *BRCA1/2*-mutated ovarian cancer; as well as TNBC, and hormone receptor-positive/ERBB2-negative/DDR-positive breast cancer [26]. In a second study, the JAVELIN BRCA/ATM trial (NCT03565991), the combination was exclusively studied in patients with *BRCA1/2*-mutated and *ATM*-mutated tumors in a Phase 2b trial, involving 200 patients (159 patients in the *BRCA1/2* cohort and 41 in the *ATM* cohort) [27].

HGSOC. In the platinum-resistant ovarian cancer arm of the TOPACIO trial [21], the niraparib and pembrolizumab combination had activity in patients with both *BRCA1/2*-wild type and mutant disease, with confirmed complete and partial responses (5 and 13%, respectively), and stable disease (47%) observed. The ORR for all participants was 18% and the disease control rate (DCR; complete response + partial response + stable disease) was 65%. Interestingly, when analyzed as subgroups based on previous bevacizumab treatment, or tumor *BRCA* or homologous recombination deficiency (HRD) status, response rates were similar between subgroups, indicating that patients with metastatic ovarian cancer may experience clinical benefit from niraparib and pembrolizumab, regardless of their biomarker status.

While BRCA status, HRD status, and prior therapy were not predictive, deeper genomic analysis performed on archival biopsies obtained at some point prior to treatment identified mutational signature 3 (Sig3) as a determinant of response to niraparib plus pembrolizumab [28]. Sig3 is a mutational signature identified to reflect HRD [29], with Sig3-positive cell lines being sensitive to PARP inhibitors. In the TOPACIO trial, 51% of ovarian cancer patients were Sig3-positive, a feature associated with longer PFS compared to that achieved by patients whose tumors were negative for Sig3 (5 months vs. 2.2 months). Significantly more Sig3-positive patients experienced stable disease or partial responses compared to Sig3-negative patients.

Additionally, components of the immune microenvironment were also examined, which demonstrated differences between gene expression patterns in chemo-naïve samples and those taken after platinum-based chemotherapy. This analysis revealed enrichment for immune related pathways in post-chemotherapy samples, along with higher immune cell-type scores and positive correlation to PD-L1 positivity. In chemo-naïve tumors, gene expression analysis revealed six pathways that were significantly enriched in patients achieving objective responses to niraparib/pembrolizumab, three of which related to Type-I interferon signaling. Samples obtained post-chemotherapy were more enriched for immune-related pathways; these samples demonstrated elevated levels of exhausted CD8+T-cells in those with an objective response, along with a higher ratio of exhausted CD8+T-cell scores to total CD8+T-cell scores in responders compared to non-responders. Immune Score (IS) positivity was designated as follows: chemo-naïve samples having the highest 25% of the pathway score for any of the interferon pathways were considered IS-positive; chemo-exposed samples having the highest 25% of the exhausted CD8+T-cell/CD8+T-cell score were also considered IS-positive.

Importantly, positivity of Sig3, IS or both were found in all patients who experienced an objective response and were also significantly associated with clinical benefit and prolonged progression-free survival (PFS) [28].

In a single-center, proof-of-concept phase 2 study of olaparib/durvalumab in 35 patients with recurrent ovarian cancer, predominantly platinum-resistant and *BRCA1/2* wild-type, the objective response rate was 14%, while DCR (partial response + stable disease) was 71%. Notably, treatment enhanced *IFNγ* and *CXCL9/CXCL10* expression, systemic IFNγ/TNFα production, and tumor-infiltrating lymphocytes in paired biopsies, indicating an immunostimulatory environment. Increased IFNγ production was associated with improved PFS, while elevated VEGFR3 levels were associated with worse PFS [30]. Taken together, the results of this trial and of the TOPACIO trial demonstrate modest activity of PARP inhibition combined with immune checkpoint blockade in platinum-resistant HGSOC. Positivity for Sig3 or a positive IS as defined in TOPACIO may be potential predictive biomarkers, serving as surrogates for HRD and for interferon-primed, CD8+-exhausted effector T-cells in the tumor microenvironment, respectively. Additionally, these results suggest that despite immunomodulatory effects of these combinations, the addition of VEGF/VEGFR blockade may improve efficacy.

Consistent with the potential benefit of addition of VEGF blockade, MEDIOLA enrolled patients with relapsed germline *BRCA1/2*-mutated platinum-sensitive ovarian cancer; 32 of whom received doublet olaparib and durvalumab and 31 of whom received triplet olaparib, durvalumab, and bevacizumab. Results showed an objective response rate (ORR) of 34% with the doublet, with median progression-free survival (PFS) 5.5 months, median OS 26.1 months and disease control rate (DCR) at 56 weeks of 9.4%. With the triplet, there was an ORR of 87%, median PFS of 14.7 months, median OS of 31.9 months and DCR at 56 weeks of 38.7% [23].

In the JAVELIN program, disease control was achieved in all patients with confirmed *BRCA1/2*-mutated platinum-sensitive disease, with an ORR of 70% and median duration of response not reached, with a range of 5.6 to at least 18.4 months (55% of patients alive and progression-free at 18 months) [26]. Despite the caveat of cross-trial comparisons, response durability compared favorably with that seen with olaparib monotherapy (e.g., median 8.2 months with olaparib monotherapy in the olaparib/cediranib program [31] and 13.2 months in the SOLO3 trial [32]). While MEDIOLA and JAVELIN are indicative of the activity of combined PARP inhibition and immune checkpoint blockade in platinum-sensitive, *BRCA1/2*-mutated disease, and suggestive of greater durability with combination treatment than with PARP inhibitor monotherapy, these results are limited by small sample sizes and non-randomized trial designs.

Breast Cancer. Of the 55 PARP inhibitor-naïve TNBC patients enrolled in TOPACIO, 47 of whom were evaluable for efficacy, there were confirmed complete and partial responses and instances of stable disease observed in 5, 5, and 13 participants, respectively. Response rates were substantially higher in in patients with *BRCA*-mutant tumors (n = 15), where the ORR was 47%, DCR 80% and median

PFS was 8.3 months, compared to an ORR of 11% a DCR of 33% and median PFS of 2.1 months in patients with *BRCA*-wild type tumors. Similarly, clinical activity was observed irrespective of PD-L1 status, though the activity was more pronounced in PD-L1-expressing TNBC [22].

In the germline *BRCA1/2*-mutated breast cancer cohort of the MEDIOLA trial, the ORR was 63% with median duration of response (DOR) of 9.2 months and median PFS of 8.2 months; twenty-four of 30 patients (80%) had disease control at 12 weeks, with median OS of 21.5 months [24]. Overall, the results of the breast cancer cohorts in these trials are in line with PARP inhibitor monotherapy [33] raising the possibility that adding immune checkpoint blockade to olaparib may not lead to improve clinical outcomes in *BRCA*-mutant breast cancer. However, there was evidence of promising DOR in early line treatment of TNBC, indicating that some subsets of breast cancer patients may benefit from olaparib and durvalumab combination therapy. Biomarker analyses indicated that PD-L1 status was not predictive of response; however, in patients with high CD8+ tumor infiltrating lymphocytes there was a modest improvement in OS, indicating that further, more selective studies may be warranted for this combination [24].

Similar to TOPACIO, in the JAVELIN program, clinical activity was primarily observed in the patients with *BRCA1/2*-mutated tumors. Response rates were similar to those reported in talazoparib monotherapy studies, although durability of response appeared to compare favorably, with DOR of 11.1 months in patients with TNBC, and 15.7 months in patients with hormone-receptor positive, ERBB2-negative, DDR+ breast cancer, compared to a median DOR of 8.6 months in the EMBRACA monotherapy study [34].

Randomized trial. The results of the TOPACIO, MEDIOLA and JAVELIN programs all point to the need for randomized studies to more definitively address whether immune checkpoint blockade improves the efficacy of PARP inhibitor monotherapy. This is also borne out by the results of the JAVELIN BRCA/ATM trial, with objective responses rates of 26.4% and 4.9% in the *BRCA1/2* and *ATM* cohorts, respectively. Although responses were more frequent and durable in tumor types associated with *BRCA1/2* mutations (median DOR 10.9 months), neither cohort met a prespecified objective response rate of 40% [27].

To date, there has only been one randomized Phase 2 trial reported involving PARP inhibition combined with immune checkpoint blockade, in which patients with metastatic *BRCA1/2*-mutated breast cancer were randomized to receive olaparib at 300 mg twice-daily versus olaparib combined with atezolizumab at 1200 mg every 21 days. This NCI-sponsored trial (NCT02849496) demonstrated no significant differences between the treatment arms. PFS and OS were 7.0 and 26.5 months in the olaparib monotherapy arm, respectively, and 7.67 and 22.4 months in the combination arm. Similar comparative results between monotherapy and combination treatment were observed in both TNBC and hormone receptor-positive subsets [35].

12.5 Effects of PARP Inhibition on the Macrophage Component of the Immune Microenvironment

The negative randomized clinical trial of olaparib versus olaparib combined with atezolizumab in *BRCA1/2*-mutated metastatic breast cancer strongly suggests that other components of immune suppression in the TME must be overcome to improve clinical outcomes. Recently, there has been significant interest in the role of tumor-associated macrophages (TAMs) [36, 37], in part because macrophages have been shown to be the predominant infiltrating immune cell type in *BRCA1/2*-associated TNBC [38]. Notably, PARP inhibitors have been shown to enhance both anti- and pro-tumorigenic features of macrophages [38, 39]. After olaparib treatment in the Brca1-deficient GEMM, F4/80 + CD45+ cells increased expression of the co-stimulatory molecule CD80, as well as that of the activation marker CD40, demonstrating potential induction of an anti-tumor phenotype, whereas levels of CD206, associated with a pro-tumor phenotype [40], did not change, so that the ratio of CD40+ anti-tumor macrophages to CD206+ pro-tumor macrophages significantly increased following olaparib exposure [38]. In line with this finding, olaparib also induced activation of the STING pathway effector TBK1 as measured by phosphorylation of Ser-172 in macrophages. Conversely, following olaparib treatment, there was also a significant increase in the frequency of F4/80 + PD-L1+ and F4/80 + CSF1R + macrophages. Therefore, these data demonstrated that PARP inhibition drives complex and opposing phenotypes, demonstrated by increased expression of functional anti-tumor markers (CD80, CD86, CD40 and pTBK1), as well as immunosuppressive markers (PD-L1 and CSF1R) [38].

These results were recapitulated in differentiating macrophages exposed to PARP inhibition *ex vivo*. In these experiments, PARP inhibitor-mediated changes in both anti- and pro-tumor features of macrophages were linked to glucose and lipid metabolic reprogramming, driven by the sterol regulatory element-binding protein 1 (SREBP1) pathway, such that SREBP1 inhibition rescued the olaparib-induced expression of PD-L1 and CSF1R [38]. Importantly, in mice bearing Brca1-deficient tumors expanded from the *K14-Cre-Brca1^{f/f};Trp53^{f/f}* GEMM, CSF-1R blockade selectively reduced the CD206+ immunosuppressive macrophage population in the tumor microenvironment and when combined with olaparib, prevented the olaparib-induced increase in expression of CSF-1R and PD-L1 in F4/80+ macrophages. As a result, the combination of CSF-1R blockade and olaparib more than doubled the median survival of mice bearing BRCA1-deficient tumors compared to olaparib alone [38]. These results have justified the development of clinical trials of combined CSF-1R blockade and PARP inhibition in patients with *BRCA1/2*-mutant breast cancer.

12.6 Combined PARP Inhibition and STING Agonism

As an alternative approach to improving the efficacy of PARP inhibitor monotherapy in *BRCA1/2*-associated breast cancer, intratumoral STING agonism has also been investigated, again utilizing the *K14-Cre-Brca1$^{f/f}$;Trp53$^{f/f}$* GEMM [41]. Compared to monotherapies, combined PARP inhibition and STING agonism results in increased STING pathway activation, greater cytotoxic T-cell recruitment and enhanced DC activation. Additionally, the combination markedly improved efficacy *in vivo*, with evidence of complete tumor clearance, prolongation of survival and induction of immunologic memory. To facilitate clinical translation, these results require confirmation with systemic STING agonism, with several agents in early phase clinical trials. Mechanistically, in addition to increased cytotoxic T-cell recruitment and activation, STING agonism may also contribute to the repolarization of tumor-associated macrophages to an anti-tumor phenotype [42] and may also contribute to the activation of NK cells in the tumor microenvironment [43].

12.7 Confirmation of Preclinical Findings on Immune Stimulation in Clinical Samples

Several studies utilizing PARP inhibition, without or with concomitant immune checkpoint blockade, have evaluated the immune microenvironment in pre- and on-treatment samples. In a pilot study in which patients with TNBC received olaparib and durvalumab, serial tumor samples obtained pre- and after a 28-day lead-in treatment of olaparib were evaluated [44]. In one patient with *BRCA1*-mutant basal breast cancer, who was an exceptional long-term survivor, tumor destruction was accompanied by a marked infiltration of immune cells containing CD8+ T-cells; in contrast, there were minimal changes in the TME of a luminal androgen receptor rapid progressor, likely due to the absence of DNA damage and tumor cell death in response to PARP inhibition. Consistent with a CD8+ T-cell infiltrate, analysis of pre- and on-treatment biopsies from 6 patients in the breast cancer cohort of the MEDIOLA trial (5 on-treatment biopsies obtained after olaparib alone and 1 obtained after combination treatment), gene set variation analysis from whole transcriptome RNA-seq demonstrated an increase in STING and Type I interferon pathway activity in 5 patients. The one patient who did not demonstrate an increase in STING pathway expression after treatment was a rapid progressor in whom a *BRCA1* reversion mutation was identified on ctDNA [45]. Finally, in the TALAVE trial, in which patients with metastatic BRCA-associated breast cancer or sporadic TNBC received a one-month lead-in of talazoparib prior to combined treatment with talazoparib and avelumab, serial biopsies procured pre- and post-talazoparib monotherapy and post-talazoparib/avelumab have demonstrated tumor cell destruction among patients with BRCA-associated disease, along with increased T-cell and CD68+CD163+ macrophage infiltrates, demonstrated by RNA-seq, as well as by cyclic immunofluorescence [46]. Taken together, these studies demonstrate that preclinical predictions emerging from immunocompetent mouse models are reflected in primary patient samples from patients with BRCA-associated breast cancer treated with PARP inhibition.

12.8 Summary

In addition to tumor cell death induced by PARP inhibition in BRCA- and other HR-deficient cancer cells based on the principles of synthetic lethality, DNA damage is associated with micronucleation, cGAS-STING pathway activation, a Type I interferon response and cytotoxic T-cell infiltration, associated with increased PD-L1 expression. Intratumoral STING pathway activation and CD8+ T-cell infiltration are required for maximal efficacy in preclinical models. PARP inhibition serves as a model for other DNA repair inhibitors targeting HR-deficient cancers, (e.g., inhibitors of polymerase θ) [47, 48], as well as for other inhibitors of the DNA damage response producing synthetic lethality in other DNA repair-deficient backgrounds [49]. Despite this biology, a randomized clinical trial combining PARP inhibition with immune checkpoint blockade in metastatic BRCA-associated breast cancer did not demonstrate combinatorial benefit compared to PARP inhibition alone. While these results do not preclude success in randomized trials in earlier stage breast cancer that may be more immunogenic [50], or in other disease types [26, 51, 52], they point to the critical need to comprehensively evaluate the immunosuppressive tumor microenvironment to fully leverage the promise of combined targeted DNA repair inhibition with immuno-oncology approaches. Addressing pro-tumorigenic macrophages in the microenvironment of BRCA-associated cancers either by depletion or repolarization is likely to be critical, as are other strategies that may correct deficiencies in the immune cycle and that may promote immunologic memory.

References

1. Pantelidou C, Sonzogni O, De Oliveria TM, Mehta AK, Kothari A, Wang D et al (2019) PARP inhibitor efficacy depends on CD8(+) T-cell recruitment via intratumoral STING pathway activation in BRCA-deficient models of triple-negative breast cancer. Cancer Discov 9(6):722–737
2. Wang Z, Sun K, Xiao Y, Feng B, Mikule K, Ma X et al (2019) Niraparib activates interferon signaling and potentiates anti-PD-1 antibody efficacy in tumor models. Sci Rep 9(1):1853
3. Jiao S, Xia W, Yamaguchi H, Wei Y, Chen MK, Hsu JM et al (2017) PARP inhibitor upregulates PD-L1 expression and enhances cancer-associated immunosuppression. Clin Cancer Res 23(14):3711–3720
4. Decout A, Katz JD, Venkatraman S, Ablasser A (2021) The cGAS-STING pathway as a therapeutic target in inflammatory diseases. Nat Rev Immunol 21(9):548–569
5. Kwon J, Bakhoum SF (2020) The cytosolic DNA-sensing cGAS-STING pathway in cancer. Cancer Discov 10(1):26–39
6. Samson N, Ablasser A (2022) The cGAS-STING pathway and cancer. Nat Cancer 3(12):1452–1463
7. Mulligan JM, Hill LA, Deharo S, Irwin G, Boyle D, Keating KE et al (2014) Identification and validation of an anthracycline/cyclophosphamide-based chemotherapy response assay in breast cancer. J Natl Cancer Inst 106(1):djt335

8. Parkes EE, Walker SM, Taggart LE, McCabe N, Knight LA, Wilkinson R et al (2017) Activation of STING-dependent innate immune signaling by S-phase-specific DNA damage in breast cancer. J Natl Cancer Inst 109(1):djw199

9. Ding L, Kim HJ, Wang Q, Kearns M, Jiang T, Ohlson CE et al (2018) PARP inhibition elicits STING-Dependent antitumor immunity in Brca1-deficient ovarian cancer. Cell Rep 25(11):2972–2980 e5

10. Kis-Toth K, Szanto A, Thai TH, Tsokos GC (2011) Cytosolic DNA-activated human dendritic cells are potent activators of the adaptive immune response. J Immunol 187(3):1222–1234

11. Poti A, Berta K, Xiao Y, Pipek O, Klus GT, Ried T et al (2018) Long-term treatment with the PARP inhibitor niraparib does not increase the mutation load in cell line models and tumour xenografts. Br J Cancer 119(11):1392–1400

12. Tobalina L, Armenia J, Irving E, O'Connor MJ, Forment JV (2021) A meta-analysis of reversion mutations in BRCA genes identifies signatures of DNA end-joining repair mechanisms driving therapy resistance. Ann Oncol 32(1):103–112

13. Zhou J, Gelot C, Pantelidou C, Li A, Yucel H, Davis RE et al (2021) A first-in-class polymerase theta inhibitor selectively targets homologous-recombination-deficient tumors. Nat Cancer 2(6):598–610

14. Zatreanu D, Robinson HMR, Alkhatib O, Boursier M, Finch H, Geo L et al (2021) Pol-theta inhibitors elicit BRCA-gene synthetic lethality and target PARP inhibitor resistance. Nat Commun 12(1):3636

15. Terrero G, Datta J, Dennison J, Sussman DA, Lohse I, Merchant NB et al (2022) Ipilimumab/nivolumab therapy in patients with metastatic pancreatic or biliary cancer with homologous recombination deficiency pathogenic germline variants. JAMA Oncol 8(6):1–3

16. Alvarado-Cruz I, Mahmoud M, Khan M, Zhao S, Oeck S, Meas R et al (2021) Differential immunomodulatory effect of PARP inhibition in BRCA1 deficient and competent tumor cells. Biochem Pharmacol 184:114359

17. Meng J, Peng J, Feng J, Maurer J, Li X, Li Y et al (2021) Niraparib exhibits a synergistic anti-tumor effect with PD-L1 blockade by inducing an immune response in ovarian cancer. J Transl Med 19(1):415

18. Wang Y, Zheng K, Xiong H, Huang Y, Chen X, Zhou Y et al (2021) PARP inhibitor upregulates PD-L1 expression and provides a new combination therapy in pancreatic cancer. Front Immunol 12:762989

19. Garcia-Diaz A, Shin DS, Moreno BH, Saco J, Escuin-Ordinas H, Rodriguez GA et al (2017) Interferon receptor signaling pathways regulating PD-L1 and PD-L2 expression. Cell Rep 19(6):1189–1201

20. Higuchi T, Flies DB, Marjon NA, Mantia-Smaldone G, Ronner L, Gimotty PA et al (2015) CTLA-4 blockade synergizes therapeutically with PARP inhibition in BRCA1-deficient ovarian cancer. Cancer Immunol Res 3(11):1257–1268

21. Konstantinopoulos PA, Waggoner S, Vidal GA, Mita M, Moroney JW, Holloway R et al (2019) Single-arm phases 1 and 2 trial of niraparib in combination with pembrolizumab in patients with recurrent platinum-resistant ovarian carcinoma. JAMA Oncol 5(8):1141–1149

22. Vinayak S, Tolaney SM, Schwartzberg L, Mita M, McCann G, Tan AR et al (2019) Open-label clinical trial of niraparib combined with pembrolizumab for treatment of advanced or metastatic triple-negative breast cancer. JAMA Oncol 5:1132–1140

23. Drew Y, Kaufman B, Banerjee S, Lortholary A, Hong SH, Park YH et al (2019) Phase II study of olaparib + durvalumab (MEDIOLA): updated results in germline BRCA-mutated platinum-sensitive relapsed (PSR) ovarian cancer (OC). Ann Oncol 30:v485–v486

24. Domchek SM, Postel-Vinay S, Im SA, Park YH, Delord JP, Italiano A et al (2020) Olaparib and durvalumab in patients with germline BRCA-mutated metastatic breast cancer (MEDIOLA): an open-label, multicentre, phase 1/2, basket study. Lancet Oncol 21(9):1155–1164

25. Krebs MG, Delord JP, Jeffry Evans TR, De Jonge M, Kim SW, Meurer M et al (2023) Olaparib and durvalumab in patients with relapsed small cell lung cancer (MEDIOLA): an open-label, multicenter, phase 1/2, basket study. Lung Cancer 180:107216

26. Yap TA, Bardia A, Dvorkin M, Galsky MD, Beck JT, Wise DR et al (2023) Avelumab plus talazoparib in patients with advanced solid tumors: the JAVELIN PARP medley nonrandomized controlled trial. JAMA Oncol 9(1):40–50
27. Schram AM, Colombo N, Arrowsmith E, Narayan V, Yonemori K, Scambia G et al (2023) Avelumab plus talazoparib in patients with BRCA1/2- or ATM-altered advanced solid tumors: results from JAVELIN BRCA/ATM, an open-label, multicenter, phase 2b, tumor-agnostic trial. JAMA Oncol 9(1):29–39
28. Farkkila A, Gulhan DC, Casado J, Jacobson CA, Nguyen H, Kochupurakkal B et al (2020) Immunogenomic profiling determines responses to combined PARP and PD-1 inhibition in ovarian cancer. Nat Commun 11(1):1459
29. Gulhan DC, Lee JJ, Melloni GEM, Cortes-Ciriano I, Park PJ (2019) Detecting the mutational signature of homologous recombination deficiency in clinical samples. Nat Genet 51(5):912–919
30. Lampert EJ, Zimmer A, Padget M, Cimino-Mathews A, Nair JR, Liu Y et al (2020) Combination of PARP inhibitor olaparib, and PD-L1 inhibitor durvalumab, in recurrent ovarian cancer: a proof-of-concept phase II study. Clin Cancer Res 26(16):4268–4279
31. Liu JF, Brady MF, Matulonis UA, Miller A, Kohn EC, Swisher EM et al (2022) Olaparib with or without cediranib versus platinum-based chemotherapy in recurrent platinum-sensitive ovarian cancer (NRG-GY004): A Randomized, Open-Label, phase III trial. J Clin Oncol 40(19):2138–2147
32. Penson RT, Valencia RV, Cibula D, Colombo N, Leath CA 3rd, Bidzinski M et al (2020) Olaparib versus nonplatinum chemotherapy in patients with platinum-sensitive relapsed ovarian cancer and a germline BRCA1/2 mutation (SOLO3): a randomized phase III trial. J Clin Oncol 38(11):1164–1174
33. Robson M, Im SA, Senkus E, Xu B, Domchek SM, Masuda N et al (2017) Olaparib for metastatic breast cancer in patients with a germline BRCA mutation. N Engl J Med 377(6):523–533
34. Litton JK, Rugo HS, Ettl J, Hurvitz SA, Goncalves A, Lee KH et al (2018) Talazoparib in patients with advanced breast cancer and a germline BRCA mutation. N Engl J Med 379(8):753–763
35. Fanucci KA, Pilat MJ, Shyr D, Shyr Y, Boerner SA, Durecki D et al (2023) Olaparib +/ − atezolizumab in patinets with BRCA-mutated locally advanced, unresectable or metastatic (advanced) breast cancer; an open-label multi-center phase II trial. Proc AACR. 2023:CT145 [abstract]
36. Campbell MJ, Tonlaar NY, Garwood ER, Huo D, Moore DH, Khramtsov AI et al (2011) Proliferating macrophages associated with high grade, hormone receptor negative breast cancer and poor clinical outcome. Breast Cancer Res Treat 128(3):703–711
37. Vitale I, Manic G, Coussens LM, Kroemer G, Galluzzi L (2019) Macrophages and metabolism in the tumor microenvironment. Cell Metab 30(1):36–50
38. Mehta AK, Cheney EM, Hartl CA, Pantelidou C, Oliwa M, Castrillon JA et al (2020) Targeting immunosuppressive macrophages overcomes PARP inhibitor resistance in BRCA1-associated triple-negative breast cancer. Nature Cancer 2(1):66–82
39. Wang L, Wang D, Sonzogni O, Ke S, Wang Q, Thavamani A et al (2022) PARP-inhibition reprograms macrophages toward an anti-tumor phenotype. Cell Rep 41(2):111462
40. Mehta AK, Kadel S, Townsend MG, Oliwa M, Guerriero JL (2021) Macrophage biology and mechanisms of immune suppression in breast cancer. Front Immunol 12:643771
41. Pantelidou C, Jadhav H, Kothari A, Liu R, Wulf GM, Guerriero JL et al (2022) STING agonism enhances anti-tumor immune responses and therapeutic efficacy of PARP inhibition in BRCA-associated breast cancer. NPJ Breast Cancer 8(1):102
42. Wang Q, Bergholz JS, Ding L, Lin Z, Kabraji SK, Hughes ME et al (2022) STING agonism reprograms tumor-associated macrophages and overcomes resistance to PARP inhibition in BRCA1-deficient models of breast cancer. Nat Commun 13(1):3022
43. Knelson EH, Ivanova EV, Tarannum M, Campisi M, Lizotte PH, Booker MA et al (2022) Activation of tumor-cell STING primes NK-cell therapy. Cancer Immunol Res 10(8):947–961

44. Labrie M, Li A, Creason A, Betts C, Keck J, Johnson B et al (2021) Multiomics analysis of serial PARP inhibitor treated metastatic TNBC inform on rational combination therapies. NPJ Precis Oncol 5(1):92
45. Staniszewska AD, Armenia J, King M, Michaloglou C, Reddy A, Singh M et al (2022) PARP inhibition is a modulator of anti-tumor immune response in BRCA-deficient tumors. Oncoimmunology 11(1):2083755
46. Lynce F, Shimada K, Geng X, Richardson ET, Mainor C, Wei M et al (2023) TALAVE: induction talazoparib followed by combined talazoparib and avelumab in patients with advanced breast cancer. Proc AACR. 2023:CT145 [abstract]
47. Li J, Ko JM-Y, Dai W, Yu VZ, Ng HY, Hoffmann J-S et al (2021) Depletion of DNA polymerase theta inhibits tumor growth and promotes genome instability through the cGAS-STING-ISG pathway in esophageal squamous cell carcinoma. Cancers 13(13):3204
48. Oh G, Wang A, Wang L, Li J, Werba G, Weissinger D et al (2023) POLQ inhibition elicits an immune response in homologous recombination-deficient pancreatic adenocarcinoma via cGAS/STING signaling. J Clin Invest 28:e165934
49. Concannon K, Morris BB, Gay CM, Byers LA (2023) Combining targeted DNA repair inhibition and immune-oncology approaches for enhanced tumor control. Mol Cell 83(5):660–680
50. Gil Del Alcazar CR, Huh SJ, Ekram MB, Trinh A, Liu LL, Beca F et al (2017) Immune escape in breast cancer during in situ to invasive carcinoma transition. Cancer Discov 7(10):1098–1115
51. Monk BJ, Coleman RL, Fujiwara K, Wilson MK, Oza AM, Oaknin A et al (2021) ATHENA (GOG-3020/ENGOT-ov45): a randomized, phase III trial to evaluate rucaparib as monotherapy (ATHENA-MONO) and rucaparib in combination with nivolumab (ATHENA-COMBO) as maintenance treatment following frontline platinum-based chemotherapy in ovarian cancer. Int J Gynecol Cancer 31(12):1589–1594
52. Fizazi K, Retz M, Petrylak DP, Goh JC, Perez-Gracia J, Lacombe L et al (2022) Nivolumab plus rucaparib for metastatic castration-resistant prostate cancer: results from the phase 2 CheckMate 9KD trial. J Immunother Cancer 10(8):e004761

Mitotic MTH1 Inhibitors in Treatment of Cancer

13

Thomas Helleday

13.1 Introduction

It is established that cancers in general have a lost redox balance [1] and in some cases show high levels of reactive oxygen species (ROS) [2]. The increased amount of ROS in cancer may also explain a general increase in the antioxidant defences system being upregulated in cancer. Also, targeting and generating high ROS levels is becoming a novel strategy for anti-cancer strategy [3].

That ROS could be potentially interesting in treatments of cancer is not entirely new. Many established treatments generate ROS either as a cell death causing agent or as a consequence of the treatment. In the case of ionizing radiation, generation of singlet oxygen or hydroxyl radicals are critical to generate DNA single- and double-strand breaks that eventually kill cells. Furthermore, inability to generate ROS in hypoxic regions is associated with resistance to ionizing radiation [4]. While it is established that cisplatin-induced DNA adducts are critical to generate toxicity in cells, cisplatin-induced ROS, unrelated to nuclear DNA damage, is also emerging to be important in the mechanism of action of cisplatin induced anti-cancer effects [5]. In spite of ROS being central in both cancer development and in the most common anti-cancer treatments, very little attention has been to inhibit repair of oxidative DNA damage in cancer, potential because knockout mice of the genes encoding oxidative DNA repair proteins have only mild phenotypes [6–8].

T. Helleday (✉)
Science for Life Laboratory, Department of Oncology-Pathology, Karolinska Institutet, Stockholm, Sweden
e-mail: thomas.helleday@scilifelab.se

Department of Oncology and Metabolism, Weston Park Cancer Centre, University of Sheffield, Sheffield, UK

223

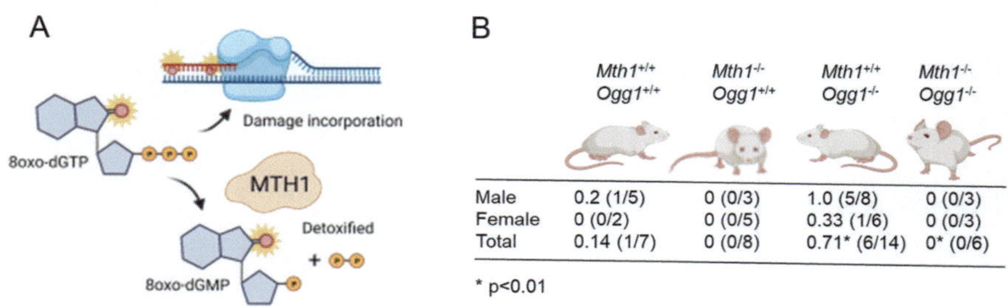

	$Mth1^{+/+}$ $Ogg1^{+/+}$	$Mth1^{-/-}$ $Ogg1^{+/+}$	$Mth1^{+/+}$ $Ogg1^{-/-}$	$Mth1^{-/-}$ $Ogg1^{-/-}$
Male	0.2 (1/5)	0 (0/3)	1.0 (5/8)	0 (0/3)
Female	0 (0/2)	0 (0/5)	0.33 (1/6)	0 (0/3)
Total	0.14 (1/7)	0 (0/8)	0.71* (6/14)	0* (0/6)

* $p < 0.01$

Fig. 13.1 **MTH1 activity prevents damage incorporation and promotes cancer survival. A,** 8oxo-dGTP can be incorporated into DNA to cause oxidative DNA damage. MTH1 enzymatic activity cleaves 8oxo-dGTP into 8oxo-dGMP, which cannot be incorporated into DNA. **B,** Cancer incidence in *Mth1/Ogg1* knockout mice. Knockout mice were examined by macroscopic procedure at 580 ($\pm$1) days after birth to identify spontaneous lung tumour development. Mean number of lung tumours/mouse for each knockout mouse is shown and the number of lung tumour-bearing mice/total mice is indicated in parentheses. Statistical differences were examined using Student's t test. Data are presented from experiment 1 in Ref. [14]

One of the oxidative DNA repair proteins is MTH1 (encoded by the *NUDT1* gene), which prevents oxidative lesions in the DNA by hydrolysing 8-oxodGTP or 2-OHdATP in the dNTP pool; cleaving off a pyrophosphate to generate 8-oxodGMP or 2-OHdAMP, respectively that cannot be incorporated into DNA [9, 10] (Fig. 1A). Since cancer cells have deregulated redox balance the MTH1 protein could be a potential anti-cancer target, to prevent incorporation of 8-oxodGTP into DNA. The rationale is that the free bases on the dNTP pool are 190–13,000 times more susceptible to damage as compared to bases in the double-stranded DNA, which are protected by being base-paired in the double helix and by being packed into nucleosomes [11]. Hence, it is plausible that the free dNTP pool in cancer cells could be particularly susceptible to a lost redox balance and high ROS. Hence, oxidized dNTPs would be potentially toxic only to replicating cancer cells. Following this, ours and other laboratories developed MTH1 inhibitors demonstrating potent anti-cancer activity [12, 13], generating a general interest in this protein as an anti-cancer target.

13.2 Biological Roles of MTH1

The Human MutT homologue 1 (MTH1) protein was originally identified as MutT in *E. coli* and shown to hydrolyse 8-oxodGTP to prevent incorporation of 8-oxodG in to DNA, which otherwise induce mutations [9, 15]. Although the bacterial MutT mutation result in a 1000-fold increase in mutation, the human MTH1 protein (catalysing the same reaction) is surprisingly not suppressing mutation rates as *Mth1-/-* knockout mice show no increase in mutations [16]. The initial hypothesis that there were backup proteins carrying out the reaction in humans appears to be incorrect [17, 18] and the likely explanation is instead that there are low levels of oxidative DNA damage in mammals. Instead, the MTH1 protein in mammalians appears to be a stress-induced protein, being required for survival under stressed conditions [19]. Also, the MTH1 protein levels are induced after treatments with ionizing radiation (IR) [20] or environmental pollutants [21, 22].

13.2.1 MTH1 in Inflammation and Cancer

MTH1 and oxidative DNA damage is associated with numerous diseases other than inflammation and cancer, and reviewed elsewhere [23]. Early on it was reported that MTH1 protein levels are potently up-regulated in phytohemagglutinin-activated T lymphocytes [24]. This is interesting and is likely related to that activated T cells have increased ROS levels which is related to the glycolytic switch in activated T cells [25], potentially resembling the same glycolytic switch in cancer [26]. Some activated T cells have high level of MTH1 [27] and another subset low MTH1 levels for unknown reasons [28]. As may be expected, the MTH1 inhibitor TH1579 only kills activated MTH1^{high} T cells at low nM concentrations by introducing oxidative DNA damage [28]. There are several reported therapeutic effects in *in vivo* models of autoimmune hepatitis [27] and experimental autoimmune encephalomyelitis [28]. While MTH1 inhibitors may have important applications in inflammatory conditions, this is outside the scope of this review.

In many cancers, both the MTH1 protein levels [29–31], as well as 8-oxodGTPase activity is upregulated [32], likely owing to the stress condition and lost redox balance. Furthermore, MTH1 is also a prognostic biomarker for survival in lung cancer [33, 34], colorectal [35, 36], pancreatic cancer [36], hepatocellular carcinoma [37]. A likely reason for MTH1 activity being high in cancer is to prevent ROS-induced senescence of cancer cells [38]. The MTH1 inhibitors developed in our laboratory have a broad anti-cancer activity in *in vitro* and *in vivo* models [27, 3940–45] and are now tested in clinical trials for treatment of solid (NCT03036228) and heamatological cancers (NCT04077307). It is interesting to note that while the mitotic MTH1 inhibitor TH1579 is highly effective anti-cancer treatment it is also highly tolerable. This inhibitor and MTH1 as a target in anti-cancer treatments is the topic of this review.

13.3 MTH1 as an Anti-cancer Target

13.3.1 Genetic Validation of MTH1 in Cancer

There is overwhelming evidence that numerous diseases and ageing are associated with oxidative stress and reactive oxygen species (ROS) [46]. Transgene expression of hMTH1 in mice increased longevity and improved cognitive ability [47]. Hence, it is surprising that *Mth1-/-* knockout mice are viable and grow old without any serious phenotype [7]. However, when grouping the incidence of lung, liver, and stomach cancers this was statistically significantly higher in *Mth1-/-* as compared to the same group of cancers in *Mth1+/+* mice [7]. This increased incidence of these particular cancers have however not been confirmed in other laboratories studying *Mth1-/-* mice (Lindahl, personal communication and unpublished results). More strikingly is that Sakumi and co-workers demonstrated that increased lung cancer incidence observed in *Ogg1-/-* mice is absent when additionally targeting MTH1 in the *Ogg1-/- Mth1-/-* double knockout mice [14] (Fig. 1B). This is *in vivo* genetic validation that the MTH1 protein is required for tumour growth. A mechanistic reason for MTH1 being important for cancer cells was first offered by Dr Priyamvada Rai in Prof Robert Weinberg's laboratory, showing that senescence in cancer was induced in the absence of MTH1 [38]. Since then, other laboratories, including our own, have demonstrated that MTH1 siRNA or shRNA targeting is toxic or arrest cancer cells both *in vitro* and *in vivo* [13, 38, 48–53] and that this toxicity is rescued by expression of RNAi resistant *MTH1* protein [12].

Since these reports, there have been other reports challenging MTH1 as an anti-cancer target by demonstrated that targeting of MTH1 by the CRISPR-Cas9 technique is compatible with survival of cancer cells [54], which is also supported by Depmap.org [55]. Several scientists suggest that this alone is sufficient evidence to de-validate MTH1 as a target. Currently, there is an urgent need for more in depth scientific understanding of the role of MTH1 in cancer, why it is upregulated and its roles also outside its enzymatic activity which is needed to get a better understanding on the role of MTH1 as potential anti-cancer target.

13.3.2 Edgetic Perturbation Limits Genetic Validation of Anti-cancer Targets

As mentioned above, many have disqualified MTH1 as an anti-cancer target based on that CRISPR-Cas9 knockout MTH1-/- cells are alive. With the same reasoning, PARP is also a de-validated anti-cancer target, as CRISPR-Cas9 targeting of PARP1 in cancer cells is well tolerated [55]. This is clearly not an accurate validation as we earlier showed PARP inhibitors are able to kill *BRCA* mutated cancer [56, 57], and the molecular explanation was later explained by PARP inhibitors being able to trap PARP1 to generate a toxic lesion [58].

Furthermore, many current DDR targets are essential for cancer cell survival following CRISPR-Cas9, e.g., ATR, CHK1, or DUT, suggesting that inhibition of any of these enzymes should work for all cancer in monotherapy. We now know that none of these inhibitors are particularly efficient in monotherapy for killing cancer. The mechanistic explanation is because of edgetic perturbation, that node removal by protein loss is not the same as an inhibitor perturbating an edge [59] (Fig. 13.2).

While the CRISPR-Cas9 technology is useful, it cannot alone be sufficient for validation of a target. In my view, full validation of a target requires a combined effort by scientists in detailed mechanistic and biological experiments along with a scientific discussion. It also requires a chemical probe. Since our original

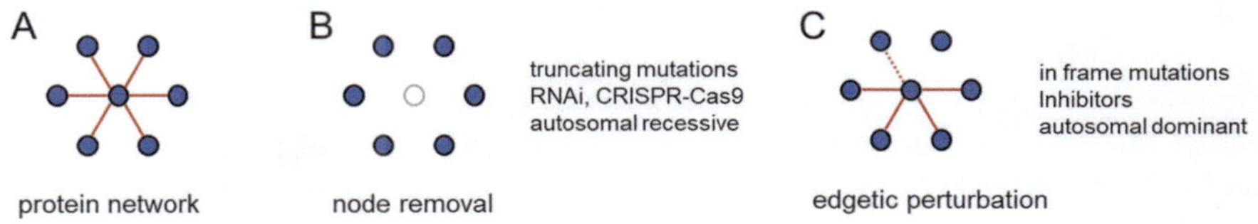

Fig. 13.2 Edgetic perturbation limits the value of CRISPR-Cas9 as a validation tool to predict drug targets. A, A protein network is made up of interactions (edges) between proteins. **B,** Protein loss result in a node removal and loss of all edges to the protein, as is the case following CRISPR-Cas9. **C,** Protein inhibition results in edgetic perturbation where some edges remain, some are lost and new ones are gained

report on PARP inhibitors killing homologous recombination defective cancers [56, 57], there has been many thousand reports on the mechanism of action and still there is not a full understanding of the process by which PARP inhibitors kill *BRCA^{mut}* cells. The incomplete understanding of PARP1 functions did not stop PARP inhibitors in clinical trials and these are now FDA/EMA approved for several cancers and saving thousands of lives.

13.3.3 Generation of MTH1 Inhibitors

The MTH1 protein belongs to the Nudix hydrolases family of enzymes, which all share a hydrolase activity to a nucleoside diphosphates linked to moiety-X [60]. Many of the enzymes in this family is now assigned to functions and there has also been comprehensive analysis of the overall function of these enzymes [18, 61–64]. Analysing the structure of MTH1 [65], it has a very large active site that is suitable to interfere with a small molecules. Hence, it has been relatively easy to generate small molecule inhibitors to MTH1 [12, 54, 66, 67], and also existing compounds, such as (S)-crizotinib, selectively targets MTH1 [13].

Interestingly, some of the MTH1 inhibitors, such as TH588, TH1579 and (S)-crizotinib, appears to have very few off-targets, as determined in protein selectively screens [12, 13]. Furthermore, in a proteome wide analysis (thermal proteome profiling) MTH1 was demonstrated to be the only statistically significant target out of 9301 proteins that was thermally stabilized by TH1579 suggesting few, if any, off target effects [53]. Although these inhibitors appear selective, it has been demonstrated that tubulin polymerisation is inhibited by both TH588 and TH1579 *in vitro* at μM concentrations [53, 66, 68] and cells expressing the TUBB L240F mutant are resistant to TH588 [69]. Hence, it is likely that the TH1579 and TH588 mediate mitotic arrest also by direct inhibition of tubulin and work as a dual inhibitor.

13.3.4 Enzymatic Inhibition of MTH1 Is Insufficient to Kill Cancer Cells

Since our original publications of TH588 and (S)-crizotinib inhibiting MTH1 and killing cancer [12, 13], there have been several reports on MTH1 enzymatic inhibitors that do not kill cancer cells [54, 66, 67]. This clearly demonstrates that MTH1 enzymatic inhibition alone is insufficient to kill cancer cells. We have analysed this in more detail and demonstrate that injection of 8-oxodGTP in zebrafish embryos makes the enzymatic MTH1 inhibitors toxic [68]. There are several conclusions that can be drawn from this: (1) incorporation of 8-oxodGTP in DNA is not only introducing mutations but is also toxic to cells through a yet unknown mechanism, (2) the overall ROS levels appears too low in cancer cells in order to make MTH1 enzyme inhibitors toxic, (3) MTH1 is likely having functions beyond hydrolysing 8-oxodGTP.

13.3.5 Mechanism of Action of MTH1 Inhibitor TH588 and TH1579

The optimised MTH1 inhibitor TH1579 (Karonudib, OXC-101) is currently evaluated in clinical trials in solid and heamatological cancer patients [53]. The mechanism of action of how TH1579 (and the structurally related compound TH588) kills cancer cells is now well established (Fig. 13.3). The TH588/TH1579 compounds stop cells in mitosis through inhibition of tubulin polymerisation, activating the spindle assembly checkpoint (SAC), which result in accumulation of ROS, oxidizing dGTP to 8-oxodGTP (Fig. 3A). It has previously been demonstrated that ROS accumulates in mitotically arrested cells following degradation of mitochondria [69, 70]. Inhibition of MTH1 enzymatic activity by TH1579 (Fig. 3B) results in 8-oxodGTP (and 2-OHdATP) being incorporated into DNA during mitotic replication (cancer-specific repair synthesis), which altogether kill cancer cells [68, 71] (Fig. 3C). Proof of this mechanism is that inhibiting the SAC with reversin or MAD2 siRNA depletion generates resistance to the inhibitors, as ROS is not generated as cells are not stopped in mitosis [68, 71].

A relevant question is how important incorporation of oxidative DNA damage is to the mechanism of action of TH588/TH1579? The bacterial MutT has an 8-oxodGTPase, but not 2-OHdATPase activity and overexpression of the bacterial MutT in human cells restores the MTH1 8-oxodGTPase, but not 2-OHdATPase or mitotic functions [12]. This MutT expression prevents incorporation of 8-oxodG into DNA [53] and partially reverse the toxic effects of TH588/TH1579 [12]. In our original publication, we suggested the partial reversion of toxicity was related to incorporation of 2-OHdATP. In hindsight, the partial rescue is likely explained because the mitotic arrest is not reversed. Further evidence that 8-oxodG damage is important for the toxic effect of TH588/TH1579 is that cells carrying an engineered error prone DNA Polδ that is able to incorporate 8-oxodGTP is more sensitive to TH588 than Polδ wild type cells [71]. An important observation is that an increase in 8-oxodGTP incorporation into DNA by error prone DNA Polδ

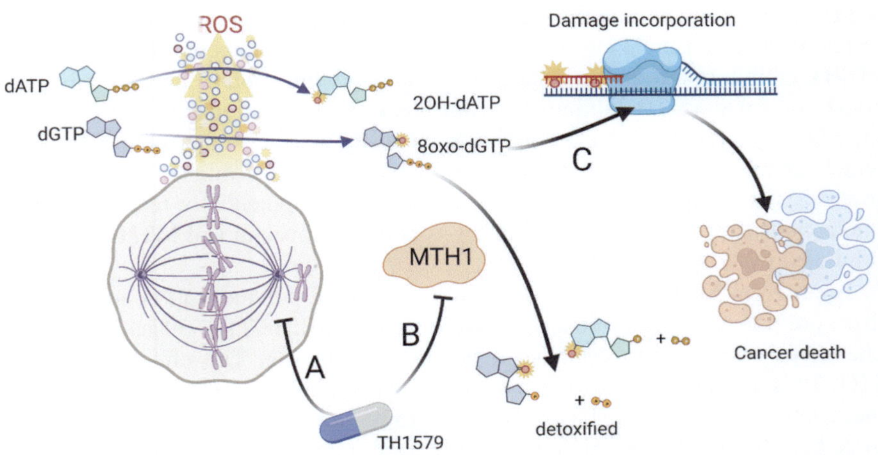

Fig. 13.3 Mechanism of action of TH1579 (OXC-101, karonudib). A, TH1579 perturbs tubulin polymerisation resulting in lagging chromosomes in mitosis that trigger the spindle assembly checkpoint that hold cells in mitosis. Reactive oxygen species (ROS) accumulates in arrested cells because of mitophagy, which in turn damage bases in the free nucleotide (dNTP) pool. **B,** TH1579 inhibits the MTH1 enzymatic activity that degrades 8oxo-dGTP and 2OH-dATP to detoxify the cell. **C,** 8oxo-dGTP and 2OH-dATP accumulates in MTH1 inhibited cells and are incorporated during repair synthesis in mitosis, occurring primarily in cancer cells because of oncogene-induced replication stress [72]. Incorporated oxidative damage in DNA kills cancer cells

is also resulting in a more profound mitotic arrest [71]. Thus, it appears that 8-oxodG in DNA is a signal for mitotic arrest, which is an area that needs to be further explored.

13.3.6 Interference of MTH1, TH588 and TH1579 on Tubulin Polymerisation

It has been suggested that the effects of TH588 and TH1579 are solely ascribed to an off-target effect on tubulin polymerisation and that essentially, TH588 and TH1579 are simple tubulin poisons [54, 66, 73, 74].

It is correct that TH588/TH1579 inhibits tubulin polymerisation also at relevant toxic concentrations in cells [68]. However, knocking down MTH1 with siRNA also has a similar effect on mitotic arrest and tubulin polymerisation in cancer cells as observed with TH588/TH1579. Both MTH1 knockdown and TH588/TH1579 has an effect on (1) mitotic arrest, (2) cellular tubulin polymerisation assay, (3) generation of a highly specific type of lagging chromosomes in mitotic spreads, (4) loss of kinetochore-microtubule attachments, and reduced inter-kinetochore distances in sister-chromatids, (5) *in vivo* evidence in tumours of mitotic arrest [68]. Hence, MTH1 itself has roles outside of 8-oxodGTPase activity. The detailed role of MTH1 in mitosis is not defined, but under investigation. However, the

MTH1 protein binds tubulin directly and low nM potent MTH1 inhibitors have different effect on breaking the MTH1-tubulin protein interaction [68]. All toxic MTH1 inhibitors are also breaking the MTH1-tubulin protein interaction, while some non-toxic MTH1 inhibitors do not break the interaction [68]. Furthermore, the MTH1 protein binds to and non-enzymatically activates other mitotic proteins which are relevant to the mitotic arrest (unpublished), suggesting the role of MTH1 in mitosis is complex and likely non-catalytic. Other potentially relevant protein interactions that disrupts MTH1 activity is between caveolin and MTH1, which is promoted by K-Ras^{G12V} [75].

Apart from MTH1 having a direct role in tubulin polymerisation and mitosis, there are numerous other data demonstrating that TH588/TH1579 have a unique phenotype compared to established tubulin poisons: (1) The effect of TH588/TH1579 is dependent on oxidative damage [76] and hypoxic signalling, being synthetic lethal with VHL [77], (2) TH588/TH1579 introduce 8-oxodG DNA damage in cells [68], (3) TH588/TH1579 synergize with tubulin poisons [68], (4) toxicity of TH588/TH1579 is dependent by the ability to introduce 8-oxodG into DNA by Polδ [71] and Polκ (Sanjiv et al, unpublished), (5) TH588/TH1579 are well tolerated *in vivo* [53] and do not cause the same toxic adverse events as tubulin poisons do, such as neuropathy.

There are also reports demonstrating TH588 induces mitotic arrest in MTH1-/- knockout cells generated by CRISPR-Cas9 [73, 74], further reinforcing the notion that TH588/TH1579 has a direct effect on tubulin polymerisation that is independent of MTH1. This is also observed from the reported *in vitro* inhibition of tubulin polymerisation [66, 68]. The conclusion from these collective results is that TH588/TH1579 have both a MTH1 dependent and MTH1 independent effects on tubulin polymerisation. Future studies on this topic could for instance exploit the TUBB L240F mutant that is resistant to TH588 to determine if it interfere with MTH1 dependent or independent effects (or both).

13.3.7 Structurally Distinct MTH1 Inhibitor AZ19 (Non-tubulin Inhibitor) Generates Mitotic Arrest

There are several structurally diverge MTH1 inhibitors (e.g., TH5769, AZ19) causes the same unique metaphase arrest with lagging chromosomes as TH588/TH1579 [68]. The AZ19 compound is a nM potent MTH1 inhibitor and is unable to interfere with tubulin polymerisation *in vitro* [54]. Yet, AZ19 interferes with tubulin polymerisation in cells, arrest cells in mitosis, generate the MTH1 characteristic type of lagging chromosomes in mitotic spreads, loss of kinetochore-microtubule attachments, and reduced inter-kinetochore distances in sister-chromatids [68]. Interestingly, AZ19 only affects tubulin mobility in G2/M cells and not in interphase cells, which is where MTH1 is active in mitosis [68]. Hence, AZ19 is likely exerting it effects on tubulin and mitosis solely through MTH1, making it likely that there may be possibilities to generate cancer killing mitotic MTH1 inhibitors that cause mitotic arrest and incorporation of 8-oxodG in cells that unlike TH588/TH1579 are not themselves interfering with tubulin polymerisation. It is worth noting that TH588/TH1579 interferes with tubulin polymerisation also in interphase cells, which is likely MTH1 independent, and suggest an off-target effect on tubulin polymerisation by TH588/TH1579 in cells.

13.4 Conclusions and a Selection of Outstanding Questions

It is clear that TH1579 (OXC-101) is a highly exciting new broad acting anticancer strategy and that it has a unique mechanism of action in DDR, exploiting oxidative DNA damage. The TH1579 has a dual mechanism of action: (1) arresting cells in mitosis by inhibiting tubulin polymerisation (also independently of MTH1) which generates ROS and 8-oxodGTP, (2) preventing incorporation of 8-oxodGTP into DNA (by targeting MTH1) which is toxic (Fig. 13.3).

There are several outstanding questions:

1. What is the detailed mechanism of action how 8-oxodG lesions in DNA are toxic?
2. Why do cancer and activated T cells overexpress MTH1?
3. Are selective MTH1 inhibitors, that both inhibits the mitotic role of MTH1 and enzymatic activity useful as anti-cancer treatments?
4. Why are TH588 and TH1579 selectively toxic to cancer and MTH1^{high} activated T-cells?
5. Why do TH588 and TH1579 specifically cause mitotic arrest in cancer and not in non-transformed cells?

13.5 Perspective

It is difficult to do translational research, going from target identification to development of a drug that eventually outperforms standard-of-care in phase III trials. The main issue is lack of basic scientific understanding on the biological pathways. Several years ago, my lab (collaborating with Nicola Curtin) and the lab of Alan Ashworth (collaborating with Stephen Jackson and KuDOS) proposed to use PARP inhibitors in killing homologous recombination (HR) defective (*BRCA^{mut}*) cancers [56, 57]. There were numerous problems developing this PARP inhibitor concept:

(1) The originally proposed mechanism, that PARP inhibitors generated a replication-associated 1-ended DNA double-strand break to trigger BRCA-dependent HR, was incomplete. It was clearly more complex than this.
(2) Highly potent nM PARP enzymatic inhibitors (such as veliparib) were unable to kill *BRCA^{mut}* cancers.

(3) siRNA treatment of PARP1 did not recapitulate what was observed with PARP inhibitors in $BRCA^{mut}$ cancers.

(4) There was a poor correlation between biochemical IC_{50} of PARP inhibition to and cellular IC_{50} killing $BRCA^{mut}$ cancer cells.

(5) With the same PARP inhibitor, there were large variation between sensitivity in $BRCA^{mut}$ cancer cell lines, which was not related to inhibition of PARP in those cells (some $BRCA^{mut}$ cancer cell lines had upfront resistance).

At the time of our discovery, it would have been extremely easy to discredit our original work and de-validate PARP inhibitors as a treatment of $BRCA^{mut}$ cancers. In fact, several labs wrote to the editors of *Nature* and demanded the retraction of our reports. Subsequently, these scientists themselves published de-validation of PARP inhibitors in $BRCA^{mut}$ cancers [78, 79], which did not obtain sufficient attention to stop further research. Because of the impressive effects on the cancers, the scientific and pharmaceutical community continued working on completing the science and pursued clinical development. Today, PARP inhibitors are approved treatments and saving many lives specifically in HR defective cancers as was originally described. However, it is worth mentioning that the clinical development were initially derailed for the wrong reasons as highlighted by a reporter in the journal *Nature* [80].

In the case of MTH1, several pharmaceutical companies spent considerable efforts in developing MTH1 inhibitors and in this process identified both compounds that killed cancer cells and also those compounds that did not. Following the first report on de-validation of MTH1 inhibitors [66], the commercial labs closed their MTH1 programs and published de-validation reports [54, 67, 81, 82]. These reports all fail to take the complex biology into account and describe a biased view with a selection of MTH1 enzyme inhibitors (not mitotic MTH1 inhibitors), defiling the MTH1 field and blocking future basic and translational research, as the topic is deemed non-fundable. Bayer presented convincing internal validation work on MTH1[83] and entered into a €190 M licensing deal for MTH1 inhibitors with a biotech company [84], which aligns poorly with their follow up publication only demonstrating negative data [82]. The scientific community would be helped if these companied would publish a complete view on the topic together with their lead candidate compounds that kill cancer cells, with biological data, to help determine potential off-target effects and also to increase our understanding of how to inhibit the mitotic function of MTH1 and if this is a relevant anti-cancer strategy.

Here I exemplify PARP and MTH1 being problematic in the validation process and also describe how CRISPR-Cas9 knockout fails to predict how enzyme inhibitors work also for other targets in the DDR field. I believe this is a general problem targeting cancer vulnerabilities, which is probably less of a problem for the cancer therapies focussed on targeting enzymatic activities in oncogenes. The science underlying the paradigm to target oncogene activity is simple, as it often is the enzymatic activity that drives the cancer and by preventing this activity the cancer growth is stopped. The underlying science in the DDR field is much more challenging as most DDR proteins are binding other DDR proteins and/or DNA. Hence, while target identification using CRISPR-Cas9 technology (node removal) may be helpful in hypothesis generation, it is likely to be flawed when trying to use it as a validation tool and edgetic pertubations need to be taken into account (Fig. 13.2). I think the lack of acknowledging these dificulties is a main reason to why we have not seen DDR inhibitors approvals, other than PARP inhibitors, for treatment in cancer.

In summary, oxygen is critical to life and oxidative DNA damage is a component of many diseases and ageing [46]. The MTH1 protein is upregulated in many cancers and certain immune cells and the overall biology is largely unknown, which really provides an opportunity. The anti-cancer and anti-inflammatory effects of TH1579 in pre-clinical models are impressive [28, 39–44, 53, 85, 86] and clinical trials are ongoing. I call for more scientists to enter the field of oxidative DDR and repair and exploit the novel inhibitors to advance science and better human health.

13.6   Conflicts of Interest

TH is listed as inventor on patents related to small molecule inhibitors of MTH1, and is a member of the board and shareholder in Oxcia AB which develops mitotic MTH1 inhibitor OXC-101.

Acknowledgements I would like to thank members of the Helleday lab for fruitful discussions. The TH laboratory currently receives funding primarily from the Swedish Research Council, the Swedish innovation agency Vinnova, the Swedish Cancer Society, and EU programs. Illustrations were created with Biorender.com.

References

1. Warburg O (1956) On respiratory impairment in cancer cells. Science 124(3215):269–270
2. Hole PS, Zabkiewicz J, Munje C, Newton Z, Pearn L, White P et al (2013) Overproduction of NOX-derived ROS in AML promotes proliferation and is associated with defective oxidative stress signaling. Blood 122(19):3322–3330
3. Trachootham D, Alexandre J, Huang P (2009) Targeting cancer cells by ROS-mediated mechanisms: a radical therapeutic approach? Nat Rev Drug Discov 8(7):579–591
4. Gray LH, Conger AD, Ebert M, Hornsey S, Scott OC (1953) The concentration of oxygen dissolved in tissues at the time of irradiation as a factor in radiotherapy. Br J Radiol 26(312):638–648
5. Marullo R, Werner E, Degtyareva N, Moore B, Altavilla G, Ramalingam SS et al (2013) Cisplatin induces a mitochondrial-ROS response that contributes to cytotoxicity depending on mitochondrial redox status and bioenergetic functions. PLoS ONE 8(11):e81162
6. Klungland A, Rosewell I, Hollenbach S, Larsen E, Daly G, Epe B et al (1999) Accumulation of premutagenic DNA lesions in mice defective in removal of oxidative base damage. Proc Natl Acad Sci U S A 96(23):13300–13305
7. Tsuzuki T, Egashira A, Igarashi H, Iwakuma T, Nakatsuru Y, Tominaga Y et al (2001) Spontaneous tumorigenesis in mice defective in the MTH1 gene encoding 8-oxo-dGTPase. Proc Natl Acad Sci U S A 98(20):11456–11461

8. Vartanian V, Lowell B, Minko IG, Wood TG, Ceci JD, George S et al (2006) The metabolic syndrome resulting from a knockout of the NEIL1 DNA glycosylase. Proc Natl Acad Sci U S A 103(6):1864–1869

9. Maki H, Sekiguchi M (1992) MutT protein specifically hydrolyses a potent mutagenic substrate for DNA synthesis. Nature 355(6357):273–275

10. Nakabeppu Y, Tsuchimoto D, Furuichi M, Sakumi K (2004) The defense mechanisms in mammalian cells against oxidative damage in nucleic acids and their involvement in the suppression of mutagenesis and cell death. Free Radic Res 38(5):423–429

11. Topal MD, Baker MS (1982) DNA precursor pool: a significant target for N-methyl-N-nitrosourea in C3H/10T1/2 clone 8 cells. Proc Natl Acad Sci U S A 79(7):2211–2215

12. Gad H, Koolmeister T, Jemth AS, Eshtad S, Jacques SA, Strom CE et al (2014) MTH1 inhibition eradicates cancer by preventing sanitation of the dNTP pool. Nature 508:215–221

13. Huber KV, Salah E, Radic B, Gridling M, Elkins JM, Stukalov A et al (2014) Stereospecific targeting of MTH1 by (S)-crizotinib as an anticancer strategy. Nature 508:222–227

14. Sakumi K, Tominaga Y, Furuichi M, Xu P, Tsuzuki T, Sekiguchi M et al (2003) Ogg1 knockout-associated lung tumorigenesis and its suppression by Mth1 gene disruption. Sakumi. 63(5):902–905

15. Bhatnagar SK, Bessman MJ (1988) Studies on the mutator gene, mutT of Escherichia coli. Molecular cloning of the gene, purification of the gene product, and identification of a novel nucleoside triphosphatase. J Biol Chem 263(18):8953–8957

16. Egashira A, Yamauchi K, Yoshiyama K, Kawate H, Katsuki M, Sekiguchi M et al (2002) Mutational specificity of mice defective in the MTH1 and/or the MSH2 genes. DNA Repair (Amst) 1(11):881–893

17. Carter M, Jemth AS, Hagenkort A, Page BD, Gustafsson R, Griese JJ et al (2015) Crystal structure, biochemical and cellular activities demonstrate separate functions of MTH1 and MTH2. Nat Commun 6:7871

18. Page BDG, Valerie NCK, Wright RHG, Wallner O, Isaksson R, Carter M et al (2018) Targeted NUDT5 inhibitors block hormone signaling in breast cancer cells. Nat Commun 9(1):250

19. Yoshimura D, Sakumi K, Ohno M, Sakai Y, Furuichi M, Iwai S et al (2003) An oxidized purine nucleoside triphosphatase, MTH1, suppresses cell death caused by oxidative stress. J Biol Chem 278(39):37965–37973

20. Bialkowski K, Szpila A, Kasprzak KS (2009) Up-regulation of 8-oxo-dGTPase activity of MTH1 protein in the brain, testes and kidneys of mice exposed to (137)Cs gamma radiation. Radiat Res 172(2):187–197

21. Kim HN, Morimoto Y, Tsuda T, Ootsuyama Y, Hirohashi M, Hirano T et al (2001) Changes in DNA 8-hydroxyguanine levels, 8-hydroxyguanine repair activity, and hOGG1 and hMTH1 mRNA expression in human lung alveolar epithelial cells induced by crocidolite asbestos. Carcinogenesis 22(2):265–269

22. Liang R, Igarashi H, Tsuzuki T, Nakabeppu Y, Sekiguchi M, Kasprzak KS et al (2001) Presence of potential nickel-responsive element(s) in the mouse MTH1 promoter. Ann Clin Lab Sci 31(1):91–98

23. Nakabeppu Y, Oka S, Sheng Z, Tsuchimoto D, Sakumi K (2010) Programmed cell death triggered by nucleotide pool damage and its prevention by MutT homolog-1 (MTH1) with oxidized purine nucleoside triphosphatase. Mutat Res 703(1):51–58

24. Oda H, Nakabeppu Y, Furuichi M, Sekiguchi M (1997) Regulation of expression of the human MTH1 gene encoding 8-oxo-dGTPase. Alternative splicing of transcription products. J Biol Chem 272(28):17843–17850

25. Nathan C, Cunningham-Bussel A (2013) Beyond oxidative stress: an immunologist's guide to reactive oxygen species. Nat Rev Immunol 13(5):349–361

26. Hanahan D, Weinberg RA (2011) Hallmarks of cancer: the next generation. Cell 144(5):646–674

27. Chen Y, Hua X, Huang B, Karsten S, You Z, Li B, et al (2021) MutT homolog 1 inhibitor karonudib attenuates autoimmune hepatitis by inhibiting DNA repair in activated T cells. Hepatol Commun

28. Karsten S, Fiskesund R, Zhang XM, Marttila P, Sanjiv K, Pham T et al (2022) MTH1 as a target to alleviate T cell driven diseases by selective suppression of activated T cells. Cell Death Differ 29(1):246–261

29. Kennedy CH, Cueto R, Belinsky SA, Lechner JF, Pryor WA (1998) Overexpression of hMTH1 mRNA: a molecular marker of oxidative stress in lung cancer cells. FEBS Lett 429(1):17–20

30. Kennedy CH, Pass HI, Mitchell JB (2003) Expression of human MutT homologue (hMTH1) protein in primary non-small-cell lung carcinomas and histologically normal surrounding tissue. Free Radic Biol Med 34(11):1447–1457

31. Zhou H, Cheng B, Lin J (2005) Expression of DNA repair enzyme hMTH1 mRNA and protein in hepatocellular carcinoma. J Huazhong Univ Sci Technolog Med Sci 25(4):389–392

32. Speina E, Arczewska KD, Gackowski D, Zielinska M, Siomek A, Kowalewski J et al (2005) Contribution of hMTH1 to the maintenance of 8-oxoguanine levels in lung DNA of non-small-cell lung cancer patients. J Natl Cancer Inst 97(5):384–395

33. Fujishita T, Okamoto T, Akamine T, Takamori S, Takada K, Katsura M et al (2017) Association of MTH1 expression with the tumor malignant potential and poor prognosis in patients with resected lung cancer. Lung Cancer 109:52–57

34. Li DN, Yang CC, Li J, Ou Yang QG, Zeng LT, Fan GQ et al (2021) The high expression of MTH1 and NUDT5 promotes tumor metastasis and indicates a poor prognosis in patients with non-small-cell lung cancer. Biochim Biophys Acta Mol Cell Res 1868(1):118895

35. Li J, Yang CC, Tian XY, Li YX, Cui J, Chen Z et al (2017) MutT-related proteins are novel progression and prognostic markers for colorectal cancer. Oncotarget 8(62):105714–105726

36. McPherson LA, Troccoli CI, Ji D, Bowles AE, Gardiner ML, Mohsen MG et al (2019) Increased MTH1-specific 8-oxodGTPase activity is a hallmark of cancer in colon, lung and pancreatic tissue. DNA Repair (Amst). 83:102644

37. Ou Q, Ma N, Yu Z, Wang R, Hou Y, Wang Z et al (2020) Nudix hydrolase 1 is a prognostic biomarker in hepatocellular carcinoma. Aging (Albany NY) 12(8):7363–7379

38. Rai P, Onder TT, Young JJ, McFaline JL, Pang B, Dedon PC et al (2009) Continuous elimination of oxidized nucleotides is necessary to prevent rapid onset of cellular senescence. Proc Natl Acad Sci U S A 106(1):169–174

39. Hua X, Sanjiv K, Gad H, Pham T, Gokturk C, Rasti A et al (2019) Karonudib is a promising anticancer therapy in hepatocellular carcinoma. Ther Adv Med Oncol 11:1758835919866960

40. Moukengue B, Brown HK, Charrier C, Battaglia S, Baud'huin M, Quillard T et al (2020) TH1579, MTH1 inhibitor, delays tumour growth and inhibits metastases development in osteosarcoma model. EBioMedicine 53:102704

41. Hansel C, Hlouschek J, Xiang K, Melnikova M, Thomale J, Helleday T et al (2021) Adaptation to chronic-cycling hypoxia renders cancer cells resistant to MTH1-inhibitor treatment which can be counteracted by glutathione depletion. Cells 10(11)

42. Oksvold MP, Berglund UW, Gad H, Bai B, Stokke T, Rein ID et al (2021) Karonudib has potent anti-tumor effects in preclinical models of B-cell lymphoma. Sci Rep 11(1):6317

43. Sanjiv K, Calderon-Montano JM, Pham TM, Erkers T, Tsuber V, Almlof I et al (2021) MTH1 inhibitor TH1579 induces oxidative DNA damage and mitotic arrest in acute myeloid leukemia. Cancer Res 81(22):5733–5744

44. Centio A, Estruch M, Reckzeh K, Sanjiv K, Vittori C, Engelhard S et al (2022) Inhibition of oxidized nucleotide sanitation by TH1579 and conventional chemotherapy cooperatively enhance oxidative DNA-damage and survival in AML. Mol Cancer Ther

45. Das I, Tuominen R, Helleday T, Hansson J, Warpman Berglund U, Egyhazi Brage S (2022) Coexpression of MTH1 and PMS2 is associated with advanced disease and disease progression after therapy in melanoma. J Invest Dermatol 142(3 Pt A):736–40 e6

46. Mittal M, Siddiqui MR, Tran K, Reddy SP, Malik AB (2014) Reactive oxygen species in inflammation and tissue injury. Antioxid Redox Signal 20(7):1126–1167

47. De Luca G, Ventura I, Sanghez V, Russo MT, Ajmone-Cat MA, Cacci E et al (2013) Prolonged lifespan with enhanced exploratory behavior in mice overexpressing the oxidized nucleoside triphosphatase hMTH1. Aging Cell 12(4):695–705

48. Burton DG, Rai P (2015) MTH1 counteracts oncogenic oxidative stress. Oncoscience 2(10):785–786
49. Giribaldi MG, Munoz A, Halvorsen K, Patel A, Rai P (2015) MTH1 expression is required for effective transformation by oncogenic HRAS. Oncotarget 6(13):11519–11529
50. Patel A, Burton DG, Halvorsen K, Balkan W, Reiner T, Perez-Stable C et al (2015) MutT Homolog 1 (MTH1) maintains multiple KRAS-driven pro-malignant pathways. Oncogene 34(20):2586–2596
51. Rai P, Young JJ, Burton DG, Giribaldi MG, Onder TT, Weinberg RA (2011) Enhanced elimination of oxidized guanine nucleotides inhibits oncogenic RAS-induced DNA damage and premature senescence. Oncogene 30(12):1489–1496
52. Helleday T (2014) Cancer phenotypic lethality, exemplified by the non-essential MTH1 enzyme being required for cancer survival. Ann Oncol (in press)
53. Warpman Berglund U, Sanjiv K, Gad H, Kalderen C, Koolmeister T, Pham T et al (2016) Validation and development of MTH1 inhibitors for treatment of cancer. Ann Oncol
54. Kettle JG, Alwan H, Bista M, Breed J, Davies NL, Eckersley K et al (2016) Potent and selective inhibitors of MTH1 probe its role in cancer cell survival. J Med Chem 59(6):2346–2361
55. Tsherniak A, Vazquez F, Montgomery PG, Weir BA, Kryukov G, Cowley GS et al (2017) Defining a cancer dependency map. Cell 170(3):564–576 e16
56. Bryant HE, Schultz N, Thomas HD, Parker KM, Flower D, Lopez E et al (2005) Specific killing of BRCA2-deficient tumours with inhibitors of poly(ADP-ribose)polymerase. Nature 434:913–917
57. Farmer H, McCabe N, Lord CJ, Tutt AN, Johnson DA, Richardson TB et al (2005) Targeting the DNA repair defect in BRCA mutant cells as a therapeutic strategy. Nature 434(7035):917–921
58. Murai J, Huang SY, Das BB, Renaud A, Zhang Y, Doroshow JH et al (2012) Trapping of PARP1 and PARP2 by clinical PARP inhibitors. Cancer Res 72(21):5588–5599
59. Zhong Q, Simonis N, Li QR, Charloteaux B, Heuze F, Klitgord N et al (2009) Edgetic perturbation models of human inherited disorders. Mol Syst Biol 5:321
60. Bessman MJ, Frick DN, O'Handley SF (1996) The MutT proteins or "Nudix" hydrolases, a family of versatile, widely distributed, "housecleaning" enzymes. J Biol Chem 271(41):25059–25062
61. Carter M, Jemth AS, Carreras-Puigvert J, Herr P, Martinez Carranza M, Vallin KSA et al (2018) Human NUDT22 Is a UDP-glucose/galactose hydrolase exhibiting a unique structural fold. Structure 26(2):295–303 e6
62. Yang JJ, Landier W, Yang W, Liu C, Hageman L, Cheng C et al (2015) Inherited NUDT15 variant is a genetic determinant of mercaptopurine intolerance in children with acute lymphoblastic leukemia. J Clin Oncol 33(11):1235–1242
63. Zhang SM, Desroses M, Hagenkort A, Valerie NCK, Rehling D, Carter M et al (2020) Development of a chemical probe against NUDT15. Nat Chem Biol
64. Carreras-Puigvert J, Zitnik M, Jemth AS, Carter M, Unterlass JE, Hallstrom B et al (2017) A comprehensive structural, biochemical and biological profiling of the human NUDIX hydrolase family. Nat Commun 8(1):1541
65. Svensson LM, Jemth AS, Desroses M, Loseva O, Helleday T, Hogbom M et al (2011) Crystal structure of human MTH1 and the 8-oxo-dGMP product complex. FEBS Lett 585(16):2617–2621
66. Kawamura T, Kawatani M, Muroi M, Kondoh Y, Futamura Y, Aono H et al (2016) Proteomic profiling of small-molecule inhibitors reveals dispensability of MTH1 for cancer cell survival. Sci Rep 6:26521
67. Petrocchi A, Leo E, Reyna NJ, Hamilton MM, Shi X, Parker CA et al (2016) Identification of potent and selective MTH1 inhibitors. Bioorg Med Chem Lett 26(6):1503–1507
68. Gad H, Mortusewicz O, Rudd SG, Stolz A, Amaral N, Brautigam L et al (2019) MTH1 promotes mitotic progression to avoid oxidative DNA damage in cancer cells. bioRxiv. https://doi.org/10.1101/575290

69. Patterson JC, Joughin BA, van de Kooij B, Lim DC, Lauffenburger DA, Yaffe MB (2019) ROS and oxidative stress are elevated in mitosis during asynchronous cell cycle progression and are exacerbated by mitotic arrest. Cell Syst 8(2):163–167 e2
70. Domenech E, Maestre C, Esteban-Martinez L, Partida D, Pascual R, Fernandez-Miranda G et al (2015) AMPK and PFKFB3 mediate glycolysis and survival in response to mitophagy during mitotic arrest. Nat Cell Biol 17(10):1304–1316
71. Rudd SG, Gad H, Sanjiv K, Amaral N, Hagenkort A, Groth P et al (2020) MTH1 inhibitor TH588 disturbs mitotic progression and induces mitosis-dependent accumulation of genomic 8-oxodG. Cancer Res 80(17):3530–3541
72. Henriksson S, Calderón-Montaño JM, Solvie D, Warpman Berglund U, Helleday T (2022) Overexpressed c-Myc sensitizes cells to TH1579, a mitotic arrest and oxidative DNA damage inducer. Biomolecules 12(12):1777
73. Patterson JC, Joughin BA, Prota AE, Muhlethaler T, Jonas OH, Whitman MA et al (2019) VISAGE reveals a targetable mitotic spindle vulnerability in cancer cells. Cell Syst 9(1):74–92 e8
74. Gul N, Karlsson J, Tangemo C, Linsefors S, Tuyizere S, Perkins R et al (2019) The MTH1 inhibitor TH588 is a microtubule-modulating agent that eliminates cancer cells by activating the mitotic surveillance pathway. Sci Rep 9(1):14667
75. Volonte D, Vyas AR, Chen C, Dacic S, Stabile LP, Kurland BF et al (2018) Caveolin-1 promotes the tumor suppressor properties of oncogene-induced cellular senescence. J Biol Chem 293(5):1794–1809
76. Wang JY, Jin L, Yan XG, Sherwin S, Farrelly M, Zhang YY et al (2016) Reactive oxygen species dictate the apoptotic response of melanoma cells to TH588. J Invest Dermatol
77. Brautigam L, Pudelko L, Jemth AS, Gad H, Narwal M, Gustafsson R et al (2016) Hypoxic signaling and the cellular redox tumor environment determine sensitivity to MTH1 inhibition. Cancer Res 76(8):2366–2375
78. Gallmeier E, Kern SE (2005) Absence of specific cell killing of the BRCA2-deficient human cancer cell line CAPAN1 by poly(ADP-ribose) polymerase inhibition. Cancer Biol Ther 4(7):703–706
79. De Soto JA, Wang X, Tominaga Y, Wang RH, Cao L, Qiao W et al (2006) The inhibition and treatment of breast cancer with poly (ADP-ribose) polymerase (PARP-1) inhibitors. Int J Biol Sci 2(4):179–185
80. Ledford H (2012) Drug candidates derailed in case of mistaken identity. Nature 483(7391):519
81. Rahm F, Viklund J, Tresaugues L, Ellermann M, Giese A, Ericsson U et al (2018) Creation of a novel class of potent and selective MutT homologue 1 (MTH1) inhibitors using fragment-based screening and structure-based drug design. J Med Chem 61(6):2533–2551
82. Ellermann M, Eheim A, Rahm F, Viklund J, Guenther J, Andersson M et al (2017) Novel class of potent and cellularly active inhibitors devalidates MTH1 as broad-spectrum cancer target. ACS Chem Biol 12(8):1986–1992
83. Glasauer A, Irlbacher H, Richter A, Toschi L, Steckel M, Haegebarth A (2015) Targeting the redox-protective protein MTH1 for cancer therapy: a novel way to exploit the unique redox status of cancer cells. Cancer Res 75
84. https://news.cision.com/se/sprint-bioscience/r/sprint-bioscience-sluter-avtal-med-bayer-healthcare,c9808303 [press release]. 2015
85. Einarsdottir BO, Karlsson J, Soderberg EMV, Lindberg MF, Funck-Brentano E, Jespersen H et al (2018) A patient-derived xenograft pre-clinical trial reveals treatment responses and a resistance mechanism to karonudib in metastatic melanoma. Cell Death Dis 9(8):810
86. Das I, Gad H, Brautigam L, Pudelko L, Tuominen R, Hoiom V et al (2020) AXL and CAV-1 play a role for MTH1 inhibitor TH1579 sensitivity in cutaneous malignant melanoma. Cell Death Differ 27(7):2081–2098

Targeting ATR in Cancer Medicine

14

Carolina Salguero, Christian Valladolid, Helen M. R. Robinson, Graeme C. M. Smith, and Timothy A. Yap

14.1 Introduction

Preserving genomic integrity is pivotal for cell survival; consequently, cells rely on a network of complex signaling pathways to facilitate faithful DNA replication and maintain genomic stability [1]. Increased proliferation rates are associated with genomic instability via the accumulation of DNA damage in the form of DNA double strand breaks (DSBs) or DNA single strand breaks (SSBs) caused by a variety of events, including replication stress induced by stalling of replication

Carolina Salguero and Christian Valladolid contributed equally.

C. Salguero · C. Valladolid · T. A. Yap (✉)
Department of Investigational Cancer Therapeutics (Phase I Program), Division of Cancer Medicine, The University of Texas MD Anderson Cancer Center, Houston, TX, USA
e-mail: tyap@mdanderson.org

C. Salguero
e-mail: csalguero@mdanderson.org

C. Valladolid
e-mail: cvbrown@mdanderson.org

H. M. R. Robinson · G. C. M. Smith
Artios Pharma, The Glenn Berge Building, Babraham Research Campus, Cambridge, UK
e-mail: hrobinson@artios.com

G. C. M. Smith
e-mail: gsmith@artios.com

T. A. Yap
The Institute for Applied Cancer Science, and Institute for Personalized Cancer Therapy, The University of Texas MD Anderson Cancer Center, 1400 Holcombe Boulevard, TX 77030 Houston, USA

T. A. Yap and G. I. Shapiro (eds.), *Targeting the DNA Damage Response for Cancer Therapy*, Cancer Treatment and Research 186,
https://doi.org/10.1007/978-3-031-30065-3_14

forks [2–4]. These events distort genetic material due to subsequent fusion of DSBs and shortening of telomeres, which can result in translocations, gene amplification, and gene mutations [5–7].

When DNA damage or replication stress is sensed, cells are prevented entry into mitosis by activating DNA Damage Response (DDR) pathways at varying phases within the cell cycle [8]. DDR signaling pathways orchestrate tightly regulated kinase cascades to resolve DNA damage and replication stress by pausing the cell cycle and initiating repair [9, 10]. Ataxia telangiectasia and Rad3-related protein (ATR) is a key PI3K-related kinase within the DDR that senses replication stress and regulates checkpoints within the cell cycle's synthesis (S) and gap 2/mitosis (G2/M) phases to preserve genomic stability [1, 10–12].

Notably, replication stress and genomic instability are hallmarks of cancer cells, making them dependent on protective DDR pathways for survival [10, 12–14]. As such, targeting ATR in cancer medicine is an attractive therapeutic approach to circumvent cancer cell survival by exploiting their dependence on ATR-driven processes.

14.2 ATR Acts as a Gatekeeper of DNA Damage Repair

Endogenous and exogenous sources of DNA damage lead to a wide variety of adducts including DSBs, SSBs, base damage, bulky adducts and base mismatches [1]. Cells have evolved complex DNA repair mechanisms designed to specifically repair these types of damage and maintain genome stability. Repair of DNA DSBs is of particular importance as it is estimated that a single unrepaired DNA DSB can initiate cell death, highlighting the critical role of DDR pathways in cell survival [16]. DSBs are repaired by a number of mechanisms: the best characterized being the error-free homologous recombination repair (HRR) pathway, the highly efficient -but error prone- nonhomologous end joining (NHEJ) pathway, and the error prone microhomology mediated end-joining pathway (regarded as a backup pathway to HRR) [15].

Repair by HRR is initiated by an upstream activator of DDR, the ataxia telangiectasia-mutated (*ATM*) PI3K-related kinase, which upon sensing DSBs triggers a cascade of events that include cell cycle arrest, repair and apoptosis [17, 18]. During S or G2-phases, exposure of single-stranded DNA can occur as an intermediate of HRR at areas of resected DNA and also at stressed replication forks. These single-stranded DNA regions quickly become coated with the high-affinity ssDNA binding protein, replication protein A (RPA), which protects against DNA degradation. The coating of single-stranded DNA by RPA recruits ATR/ATR-interacting protein (ATRIP) complexes to sites of damage [1, 16]. Following localization to sites of damage, ATR is activated by either topoisomerase II binding protein (TopBP1) or Ewing tumour-associated antigen 1 (ETAA1) [17]. Moreover, recruitment of TopBP1 is mediated by Rad17, which loads the 9-1-1 (Rad9-Hus1-Rad1) complex onto chromatin, binds to TopBP1, and results in ATR activation [4]. Once activated, ATR proceeds to phosphorylate a series of downstream targets; however, its activation of checkpoint kinase 1 (CHK1) is integral to its regulation of cell cycle checkpoints (Fig. 14.1) [16].

ATR commands control over the S and G2/M checkpoints by phosphorylating and activating CHK1 [1, 18]. Active CHK1 kinase in turn phosphorylates and inactivates the cell division cycle 25A/25C (CDC25A/CDC25C) phosphatase proteins, leading to their respective degradation [1]. Degradation of CDC25A thereby renders CDK2 and its associated complexes inactive by removing an inhibitory phosphorylation present on CDK2 [19]. Consequently, progression to S phase is interrupted, preventing DNA replication and promoting DNA repair [16]. ATR-mediated activation of CHK1 also interrupts the G2/M checkpoint in a Wee1-like protein kinase (WEE1) dependent manner. Active CHK1 phosphorylates and stabilizes WEE1, enhancing its activity toward CDK1 [19]. Both CDK1 and CDK2 remain in inactive states induced by WEE1's inhibitory phosphorylation [19]. Inactivation of CDC25C by CHK1 prevents the removal of the inhibitory phosphorylation on CDK1, which halts the G2/M checkpoint to allow time for post-replicative DNA repair and prevent replication of unrepaired DNA [16].

Additionally, ATR also plays a role in regulating replication forks through multiple mechanisms [1]. One mechanism involves ATR-mediated fork remodeling: ATR phosphorylates the helicase SWI/SNF-related, matrix associated, actin dependent regulator of chromatin, subfamily-A-like 1 (SMARCAL1), promoting maintenance of fork stability and fork restart in cooperation with RAD51 and zinc-finger RANBP2-type containing 3 (ZRANB3) [20]. Another known mechanism underscores the importance of the ATR-CHK1 axis in resolving replication stress during the formation of R-loops, which are RNA–DNA hybrid transcription intermediates that induce genome instability. Here, the ATR-CHK1 pathway is activated by R-loop induced reversed replication forks. Upon activation, ATR protects the genome by regulating the activity of the MUS81 endonuclease, preventing excess nucleolytic degradation of reversed forks. Active ATR also suppresses R-loop accumulation and enables replication recovery, while promoting arrest of the cell cycle at the G2/M-phase [21]. Resolution of replication stress triggers ATR to resume HRR activities by promoting fork reversal and restart, a process involving the recruitment of *BRCA2* and RAD51 to sites of damage [11, 22].

In addition to its role in HRR, ATR has further roles in DNA repair through its involvement in the inter-strand crosslink repair (ICLR) and nucleotide excision repair (NER) pathways. ICLR removes toxic inter-strand DNA crosslinks (lesions involving both strands of DNA that can result in replication fork-stalling and inhibition of transcription). The presence of ICLs activates ATR and requires ATR-mediated phosphorylation of Fanconi Anemia proteins, which are key players in mediating ICLR [23, 24]. Lastly, NER is a critical mechanism that repairs a wide variety of DNA lesions caused by chemical agents or environmental factors (particularly UV radiation) [25]. In this repair mechanism, ATR phosphorylates and stabilizes Xeroderma pigmentosa group A (XPA), thereby recruiting the protein to sites of damage during the S-phase of the cell-cycle and aiding in the activation of the NER pathway [26]. As a key player in multiple processes, ATR

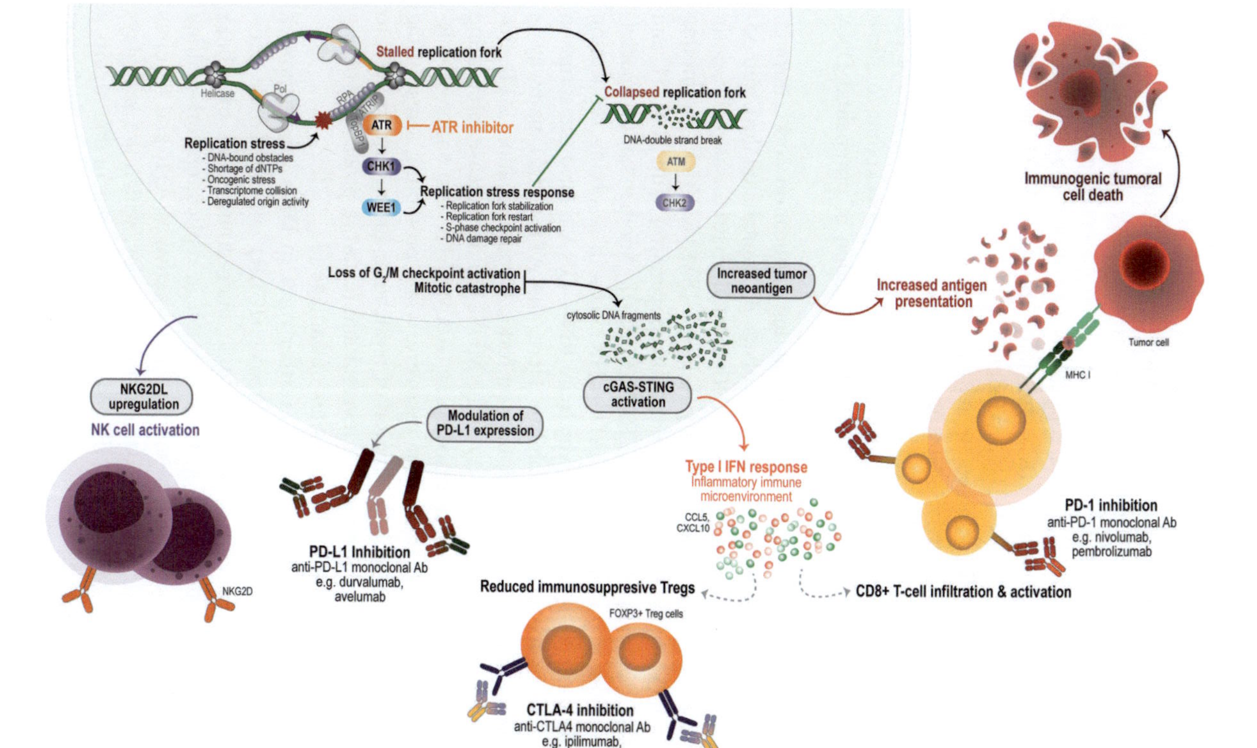

Fig. 14.1 **ATR activation, inhibition and modulation of antitumor immunity**. ATR is activated in response to replication stress, single-stranded DNA, and increased R-loops. ATR activation triggers a kinase cascade of CHK1 and WEE1, resulting in checkpoint activation and cell cycle arrest for DNA repair. ATR inhibition induces inappropriate mitotic entry that culminates in mitotic catastrophe and the release of DNA fragments into the cytosol, which in turn activate the cGAS-STING pathway and a type I IFN response. DDR may also be a means of increasing tumor mutational burden and therefore the generation of neoantigens

is a master regulator of DNA repair and more broadly in the replication stress response.

14.3 ATR Signaling Fosters Cancer Cell Survival

Activation of DDR in normal cells can either resolve DNA damage and/or replication stress to promote cell survival, or it can trigger programmed cell death when DNA damage cannot be removed, inhibiting tumorigenesis and preventing inheritance of DNA mutations in daughter cells [28–31]. Since DDR is often dampened in cancer cells, these cells present increased DNA damage that is tolerated due to a simultaneous amelioration of unrepaired DNA damage response. In this way, DDR is used by cancer cells as a decoy mechanism to shield against cell death and allow genomically unstable cells to traverse the cell-cycle unscathed, making cancer cells dependent on DDR for survival. That is, tolerance of replication stress is crucial for tumor viability, and oncogene-induced dysregulation of DNA replication generates high levels of replication stress in cancer cells [27–29]. Furthermore, most cancers also feature defective G1 checkpoints, largely due to *p53* signaling loss [30], rendering cancel cells dependent on S- and G2-phase checkpoints, which are ATR-regulated processes [30].

Frequent mutations in DDR genes also increase dependency on ATR signaling [28, 31]. In these situations, cancer cells rely on ATR to respond to and resolve replication stress and repair DNA damage in order to bypass cell death [27]. Given that ATR function is conserved in the vast majority of cancers, it is has emerged as a favorable target in cancer medicine [32]. ATR inhibition in normal cycling cells, with intact cell-cycle checkpoints, leads to moderate cytotoxicity due to replication fork stalling and collapse; however, as cancer cells have high replication stress, they are more dependent on ATR for survival and as a result are more sensitive to its inhibition than normal cells [27, 28]. Furthermore, in-vitro data suggests that chronic use of ATR inhibitors impairs the cell's ability to repair damage by HRR while also impacting the availability of necessary HRR proteins, such as TopBP1, *BRCA1*, and RAD51 [28]. This targeted approach has culminated in the development of many clinical studies aimed at evaluating the clinical efficacy of ATR inhibition as both a monotherapy in certain DDR defective cancer backgrounds and in combinational approaches [19, 33].

14.4 Early Development of ATR Inhibitors

The development of potent and selective ATR kinase inhibitors has been closely related to (1) the availability of well-characterized assays that permit accurate measurements of selective kinase activity, (2) the availability of structural and functional insights to guide a drug design strategy that maximizes selectivity, and (3) the development of screening tools and biomarkers that can identify suitable patients. Notably, the first generation of small molecule ATR inhibitors struggled to find balance between potency and selectivity to reach clinical usage. For instance, while Schisandrin B, an active ingredient of the magnolia berry (*Schisandra chinensis*), inhibited ATR kinase activity at high concentrations leading to off-target effects and toxicity, the small molecule NU6087 demonstrated moderate selectivity over *ATM* homologs, but did not display selectivity over the wider kinase family [34]. With the development of a cell-screening assay that measured ATP-dependent phosphorylation of H2AX as a more accurate quantification of ATR kinase activity in experimental conditions, the small molecule ETP-46464 was selected from a library of compounds based on its increased selectivity over other ATR homologs. Although poor pharmacological properties in mice prevented ETP-46464 from advancing to clinical studies, the discovery of this compound provided proof of concept for a more reliable biomarker of replication stress that accounts for double stand breaks and has become the standard marker for quantifying DNA damage [35]. Based on recent advances in the development of well-characterized assays, as well as new insights in the structure–function relationship of ATR, many pharmaceutical companies have taken on the challenge to design and develop potent and selective ATP competitive inhibitors of ATR with the most advanced targeted therapies described here.

14.5 ATR Inhibitors in the Clinic

14.5.1 Berzosertib (M6620/VX-970/VE-822)

Shortly after the development of the assay that measured ATR-dependent phosphorylation of γH2AX, a high throughput screen that combined structure–activity relationship with homology modeling led to the discovery of VE-821, a selective inhibitor with 600-fold selectivity for ATR over *ATM*, DNA-PK, mTOR, and PI3K [36]. In addition to increased selectivity, VE-821 also showed strong inhibition of CHK1 phosphorylation in cellular models of *ATM* and/or *p53* deficiency [37]. In-vitro experiments showed that VE-821 sensitized ovarian cancer cells to DNA damaging agents such as cisplatin and gemcitabine, and the effects of gemcitabine were potentiated when combined with VE-821 in pancreatic cancer cells [38]. It was also observed that VE-821 could further sensitize *BRCA1*-depleted cells to DNA damaging agents [44]. Such synergistic effects appear to be stronger with DNA-damaging agents, such as cisplatin and carboplatin, since DNA crosslinking triggers early activation of ATR and the DDR machinery. Interestingly, *p53*-deficient cancer cell lines were shown to be more sensitive to the combination of VE-821 and cisplatin than normal cell lines, and significant synergistic activity was observed in *ATM*-deficient cell lines [43]. These results were further confirmed by treating *ATM*-proficient cells with the triple combination of VE-821, cisplatin, and a highly selective *ATM* inhibitor (KU-55933) [37]. Taken together, these results suggested that cancer cells with defective *ATM* signaling are more reliant on ATR; hence, demonstrating a synthetic lethal interaction between the S-phase specific

ATR and the *ATM-p53* pathway mediating the G1 checkpoint [39]. However, it must be noted that recent studies have shown that *ATM* mutations and *p53* status are not enough to predict clinical benefit to ATR inhibition, and mutations in other DDR genes—such as *PTEN, XRCC1, BRCA1, BRCA2*, and *ARID1A*—may promote synthetic lethality with ATR inhibitors [40].

Based on promising pre-clinical data, VE-822, an optimized analog of VE-821 with increased potency and selectivity for ATR, became the first inhibitor to enter clinical trials labeled as VX-970, later named M6620 and berzosertib [41]. Berzosertib alone was found to sensitize multiple lung cancer cell lines to a wide variety of DNA-damaging chemotherapeutic agents (cisplatin, oxaliplatin, gemcitabine, etoposide, and the active metabolite of irinotecan, SN38), and the combination of berzosertib and cisplatin showed sustained tumor regression in non-small cell lung cancer (NSCLC) patient-derived xenograft models [42]. A recent CRISPR-Cas9 screen suggested that the ATR-CHK1 pathway has the potential for synthetic lethality in small cell lung cancer (SCLC) [43]. In that study, the combination of berzosertib with cisplatin displayed greater synergistic activity in different SCLC cell lines and primary lung fibroblasts when compared to treatment with the combination of cisplatin and etoposide. Interestingly, while SCLC cell-derived xenografts showed that the combination of berzosertib with cisplatin inhibited tumor growth, other studies showed that pediatric solid tumor xenografts treated with berzosertib and cisplatin displayed a larger event free survival relative to those treated with cisplatin monotherapy [44, 45]. Together, these studies were the first to confirm the clinical potential of berzosertib as a chemo-sensitizer of DNA damaging agents in lung cancer patients, as well as in pediatric solid tumors, setting the stage for several other studies that also showed the clinical potential of berzosertib in combination with cisplatin in other cancer types, including colon cancer, triple negative breast cancer (TNBC), and esophageal tumors, amongst others [44–47].

Berzosertib monotherapy has already advanced to a phase II clinical trial investigating antitumor activity in molecularly selected solid tumors, leiomyosarcoma and osteosarcoma (NCT03718091). Although clinical trials are currently studying the combination of berzosertib with radiotherapy, chemo-radiotherapy agents, PARP inhibitors, VEGF inhibitors, as well as with anti-PD-L1 antibodies, such as avelumab, the most common strategy for berzosertib treatment combinations in registered clinical trials appears to be with DNA damaging agents such as cisplatin, carboplatin, gemcitabine, topotecan, irinotecan, and paclitaxel, amongst others (Table 14.1).

The first-in-human trial of berzosertib in combination with cytotoxic chemotherapy agents in patients with advanced solid tumors started with a lead-in safety phase of berzosertib monotherapy, followed by three dose escalation arms aimed to determine the safety profile and recommended phase 2 dose (RP2D) of the combinations of berzosertib with (1) cisplatin, (2) gemcitabine with and without cisplatin, and (3) irinotecan. This trial also included 3 expansion cohorts to further elucidate preliminary anti-tumor activity for the combination of berzosertib and gemcitabine in NSCLC patients harboring *p53* mutations and/or loss of *ATM*

Table 14.1 Trials investigating berzosertib combinational strategies

ATR inhibitor	Phase	Combination strategy	Schedule	Study population	Safety	Efficacy	References
Berzosertib (M6620, VX-970, VE-822) Berzosertib (M6620, VX-970, VE-822)	I	Cisplatin Gemcitabine Gemcitabine + Cisplatin Carboplatin	Lead-in monotherapy Part A: combination with gemcitabine as well as gemcitabine and cisplatin Part B: combination with cisplatin as well as cisplatin and etoposide Part C1: combination with gemcitabine in patients NSCLC Part C2: combination with cisplatin in subjects with advanced TNBC Part C3: combination with cisplatin or carboplatin in subjects with platinum-resistant advanced SCLC	Advanced solid tumors	Part A (berzosertib + gemcitabine) RP2D: 210 mg/m^2 of berzosertib and 1000 mg/m^2 of gemcitabine Grade $\geq$ 3 AE: neutropenia, increased ALT and fatigue (16% each), anemia and thrombocytopenia (10% each) Part B RP2D: 140 mg/m^2 of berzosertib and 75 mg/m^2 of cisplatin Grade $\geq$ 3 AE: neutropenia (21.7%), anemia (4.3%), and thrombocytopenia (4.3%)	Part A (berzosertib + gemcitabine) 60.4% of patients achieved SD and 8.3% PR as best response Part B (berzosertib + cisplatin) 57.7% of patients achieved SD and 15.4% PR as best response	NCT02157792 [48, 53]

(continued)

Table 14.1 (continued)

ATR inhibitor	Phase	Combination strategy	Schedule	Study population	Safety	Efficacy	References
	II	Gemcitabine	Gemcitabine 1000 mg/m^2 (D1, D8) $\pm$ berzosertib 210 mg/m^2 (D2, D9)—21-day cycles	Platinum-resistant ovarian cancers	Gemcitabine + berzosertib Grade $\geq$ 3 AE: Neutropenia (47%), thrombocytopenia (24%)	PFS: 22.9 weeks for the gemcitabine + berzosertib arm versus 14.7 weeks gemcitabine alone (HR, 0.57; 90% CI, 0.33–0.98; p = 0.044)	NCT02595892 [51]
	II	Gemcitabine	Gemcitabine 1000 mg/m^2 (D1, D8) $\pm$ berzosertib 210 mg/m^2 (D2, D9)—21-day cycles	Leiomyosarcomas	N/A	Active, not recruiting	NCT04807816
	I/II	Topotecan	Phase I: Topotecan (D1–5) + berzosertib (D5 or D2 and D5 at escalating doses)—21-day cycles Phase II: 210 mg/m^2 of berzosertib and 1.25 mg/m^2 of topotecan	SCLCs and extrapulmonary small-cell cancers	Phase I Grade $\geq$ 3 AE: Anemia, leukopenia, and neutropenia (19% each); lymphopenia (14%); and thrombocytopenia (10%)	Phase II Objective response rate among patients with SCLC was 36% (9/25)	NCT02487095 [54, 55]

(continued)

Table 14.1 (continued)

ATR inhibitor	Phase	Combination strategy	Schedule	Study population	Safety	Efficacy	References
	II	Topotecan	210 mg/m2 of berzosertib (D5 or D2) and 1.25 mg/m^2 of topotecan (D1-D5), 21-day cycles	Relapsed platinum-resistant SCLCs	N/A	Active, not recruiting	NCT04768296
	I	Irinotecan	Irinotecan + berzosertib (D1, D15)—28-day cycles	Advanced, unresectable solid tumors	N/A	Active, not recruiting	NCT02595931
	II	Irinotecan	Irinotecan + berzosertib (D1, D15)—28-day cycles	Metastatic or unresectable gastric harboring *p53* mutations	N/A	Active, not recruiting	NCT03641313

(continued)

Table 14.1 (continued)

ATR inhibitor	Phase	Combination strategy	Schedule	Study population	Safety	Efficacy	References
	I/II	Sacituzumab govitecan	Sacituzumab govitecan (D1, D8) + berzosertib (escalating doses)—21-day cycles	SCLCs and HRD cancers resistant to PARPi. Pathogenic mutations in *BRCA1, BRCA2, ATM, BRIP1, BARD1, CDK12, CHEK1, CHEK2, FANCL, PALB2, PPP2R2A, RAD51B, RAD51C, RAD51D*, or *RAD54L*	N/A	Active, not recruiting	NCT04826341
	II	Carboplatin Docetaxel + Carboplatin	Berzosertib 90 mg/m^2 (D2, D9) + carboplatin (D1)—21-day cycles Docetaxel 60 mg/m^2 (D1) + carboplatin (D1)—21-day cycles	Metastatic castration-resistant prostate cancers	N/A	Active, not recruiting	NCT03517969

(continued)

C. Salguero et al.

Table 14.1 (continued)

ATR inhibitor	Phase	Combination strategy	Schedule	Study population	Safety	Efficacy	References
	I	Carboplatin + Gemcitabine	Carboplatin (D1) + Gemcitabine (D1, D8) + berzosertib (D2, D9)—21-day cycles	Metastatic Ovarian, Primary Peritoneal, or Fallopian Tube Cancer	N/A	Active, not recruiting	NCT02627443
	I	Veliparib + Cisplatin	Berzosertib (D2, D9) + veliparib BID (D1-3 and 8–10) + cisplatin (D1, D8)—21-day cycles	Advanced solid tumors	N/A	Active, not recruiting	NCT02723864
	I/II	Carboplatin + Gemcitabine + Pembrolizumab	Carboplatin (D1) + Gemcitabine (D1, D8) + berzosertib (D2, D9) + Pembrolizumab (D1) during 4, 21-day cycles. After cycle 4 berzosertib (D2, D9) + Pembrolizumab (D1)	Lung non-small cell squamous carcinoma	N/A	Active, not recruiting	NCT04216316

(continued)

Table 14.1 (continued)

ATR inhibitor	Phase	Combination strategy	Schedule	Study population	Safety	Efficacy	References
	I	Avelumab	Avelumab (D1, D15) + berzosertib (D1, D8, D15, D22)—28 day cycles	Advanced solid tumors	N/A	Active, not recruiting	NCT04266912
	Ib/II	Avelumab	Part A: safety run-in of carboplatin AUC 5 (D1) + avelumab 1600 mg (D1) + berzosertib 90 mg/m2 (D2)—21 day cycles	Recurrent platinum-sensitive ovarian cancers resistant to PARPi	N/A	Completed	NCT03704467

expression, the combination of berzosertib and cisplatin in TNBC patients with germline (*g*) *BRCA* wild type status, and the combination of berzosertib and cisplatin or carboplatin in patients with platinum-resistant advanced SCLC.

Recent results from two dose escalation arms of this first-in-human trial demonstrated preliminary antitumor activity for berzosertib when combined with gemcitabine and/or cisplatin [48]. That is, most patients who received berzosertib in combination with cisplatin (73.1%), and those who received berzosertib in combination with gemcitabine (68.7%) or berzosertib in combination with gemcitabine and cisplatin (71.0%) achieved disease control with partial response (PR) or stable disease (SD) as their best response per RECIST v1.1 [48]. Interestingly, all patients who received prior platinum-based chemotherapy, and had experienced disease progression, achieved PR when treated with berzosertib in combination with cisplatin. Since ATR inhibition can disrupt DNA replication fork stability and homologous recombination repair (the two major mechanisms of PARP inhibitor resistance), preliminary results from this trial suggest that berzosertib inhibition may contribute to re-sensitizing solid tumors to cisplatin [49].

The RP2D for the combination of berzosertib and cisplatin was determined as 140 mg/m^2 of berzosertib (administered on days 2 and 9), and 75 mg/m^2 of cisplatin administered every 3 weeks (Q3W) on day 1. This RP2D was generally well tolerated, and the safety profile of this combination was consistent with that of cisplatin alone. Importantly, while the human equivalent dose required for berzosertib target engagement was estimated from preclinical models to be ~60 mg/m^2, results from the first-in-human trial show that dosing berzosertib at 140 mg/m^2 induces a reduction in serine 345-phosphorylated CHK1, without evidence of PK interactions in a range of malignancies, including ovarian, breast, thyroid, and pancreatic cancers [50]. In a similar manner, the RP2D combination of berzosertib and gemcitabine, which is currently being evaluated in patients with advanced NSCLC in an expansion arm of this trial, was established as 210 mg/m^2 of berzosertib (administered on days 2 and 9), and 1000 mg/ m^2 of gemcitabine, administered Q3W on days 1 and 8. Yet, the dose escalation for berzosertib in combination with both gemcitabine and cisplatin was terminated after two patients experienced febrile neutropenia or neutropenia as dose limiting toxicities (DLTs). Taken together, results from the first two arms of the first-in-human trial of berzosertib demonstrate that a tolerable safety toxicity profile is observed when berzosertib is combined with either gemcitabine or cisplatin, but not when combined with both agents [48].

The pharmacokinetic (PK) profile of a berzosertib monotherapy lead-in was determined across the dose range of 18–210 mg/m^2 (n = 30), and it was characterized by biphasic decline with a moderate-to-high clearance, a high distribution volume, and an apparent terminal half-life of approximately 17 hours [48]. While the PK characteristics of berzosertib in combination with either gemcitabine or cisplatin were consistent with the corresponding doses of berzosertib monotherapy, the collective PK data from these two arms suggest that pre-administration of cisplatin 24 hours before berzosertib administration does not affect the PK profile of berzosertib.

Another trial that is currently investigating the combination of berzosertib and gemcitabine is a multicenter, randomized, phase II study that recently published preliminary efficacy and safety data suggesting that this combination provides clinical benefit to platinum-resistant high-grade serous ovarian cancer (HGSOC) patients. At the cutoff date of publication, 70 patients had been randomly assigned to either receive treatment with the berzosertib and gemcitabine combination (n = 34) and achieved a median profession-free survival (PFS) of 22.9 weeks (90%, CI 17.9–72.0), or they were assigned to receive treatment with gemcitabine alone (n = 36) and achieved a median PFS of 14.7 weeks (90%, CI 9.7–36.7). Yet, while the combination of berzosertib and gemcitabine displayed a promising PFS with a hazard ratio of 0.57 (90%, CI 0.33–0.98), a higher objective response was observed for the group of patients who received treatment with gemcitabine alone. According to the authors, discrepancies between ORR and PFS are not uncommon in platinum-resistant ovarian cancer patients [51]. A sub-analysis of the patient population based on the length of the platinum-free interval also showed that patients who are treated with the berzosertib and gemcitabine combination, and who have had a platinum-free interval of 3 months or less, have a 30% increase in median PFS (27.7 weeks compared to 18.6 weeks in patients with intervals larger than 3 months). Since the PFS benefit observed for patients with a platinum-free interval of 3 months or less may be related to the enrichment for biomarkers of replicative stress, the authors followed up on this finding with further correlative assays [51]. Interestingly, results from follow-up studies using the same replication stress signature show that the combination of berzosertib and gemcitabine benefited more patients with tumors displaying low replication stress (RS-low) in contrast to patients with high replication stress tumors (who appeared to receive a greater benefit from the increase of replication stress caused by gemcitabine monotherapy [52]. Based on these results, it is suggested that increasing replication stress in RS-loss with gemcitabine concomitant with ATR inhibition by berzosertib is necessary for lethality [52].

Finally, a few clinical trials have published results about the preliminary efficacy and safety profile of the combination of berzosertib with topotecan in patients with lung cancers. A proof-of-concept phase I clinical trial that investigated the combination of berzosertib with topotecan in patients with platinum-resistant small cell lung cancer (SCLC) showed that 60% (3/5) of the patients treated achieved a PR or prolonged SD lasting ≥6 months, and the combination seemed to be well tolerated with no additive toxicity observed [54]. Yet, shortly after the interim results of the DDRiver SCLC 250 phase II trial investigating the combination of berzosertib with topotecan in platinum-resistant SCLC patients reported an objective response rate of 36% (9/25) and a median duration of response of 6.4 months, the trial was discontinued based on a low probability of meeting the primary objective [55, 56]. Further results from ongoing clinical trials are needed to demonstrate whether treating patients with advanced cancers, whose tumors are undergoing high replicative stress, with the combination of berzosertib and DNA-damaging chemotherapeutic agents may potentially help overcome platinum and/or PARP inhibitor resistance.

14.5.2 Ceralasertib (AZD6738)

Ceralasertib is a potent and selective ATR inhibitor with a promising preclinical data package showing efficacy in DDR-deficient settings [57]. Early preclinical studies showed that ceralasertib increases γH2AX phosphorylation, while inhibiting phosphorylation downstream of CHK1 in a variety of *ATM*-deficient cell lines and inducing accumulation of unrepaired DNA damage and cell death in *ATM/p53*-deficient leukemia cells [58, 59]. Recently, a growth inhibition assay assessing the sensitivity of 276 cancer cell lines to ceralasertib reported that cell lines harboring CCNE1 amplification or *ARD1A*, *ATRX*, and *SETD2* mutations were associated with sensitivity. At first sight, cancer cell lines harboring *ATM* mutations were not associated with sensitivity; yet, upon stratifying the cancer cells based on *ATM* expression levels, it was shown that complete absence of *ATM* function is significantly associated with sensitivity to ceralasertib [60]. This finding, along with previous observations of antitumor responses from patients harboring *ATM* loss-of-function, supports the idea that patient selection for ATR inhibitors should consider biallelic deleterious mutations and *ATM*-null expression [61].

Preliminary results from the dose escalation and expansion monotherapy arms of the PATRIOT phase I clinical trial reported that ceralasertib was better tolerated when administered at an intermittent schedule of 2-weeks-on/2-weeks-off because only 20% of the patients experienced grade ≥ 3 treatment related adverse events (TRAEs) compared to 67% of patients when ceralasertib was administered in a continuous schedule (NCT02223923). Although it was previously shown that ceralasertib monotherapy in-vivo only induces significant tumor control/stasis and that the synergistic effects resulting in tumor regression are pronounced when ceralasertib is combined with DNA damaging agents or certain targeted small molecules, preliminary antitumor activity of the ceralasertib monotherapy arms of the PATRIOT trial show that 7% of patients achieved PR and 48% of them achieved SD as best overall response [60, 62, 63].

In-vivo, the combination of ceralasertib and cisplatin induced significant tumor reduction in HER2-positive breast cancer cells, as well as tumor regression in *ATM*-deficient lung cancer xenograft models and synergistic effects in *ATM*-deficient NSCLC cell lines [64, 65]. Results from a phase I trial investigating the combination of ceralasertib and carboplatin in advanced solid tumor patients reported that 2 (6%) of patients with low *ATM* or SLFN11 expression achieved PR as best response by RECIST v1.1, while 53% patients (including two unconfirmed PRs) achieved SD for ≥ 35 days (NCT02264678) [66]. Although no association between *ATM* and SLFN11 expression level and antitumor activity was reported, likely due to the sample size, these findings support the notion that further investigations on the interaction between ATR and loss of *ATM* function are needed. In contrast, a phase I clinical trial investigating the safety and antitumor activity of the ceralasertib and paclitaxel combination in advanced solid tumors (enriched for melanoma patients) reported one patient achieved complete response (CR), while 21% achieved PR and 32% achieved SD. Even though the ORR for the entire population was 22.6% (95% CI, 12.5–35.5), an ORR of 33.3% (95% CI, 10.8–51.8) was reported for the subset of melanoma patients resistant to PD1/L1 treatment [67].

Although both phase I trials studying the combinations of ceralasertib with chemotherapy agents reported that the combinational strategies are safe and well tolerated, thrombocytopenia, neutropenia and anemia were reported as the most common grade ≥ 3 TRAEs, with schedule limiting consequences observed with the combination of ceralasertib and carboplatin. Since toxicity may be one of the major challenges in the implementation of ATR inhibitor combinations with DNA damaging agents and other targeted small molecules, the success of clinical trials investigating ceralasertib combinations depends on the optimization of the dose scheduling sequences and targeted genetic tumor aberrations. For instance, recent in-vivo studies suggest that to achieve tumor regressions, concurrent dosing for the ceralasertib and irinotecan combination should be extended at least one day, while a few days of ceralasertib dosing should be included after concurrent dosing with carboplatin [60]. In a similar fashion, the ATRiUM phase I clinical trial is investigating the safety and antitumor activity of ceralasertib with either intermittent or continuous gemcitabine dosing in advanced solid tumors, particularly in patients with advanced pancreatic ductal adenocarcinoma with *ATM*-loss-of-function [68, 69]. In all, results from an ongoing phase II trial investigating ceralasertib monotherapy in advanced solid tumors (enriching for mCRPC with low *ATM* expression), as well as results from the remaining arms of the PATRIOT phase I clinical trial and the ATRiUM phase I are required to further assess the clinical efficacy of ceralasertib monotherapy and in combination with chemotherapy agents in a molecularly targeted population.

Although synergistic effects in-vivo were observed when combining ceralasertib with either PARP or WEE1 inhibitors, only the PARP inhibitors and ceralasertib combination has successfully reached phase II clinical trials. Out of the six clinical trials that are currently investigating the combination of ceralasertib and olaparib in the advanced cancer setting, one phase I study reported on safety and preliminary antitumor efficacy, as well as established the RP2D of the ceralasertib and olaparib combination in patients with advanced solid tumors, and two Phase II trials have presented contrasting preliminary results based on patient selection (Table 14.2) [63, 70, 71]. Briefly, results from one of the first modular phase I clinical trials to test the combination of ceralasertib and olaparib established a concurrent RP2D of ceralasertib at 160 mg QD on days 1–7 and olaparib at 300 mg twice daily (BID) on days 1–28, with thrombocytopenia and neutropenia defined as dose limiting toxicities [72]. Within the module that tested the dose escalation of ceralasertib and olaparib, antitumor responses were observed in patients with advanced breast, ovarian, prostate, pancreatic, and ampullary cancer. Interestingly, while some of the responding tumors had *BRCA1/2* mutations, antitumor responses were independent of *ATM* status [72]. Such results are in accordance with recent preclinical studies suggesting that the combination of ceralasertib and olaparib in a concurrent schedule induces tumor regression in TNBC *BRCA*-wild type and *BRCA2*-mutated xenograft models [60], and the development of a phase II clinical trial currently recruiting patients to investigate the combination of ceralasertib and olaparib in advanced germline *BRCA* mutated breast cancer (NCT04090567).

Although differences in study design preclude us from direct comparisons, preliminary antitumor activity from two phase II clinical trials investigating the combination of ceralasertib and olaparib seemed to be influenced by the selection of targeted genetic tumor aberrations. That is, the phase II clinical trial investigating the clinical benefit of this combination in patients with advanced solid tumors with or without ARID1A-deficiency (defined as lack of expression of BAF250a by IHC) reported an ORR of 20% for patients with ARID1A-deficiency, including two patients that achieved sustained CRs, while no objective responses were observed in the cohort of patients with active ARID1A function [73]. In contrast, the phase II clinical trial investigating signals of activity of the ceralasertib and olaparib combination in patients with HGSOC reported no partial or complete responses in a PARP naïve, genetically unselected, platinum-resistant cohort of 12 patients. Nonetheless, 75% of the patients in that trial achieved SD as best overall response by RECIST v1.1 and 27% of the patients achieved $\geq 50\%$ decrease in CA-125, most of them harboring tumors with somatic *BRCA1* mutations [74].

As mentioned by investigators of the HGSOC phase II trial, it is likely that more responses may have been achieved by focusing the patient population to ovarian cancer patients harboring tumors with *BRCA1/2* mutations and/or CCNE1 copy number amplification [74]. Taking it all together, the ceralasertib and olaparib combination appears to be well tolerated, but it is necessary to continue optimizing patient selection strategies based on the selection of genetic aberrations that induce synthetic lethality in different types of cancer types. Such concept seems to be reflected in recent preliminary results from the HUDSON trial, a phase II multidrug, biomarker selected umbrella study investigating the combination of multiple targeted small molecules with durvalumab, including ceralasertib for NSCLC patients who progressed after anti-PD-1/PD-L1 and platinum therapy (NCT03334617). Although no correlation was found between *ATM* biomarker status and clinical responses by RECIST 1.1, the HUDSON trial reported an improved ORR (11.1%) and longer PFS (7.43 months) for patients whose tumors harbored *ATM* mutations or low protein expression -when compared to an ORR of 8.3% and PFS of 4.96 months for NSCLC patients with acquired resistance to prior immunotherapy, regardless of *ATM* status [75].

By comparing gene expression profiles in paired blood samples from patients with controlled disease and patients whose disease progressed with the ceralasertib monotherapy run-in, the HUDSON trial showed increases in an antigen presentation gene signature and decreases in exhausted T-cell and NK-cell signatures, supporting a model in which ceralasertib also has an active role in the immune activation caused by the combination of ceralasertib with durvalumab [77]. These findings are also in agreement with results from a phase II clinical trial investigating the clinical activity of the ceralasertib and durvalumab combination in advanced gastric cancer patients, which reported (1) significantly longer PFS for patients whose tumors harbored *ATM*-deficiency and/or HRD-deficiency when compared to patients with active *ATM* function and HRD-proficient (5.60 months

Table 14.2 Trials investigating ceralasertib combinational strategies

ATR inhibitor	Phase	Combination strategy	Schedule	Study population	Safety	Efficacy	References
Ceralasertib (AZD6738) Ceralasertib (AZD6738) Ceralasertib (AZD6738)	I	Monotherapy	Dose escalation and dose expansion	Advanced solid tumors	Grade $\geq$3 TRAEs in 67%	21% of patients in dose escalation and 25% in dose expansion had SD$\geq$16 weeks (n = 46) 3 PR (7%) 22 SD (48%)	NCT02223923 [62]
	II	Monotherapy	Ceralasertib monotherapy, 28-day cycles	Advanced solid tumors and mCRPC; target 60% with low *ATM* expression	N/A	Recruitment ongoing	NCT04564027
	I	Carboplatin	Dose escalation (ceralasertib 20 mg -60 mg) sequential and concurrent dosing	Advanced solid tumors	RP2D ceralasertib 40 mg QD (D1-D2) + carboplatin AUC5 Q3W, q21d Toxicities of grade $\geq$3 were neutropenia, anemia, and thrombocytopenia	2 PR (6%) 18 SD (53%)	NCT02264678 [66]
	I	Paclitaxel	Paclitaxel 80 mg/m^2 (D1, D8, D15) + ceralasertib at escalating doses 40 mg OD – 240 mg BID, 28-day cycles	Advanced solid tumors	RP2D ceralasertib 240 mg BID (D1–14) + paclitaxel at 80 mg/m^2 (D1, 8, 15), q28w Toxicities of grade $\geq$3 were neutropenia, anemia, and thrombocytopenia	ORR 25.6% (n = 57) 1 CR (1.9%) 12 PR (21.1%) 18 SD (31.6%)	NCT02630199 [67]

(continued)

Table 14.2 (continued)

ATR inhibitor	Phase	Combination strategy	Schedule	Study population	Safety	Efficacy	References
	I	Gemcitabine	Gemcitabine at escalating doses 500–1000 mg/m^2 (D3, D10, D17) + ceralasertib at escalating doses 40–120 mg (D1–21), 28-day cycles Gemcitabine at escalating doses 500–1000 mg/m^2 (D3, D10, D17) + ceralasertib at escalating doses 40–120 mg, for up to 12 days, 28-day cycles	Advanced solid tumors	N/A	Recruitment ongoing	NCT03669601
	I	Trastuzumab deruxtecan	Trastuzumab deruxtecan (D1) + ceralasertib BD (D1-7)	Advanced solid tumors with HER2 expression	N/A	Recruitment ongoing	NCT04704661

(continued)

Table 14.2 (continued)

ATR inhibitor	Phase	Combination strategy	Schedule	Study population	Safety	Efficacy	References
	I	Carboplatin Olaparib Durvalumab	Dose escalation and dose expansion	Advanced solid tumors: Head & Neck, SCC, *ATM* proficient and deficient NSCLC, Gastric, Breast and Ovarian Cancer	RP2D for olaparib combination: ceralasertib 160 mg QD (D1 D7) + olaparib 300 mg BID (D1-D28) Olaparib combination: DLT thrombocytopenia and neutropenia. Toxicity, including grade ≥ 3: thrombocytopenia, anemia, neutropenia, fatigue, decreased appetite, nausea, vomiting, constipation, diarrhea and cough Durvalumab combination: DLT thrombocytopenia Toxicity, including grade ≥ 3: anemia, fatigue, nausea, decreased appetite, cough, vomiting, dizziness, pruritus, constipation, diarrhea, musculoskeletal chest pain and dyspnea	Tumor activity for olaparib combo: 1 CR (2.5%) 5 PR (12.8%) Independent of *ATM* status Tumor activity for durvalumab combo: 1 CR (4.8%) 2 PR (9.5%) Independent of PD-L1 expression	NCT02264678 [72]

(continued)

Table 14.2 (continued)

ATR inhibitor	Phase	Combination strategy	Schedule	Study population	Safety	Efficacy	References
	II	Olaparib	Olaparib BID (D1-D28) + Ceralasertib QD(D1-D7), 28-day cycles	Advanced metastatic *gBRCAm* breast cancer	N/A	Recruitment ongoing	NCT04090567
	II	Olaparib	Ceralasertib monotherapy Olaparib 300 mg BID (D1-D28) + Ceralasertib 160 mg QD(D1-D7), 28-day cycles	Advanced pancreatic, clear cell renal and urothelial carcinoma with *ARD1A* and *ATM* mutations	N/A	Recruitment ongoing	NCT03682289 (73)
	II	Olaparib	Olaparib 300 mg BID (D1-D28) + Ceralasertib 160 mg QD (D1-D7), 28-day cycles	Recurrent HGSOC, primary peritoneal, or fallopian cancer	Toxicity, including grade $\geq$ 3: nausea, fatigue, anorexia and anemia	Recruitment ongoing No objective responses in the platinum resistance HGSOC cohort 9 SD (75%)	NCT03462342 [74]
	II	Olaparib	Olaparib BID (D1-D28) + Ceralasertib QD (D1-D7), 28-day cycles	*IDH* mutant cholangiocarcinoma or solid tumors	N/A	Recruitment ongoing	NCT03878095

(continued)

Table 14.2 (continued)

ATR inhibitor	Phase	Combination strategy	Schedule	Study population	Safety	Efficacy	References
	II	Olaparib	Olaparib BID (D1-D28) + Ceralasertib QD (D1-D7), 28-day cycles	Recurrent osteosarcoma	N/A	Recruitment ongoing	NCT04417062
	II	Durvalumab	Ceralasertib 240 mg BID (D15-D28) + Durvalumab IV at 1500 mg Q4W, 28-day cycles	Advanced biliary track cancers with prior immunotherapy	N/A	Recruitment ongoing	NCT04298008
	II	Durvalumab	Ceralasertib 240 mg BID (D15-D28) + Durvalumab IV at 1500 mg Q4W, 28-day cycles	Advanced gastric cancer	AEs manageable with dose modification	ORR overall: 22.6% PFS: 3 months OS: 6.7 months	NCT03780608 [76]

(continued)

Table 14.2 (continued)

ATR inhibitor	Phase	Combination strategy	Schedule	Study population	Safety	Efficacy	References
	II	Durvalumab	Ceralasertib 240 mg BID (D1-D7, D22-D28) + Durvalumab IV at 1500 mg Q4W, 28-day cycles Ceralasertib 240 mg BID (D15-D28) + Durvalumab IV at 1500 mg Q4W, 28-day cycles Ceralasertib 240 or 160 mg BID (D22-D28) + Durvalumab IV at 1500 mg Q4W, 28-day cycles	NSCLC who progressed on anti-PD-1/PD-L1, with and without *ATM*-loss-of-function or *ATM* mutations	N/A	ORR overall: 8.7–11.1% $PFS_{6months}$: 37.0–53.8% $OS_{6months}$: 74.8–77.3% For population with *ATM* aberrations ORR: 13.3% $PFS_{6months}$: 61.2% $OS_{6months}$: 100%	NCT03334617 [75]
	II	Durvalumab	Ceralasertib 240 mg BID (D1-D7 cycle 1 and D22-D28 subsequent cycles) + durvalumab IV at 1500 mg Q4W, 28-day cycles versus docetaxel standard of care	NSCLC who progressed on anti-PD-1/PD-L1	N/A	Recruitment ongoing	NCT03833440

versus 1.65 months, HR 0.13., 95% CI 0.045–0.39, $p < 0.001$), as well as, (2) upregulation of the innate immune response, (3) activation of intratumoral lymphocytes, and (4) increase of tumor reactive CD8+ T-cells in patients who responded to treatment [76].

Finally, a phase III clinical trial (LATIFY, NCT05450692) will compare the clinical benefit of the ceralasertib and durvalumab combination versus docetaxel monotherapy in NSCLC patients who progressed after anti-PD-1/PD-L1 and platinum therapy. This is based on the finding that NSCLC patients with primary resistance to immunotherapy only responded to the combination of ceralasertib and durvalumab in the HUDSON trial [75].

14.5.3 Elimusertib (BAY1895344)

By evaluating the molecular interactions of available ATR inhibitors within the binding pocket of an ATR homology model created using the crystal structure of a PI3K kinase and performing a high-throughput screen, Bayer identified a lead compound that was further optimized to reduce potential off-target toxicity [78]. BAY1895344, also called elimusertib, is a potent and selective ATR inhibitor shown to increase γH2AX phosphorylation in HT-29 cells and inhibit cell proliferation in a variety of cancer cell lines, including different lymphoma cells and cell lines harboring mutations that affect the *ATM* pathway, Elimusertib induced stronger antitumor activity than ceralasertib and berzosertib in a lymphoma cell line-derived xenograft (CDX) model, with antitumor activity also observed in ovarian, prostate and colorectal CDX models harboring DDR defects [40]. In addition, elimusertib treatment inhibited neuroblastoma cell growth and induced strong tumor growth inhibition in neuroblastoma xenograft and ALK-driven genetically modified mice models [79]. Interestingly, RNA-seq data from mice who achieved tumor size decrease after elimusertib treatment revealed expression of inflammatory response and immune tumor infiltration, suggesting that ATR inhibition by elimusertib positively impacts the tumoral immune response [79].

Synergistic antitumor efficacy for the combination of elimusertib and DNA-damaging treatments was observed in colorectal cancer cells treated with elimusertib and cisplatin, as well as in colorectal xenograft models treated with elimusertib and radiation therapy [40]. In contrast, antagonistic interactions were observed with the combination of elimusertib and docetaxel [40].

Treatment with elimusertib and olaparib displayed strong antitumor efficacy and a tolerable profile in a TNBC xenograft model and delayed tumor growth in a PARP inhibitor resistant prostate cancer xenograft model [40]. In a similar manner, synergistic antitumor activity was also observed with sequential dosing of anti-PD-1/PD-L1 antibodies and elimusertib in immunocompromised and lymphoma mice models [40]. Taken together, preclinical studies suggest that combining elimusertib with certain DNA damaging agents, as well as with DDR and checkpoint inhibitors, may result in synergistic antitumor activity when compared to the respective singe-agent treatments.

Further studies are currently being conducted to determine the precise combination schedules that are safe and well-tolerated in humans. For instance, results from the dose escalation of the first-in-human trial of elimusertib in patients with advanced solid tumors determined that intermittent dosing of 40 mg BID 3 days on/4 days off is the maximum tolerated dose (MTD) of single-agent elimusertib, with pharmacodynamic data showing on-treatment tumor increases in γH2AX levels (NCT03188965) [80]. The most frequently observed adverse events (AE) in the dose escalation was grade 3 anemia, likely due to limited differentiation and expansion of erythrocyte precursors that are sensitive to replication stress [81]. Based on the safety results from the first elimusertib monotherapy trial, combinational strategies with chemotherapy agents may induce overlapping hematologic toxicity and dose escalations should be approached with caution.

Nonetheless, this trial provided proof-of-concept for the clinical antitumor activity of elimusertib: 4 patients achieved PRs, while 8 achieved SD with a median duration of response of 11.25 months and resulting in 69% disease control rate in patients treated at MTD or above [80]. More importantly, 3 of the 4 patients that achieved PRs had tumors with low *ATM* expression by IHC, with two of them harboring deleterious *ATM* mutations. Albeit a small sample size, an ORR of 33.3% was reported for the subgroup of patients with *ATM* protein loss, and an ORR of 37.5% was calculated for the subgroup of patients harboring *ATM* deleterious mutations [80]. Within the responders for this trial, the investigators noted one heavily pretreated ovarian cancer patient who had received 9 chemotherapy lines, as well as prior PARP inhibitor and immunotherapy, achieved SD for more than year [80]. The clinical benefit observed for this PARP-resistant ovarian cancer patient harboring a *BRCA1* deleterious mutation seem to suggest that PARP inhibitor resistance may be mediated by protection of the DNA replication fork by ATR, opening the possibility of expanding ATR inhibitor treatments to PARP inhibitor-resistant patient population and providing clinical rationale for a phase I clinical trial that investigates the combination of elimusertib and niraparib in patients with advanced ovarian cancer and other solid tumors (Table 14.3, NCT04267939) [80].

14.5.4 Gartisertib (M4344/VX-803)

As an ATP-competitive inhibitor, gartisertib is a selective ATR inhibitor with 100-fold selectivity over a wide range of kinases and strong potency demonstrated by suppression of ATR-driven checkpoint kinase-1 (CHK1) phosphorylation in a prostate cancer cell line, as well as by induction of γH2AX phosphorylation in a small-cell lung cancer cell line [82]. Remarkably, sensitivity assays and gene expression analysis of a variety of cancer lines showed that cancer cells with higher replication stress and high neuroendocrine expression signatures are highly sensitive to gartisertib treatment, suggesting that those genomic signatures may be useful for patient selection and as biomarkers of response [82].

Table 14.3 Trials investigating elimusertib combinational strategies

ATR inhibitor	Phase	Combination strategy	Schedule	Study population	Safety	Efficacy	References
Elimusertib (BAY1895344)	I/Ib	Monotherapy	Dose escalation and dose expansion	Advanced solid tumors and lymphoma, enriching for *ATM* mutations and loss-of-function	MTD 40 mg twice daily 3 days on/ 4 days off Grade ≥4 TRAEs neutropenia (33% in 80 mg cohort, 17% in 60 mg cohort), thrombocytopenia (17% in 80 mg cohort)	ORR: 30.8% in patients treated with ≥40 mg BID 4 PR (19%) 8 SD (38%)	NCT03188965 [80]
	I/II	Monotherapy	Dose escalation and dose expansion	Advanced solid tumors; sarcoma and lymphoma	N/A	Recruitment ongoing	NCT05071209
	I	FOLFIRI	Dose escalation and dose expansion	Advanced gastrointestinal cancers	N/A	Recruitment ongoing	NCT04535401
	I	Gemcitabine	Dose escalation and dose expansion	Advanced solid tumors; pancreatic and ovarian	N/A	Recruitment ongoing	NCT04616534
	I	Cisplatin Cisplatin + Gemcitabine	Dose escalation and dose expansion	Advanced solid tumors, enriching for urothelial cancer	N/A	Recruitment ongoing	NCT04491942
	I	Irinotecan Topotecan	Dose escalation and dose expansion	Advanced SCLC, neuroendocrine and pancreatic cancer	N/A	Recruitment ongoing	NCT04514497

(continued)

Table 14.3 (continued)

ATR inhibitor	Phase	Combination strategy	Schedule	Study population	Safety	Efficacy	References
	I	Niraparib	Dose escalation and dose expansion	Ovarian cancer and advanced solid tumors (excluding prostate)	N/A	Recruitment ongoing	NCT04267939
	Ib/II	Pembrolizumab	Dose escalation and dose expansion	Advanced solid tumors with DDR deficiency	N/A	Recruitment ongoing	NCT04095273
	I	Pembrolizumab + Radiation	Dose escalation and dose expansion	Recurrent head and neck	N/A	Recruitment ongoing	NCT04576091

As a single-agent, gartisertib was shown to suppress proliferation in prostate cancer cells at a lower concentration and at a higher rate than berzosertib and ceralasertib, and it was shown to induce tumor stasis and tumor regression in ALT mice models [83, 84]. A variety of preclinical models also demonstrated synergistic effects of different gartisertib combination strategies. For instance, the combination of gartisertib and TOP1 inhibitors showed synergistic antitumor activity in several small-cell lung cancer cell lines and cell-derived mouse xenografts, as well as in prostate cancer patient-derived tumor organoids [85]. In addition, combining gartisertib with DNA damaging agents such as gemcitabine and cisplatin, as well as with PARP inhibitors such as talazoparib, displayed synergy at noncytotoxic concentrations in a small-cell lung cancer cell line.

14.5.5 Camonsertib (RP-3500)

Camonsertib, developed by Repare Therapeutics and recently licensed to Roche, is a highly selective ATR inhibitor that demonstrated potent single-agent efficacy by a dose-dependent inhibition of CHK1 phosphorylation and induction of γH2AX, DNA-PK and KAP1 phosphorylation in-vivo [86]. Camonsertib monotherapy induced significant tumor growth inhibition in an *ATM*-deficient colorectal xenograft model and also induced complete tumor regression in a gastric xenograft model [86]. Unlike other ATR inhibitors, tumor growth inhibition with minimal hematological adverse effects was observed with intermittent camonsertib treatment in *ATM*-deficient mouse models [86]. In line with preclinical data suggesting that intermittent camonsertib dosing schedules with dose holidays of at least 4 consecutive days allow for reticulocyte regeneration to avoid hematological toxicities in-vivo, recent preliminary data from the TRESR phase I/IIa clinical trial investigating the safety and preliminary efficacy of camonsertib showed a significant reduction of grade 3 anemia in advanced cancer patients (NCT04497116) [87]. In this study, 14.5% of patients treated with intermittent camonsertib dosing experienced grade 3 anemia, compared with 65.7% of patients who experienced grade 3 anemia after intermittent elimusertib treatment [87, 88]. Preliminary data from the TRESR trial also showed clinical activity across different tumor types, with meaningful clinical benefit in 49% of evaluable patients and an ORR of 25% [87]. Aligned with preclinical data, clinical activity was observed in CRPC patients whose tumors harbored *ATM* and *CDK12* mutations, ovarian cancer with *BRCA1* and *RAD51C* mutations, as well as breast cancer, melanoma, and HNSCC patients with tumors harboring *BRCA1* and *BRCA2* mutations. Notably, 37 patients whose tumors harbored relevant genomic mutations achieved molecular responses in ctDNA, suggesting that ctDNA responses may predict clinical benefit [87].

Intermittent concomitant rather than sequential administration of camonsertib and PARP inhibitors in different *ATM* and *BRCA1* deficient models led to stronger synergistic antitumor activity without increases in hematological toxicity [86]. Along with the additional modules of the TRESR clinical trial that are currently investigating the combination of camonsertib and talazoparib, the ATTACC phase

I/IIa clinical trial investigating the safety and preliminary efficacy of camonsertib in combination with either olaparib or niraparib is currently recruiting patients (NCT04972110).

14.5.6 M1774

Building on learnings from berzosertib, Merck KGaA developed M1774 as a potent and selective ATR inhibitor that has demonstrated antitumor activity in PDX models. The modular DDRiver Solid Tumors 301 clinical trial is currently investigating the safety and tolerability and preliminary efficacy of M1774 in patients with advanced solid tumors harboring selected mutations, including deleterious mutations in *ATM, ARID1A, ATRX* and/or *DAXX* (NCT04170153) [89]. Recent results from the dose escalation of this trial suggested an MTD of 180 mg QD continuous dosing and a recommended dose for expansion of 180 mg 2 weeks on/1 week off, with modulation of γH2AX in peripheral blood mononuclear cells achieved in doses starting at 130 mg QD [89]. While the DDRiver 301 trial is currently recruiting patients for two dose expansion modules in biomarker selected cohorts and food effects cohort, it is also recruiting patients in a module investigating the safety and tolerability of the combination of M1174 and niraparib. In addition, a recent clinical trial investigating the safety and tolerability of M1774 in combination with a DDR inhibitor or an immune checkpoint inhibitor has recently started to recruit patients (NCT05396833).

14.5.7 ART0380

ART0380, licensed by Artios Pharma Ltd from The University of Texas MD Anderson Cancer Center and ShangPharma Innovation, demonstrated target engagement by γH2AX and pKAP1 modulation in-vivo and, is currently being investigated as monotherapy and in combination with gemcitabine or irinotecan in a modular phase I/IIa clinical trial for advanced solid tumor patients (NCT04657068). In order to measure target engagement, Artios has developed an assay in normal peripheral blood mononuclear cells (PMBCs) and in circulating tumor cells (CTCs) [90]. Although interim results for this trial have not been presented thus far, Artios recently mentioned in a press release that upon treatment with single-agent ART0380, modulation of γH2AX in patient blood samples is observed at a larger magnitude in CTCs than in PBMCs, and that based on preliminary results from the dose escalation phase of the trial, ART0380 has a safe and tolerable profile. Therefore, the intermittent dose escalation ART0380 has progressed to the dose expansion phase in patients with *ATM*-deficient tumors.

14.6 ATR and PARP Inhibitor Combination Strategies

Synthetic lethal strategies for cancer treatment, where cell death is induced by targeting proteins or pathways that are redundant in normal cells but not cancer cells, are showing clinical promise. Inhibitors of PARP1 (Poly (ADP)-ribose polymerase 1, a key DDR enzyme) are prime examples of anti-cancer therapeutics capable of harnessing the synthetic lethal mechanism and have revolutionized the field of cancer therapeutics. Seminal work led by multiple teams in the early 2000s identified HR-deficient *BRCA1/2*-mutated cancers as selective targets for PARP inhibitor-induced lethality [91–93]. Today, several PARP inhibitors are FDA-approved for the treatment of *BRCA1/2*-mutated cancers, including in multiple settings of ovarian cancer, metastatic breast cancer, pancreatic cancer, and advanced castration-resistant prostate cancer (CRPC) [94–97]. Unfortunately, PARP inhibitor resistance is ubiquitous in the clinic. Acquired PARP inhibitor resistance can occur following prolonged treatment, whereas primary PARP inhibitor resistance is observed in many patients with *BRCA1/2*-mutated cancers and fail to respond at treatment initiation [98]. One strategy to overcome PARP inhibitor resistance is to develop rational combination treatments to sensitize cells to PARP inhibitors.

Growing evidence suggests that ATR inhibition may help to overcome PARP inhibitor resistance [99, 100]. The *ATR* gene was identified as a mediator of PARP inhibitor sensitivity in a synthetic lethal siRNA screen [92]. DNA DSBs that are produced following exposure to PARP inhibitors renders cells dependent on ATR for DNA repair [8]. As such, exposure to an ATR inhibitor disables ATR-mediated repair pathways and promotes cell death. Additionally, a known mechanism of PARP inhibitor resistance involves restored replication fork stabilization that may involve ATR, as well as other DDR proteins, such as CHK1 and WEE1 [99]. Preclinical studies have demonstrated that ATR inhibition leads to replication fork collapse that produces irreparable DNA DSBs [101, 102]. Building on this, the rationale for the combination of PARP and ATR inhibitors was demonstrated in another preclinical study in which PARP inhibitor resistant cells exhibited enhanced sensitivity in response to dual ATR and PARP inhibition in ovarian cancer patient-derived xenograft (PDX) models [103]. Furthermore, there are multiple ongoing clinical trials currently evaluating this drug combination, with at least 10 active studies taking place world-wide at the time of publication (Table 14.4).

With an expansive landscape of trials evaluating ATR and PARP inhibitor combinations, it is important to understand the tolerability and clinical efficacy of this approach. Overlapping toxicities stemming from combined ATR and PARP inhibition may be an issue for this drug combination. One example of such toxicity was reported in a dose-finding phase I trial in which ceralasertib was combined with the olaparib PARP inhibitor, which resulted in dose limiting toxicities (DLTs) in the form of thrombocytopenia and neutropenia that restricted continuous concurrent dosing of these agents [104].

Nonetheless, promising clinical activity produced by this drug combination was reported in a separate phase II trials evaluating a cohort of patients with recurrent

Table 14.4 Ongoing clinical trials combining ATR and PARP inhibitors

ATR inhibitor	PARP inhibitor	Trial phase	Status	Indication	References
RP-3500	Niraparib or olaparib	I and II	Recruiting	Advanced solid tumor	NCT04972110
RP-3500	Talazoparib	I and II	Recruiting	Advanced solid tumor	NCT04497116
Elimusertib	Niraparib	I	Recruiting	Advanced solid tumors (excluding prostate cancer) Ovarian cancer	NCT04267939
IMP9064	Senaparib	I	Recruiting	Solid tumor Advanced solid tumor	NCT05269316
M1774	Niraparib	I	Recruiting	Metastatic or locally advanced unresectable solid tumors	NCT04170153
Ceralasertib	Olaparib	II	Recruiting	High grade serous carcinoma	NCT03462342
		II	Recruiting	Gynecological cancers	NCT04065269
		II	Active, not recruiting	Prostate cancer	NCT03787680
		II	Recruiting	Clear cell renal cell carcinoma Locally advanced pancreatic cancer Locally advanced malignant solid neoplasm Metastatic renal cell carcinoma Metastatic urothelial carcinoma Metastatic pancreatic cancer Stage III pancreatic cancer Stage III renal cell cancer Stage IV pancreatic cancer Stage IV renal cell cancer	NCT03682289
		II	Recruiting	Anatomic stage IV breast cancer Metastatic triple negative breast carcinoma	NCT03801369

ovarian cancer who had progressed on prior PARP inhibitor treatment [105]. In a cohort of thirteen patients, the reported objective response rate (ORR) was 46% across six patients who had achieved radiologic PR [105]. Of these patients, 69% had germline *BRCA* mutations, 23% had somatic *BRCA* mutations, and 8% had other homologous recombination deficient mutations [105]. Although no patient discontinued treatment due to toxicity, reported adverse events included thrombocytopenia, anemia, and neutropenia, with dose reductions reported for both ceralasertib and olaparib [105]. Interestingly, this same study reported no objective responses in a cohort of PARP inhibitor naïve patients with platinum-resistant ovarian cancer [106]. Enrichment of therapeutic responses in the cohort of patients with past PARP inhibitor exposure further supports the notion that combined ATR and PARP inhibitor strategies may be key to overcome PARP inhibitor resistance in the clinic [106].

14.7 ATR and Immune-Checkpoint Inhibitor Combination Strategies

An emerging body of preclinical and clinical evidence supports the immunomodulatory role of ATR inhibitors in the tumor microenvironment. For instance, a recent single DNA fiber analysis after ATR inhibition showed induction of chromatin bridge formation and chromosome lagging, which in turn accelerated mitotic entry and further activated the cyclic GMP-AMP synthase-stimulator of interferon genes (cGAS-STING) tumor sensing axis [107]. Since genotoxic stress also induces the release of cytosolic DNA fragments that activate the cGAS-STING pathway, the combination of ATR inhibition with chemotherapeutics seems a rational combination to activate the innate immune response [111, 112].

It was also recently shown that treating prostate cancer cell lines with elimusertib induced S-phase DNA damage, activation of cGAS-STING signaling, as well as upregulation of *CCL5* (chemokine ligand 5) and *CXCL10* (C-X-C motif chemokine ligand 10) expression that culminated in activation of innate immunity [108, 109]. This is further supported by the increase in activated cGAS-STING and TBK1 levels, CD8+ T-cell infiltration, reduction of regulatory T-cell infiltration, and T-cell exhaustion observed in immunocompetent hepatocellular carcinoma mouse models treated with the triple combination of radiation, followed by ceralasertib and PD-L1 inhibition [110]. In addition, shortly after treatment with ceralasertib there was a modest increase in the intratumoral concentration of IFN-γ and proliferating CD8+ T-cells that was accompanied by a reduction of the PD-L1 tumor upregulation induced by radiation. At later time points, the combination of ceralasertib and radiation induced an increase in infiltrating CD8+ T-cells, as well as production of INF-γ and tumor necrosis factor α [110]. Similar results were obtained by studying the combination of ceralasertib and radiation on immunocompetent mouse models of HPV-driven cancer, where a signature of type I and II IFN gene expression and modulation of cytokine gene expression (including *CCL3* and *CXCL10*) were associated with treatment. Interestingly, increased antigen presentation and levels of major histocompatibility complex class I were also observed in vivo with the combination of ceralasertib and radiation [111]. Taken together, results from multiple preclinical studies suggest that the combination of radiation and ATR inhibitors stimulates IFN response and triggers antigen presentation.

ATR inhibition has also been shown to suppress upregulation of the natural killer group 2D (NKG2D) cell surface ligand that binds to activated CD8+ T-cells to trigger pro-inflammatory cytokine production [112]. It has also been suggested that *ATM*/ATR/CHK1 signaling upregulation leads to transcriptional activation of PD-L1 via the signal transducer and activators of transcription STAT1 and STAT3 and the IFN regulatory factor (IRF1) pathway [113]. In fact, an increase in PD-L1 expression, accompanied by increased infiltrating macrophages and reduced infiltrating CD3+ T-cells, was observed in ATR deficient melanoma models (Fig. 14.1) [114]. Remarkably, such preclinical data is supported by results from the phase I clinical trial investigating elimusertib monotherapy, where paired tumor samples from patients with PD-L1 positive tumors revealed upregulation of PD-L1 [80]. Interestingly, patients with metastatic melanoma that were previously resistant to PD-L1 inhibitors achieved durable responses when treated with the combination of ceralasertib and paclitaxel [115]. In this combinational trial, interlukin-12 fluctuations were also observed in patients that received clinical benefit suggesting activation of the innate immune response [115].

14.8 Candidate Biomarkers of ATR Sensitization

Therapeutic biomarkers are used as indicators of disease prognosis and predictive measures of treatment response [116]. Emerging data from various preclinical and clinical studies that evaluating ATR inhibitors as monotherapy or in combination strategies have identified candidate predictive biomarkers that may indicate sensitivity to ATR inhibition. Here, we summarize key genetic biomarkers and discuss their role in defining target patient populations that may respond best to ATR inhibitors.

ATM is a DDR kinase that senses and repairs dsDNA breaks and whose mutation may confer dependency on the ATR-CHK1 axis, offering an exploitable target for ATR inhibitors [117]. Although *ATM* is frequently mutated in cancer, the functional impact of many *ATM* variants is not well established [118]. Furthermore, there is significant overlap between *ATM* and ATR signaling pathways, as supported by various preclinical and clinical studies evaluating various cancer types including hematological and solid tumors [8, 12, 119]. Clinical responses have been reported from phase I studies of ATR inhibitors specifically in patients with *ATM* aberrations, including *ATM* deleterious mutations or protein loss [12, 16, 120]. Although *ATM* is frequently mutated in cancer, the functional impact of many *ATM* variants is not well established [118]. However, a large proportion of *ATM* mutations derive from missense variants, which can lead to a reduction in

ATM protein expression levels [31]. This highlights the potential use of immuno-histochemistry (IHC) analysis as a clinical tool to probe *ATM* expression levels and identify those who could benefit from ATR inhibition [31]. Pilie et al., further demonstrated the utility of IHC to understand *ATM* mutation annotations reported as variants of unknown significance (VUS), in which IHC analysis reported loss of protein in up to 25% of *ATM* VUS mutations, thus clarifying their functional impact [118]. This study also identified *ATM* loss of protein in patient tumor samples without identified *ATM* mutations, which points to the involvement of other mechanisms such as epigenetic or post-translational loss [118].

Another widely evaluated biomarker of ATR inhibitor sensitivity is *p53*, which plays a prominent role in G1 checkpoint control and whose loss comprises a high proportion of cancer cases [31]. Although there is preclinical data to support *p53*'s role as a predictive biomarker, the data remains inconsistent. For instance, Toledo et al., showed that cells with defective *p53* had augmented replication stress in response to ATR inhibitors compared to cells with wildtype *p53* [35]. A similar finding was reported in Kwok et al., in which treatment with the ATR inhibitor AZD6738 resulted in selective toxicity in *p53* defective xenografts and cell lines [121]. In contrast, another study showed no increase in sensitivity to single agent ATR inhibition with VE-821 in *p53* mutant cell lines compared to matched wildtype *p53* cells [122]. Although Dillion et al., reported radio-sensitization by AZD6738 to single radiation fractions in a panel of cell lines, the narrow sensitivity range to AZD6738 was independent of *p53* status [123]. Cumulatively, despite strong rationale supporting the use of ATR inhibitors to treat *p53* deficient tumors, the conflicting data suggests further studies are necessary to assess its utility as a predictive biomarker of response. Although data is still pending, multiple clinical trials are underway to evaluate ATR inhibitors as monotherapy or in combination strategies in patients with solid tumors harboring *TP53* mutations [48, 124].

A link between ATR sensitivity and deficiency of the BAF complex component AT-Rich Interactive Domain-containing protein 1A (*ARID1A*) was established in a large-scale genetic screen reported in Williamson et al. [125]. In this study, both in-vitro and in-vivo models were used to demonstrate wide-ranged genomic instability and cell death in *ARID1A* mutant cancer cell lines and tumors in response to ATR inhibition [125]. The clinical significance of this finding is highlighted by the fact that up to 7% of all cancers are associated with ARID1A loss and the frequency of loss is increased in certain cancers, for example, ARID1A loss is reported in up to 50% of clear cell ovarian carcinoma cases [126]. Further support for ATR inhibition in the setting of ARID1A loss was demonstrated in Tsai et al., in which an accumulation of R-loop formation was identified as a driver of replication stress in an ovarian cancer line with *ARID1A* knockout [126]. Translation of these data to the clinical setting has also produced compelling results. Antitumor activity was observed in patients with ARID1A-deficient solid tumors treated with the single-agent ATR inhibitor ceralasertib, including two patients that achieved RECIST-confirmed complete responses [127]. In addition, treatment with M6620 monotherapy resulted in a RECIST-confirmed complete response after 16 cycles in a patient with metastatic colorectal cancer with *ARID1A* mutation and IHC confirmed loss of both ARID1A and *ATM*, with a reported progression free survival of 29 months at their last assessment [128]. The use of cell-free DNA (cfDNA) as an indicator of treatment response was also evaluated in this study, which revealed declining levels of allele frequencies for *ARID1A*, among other identified mutations, to undetectable levels after 9 cycles of treatment with M6620 compared to baseline [128].

Targeting deficiencies in homologous recombination DNA repair (HRR) also offers a potential opportunity for ATR inhibition [129, 130]. For example, Krajewska et al., demonstrated sensitivity of the breast cancer cell line MCF-7 to ATR inhibitors upon inactivation of RAD51 in the HRR pathway [129]. Other studies have since further elucidated the major role ATR plays in regulating homologous recombination processes. For instance, Kim et al., showed that increased ATR signaling promotes the capacity of HRR in cancer cells by regulating the abundance of homologous recombination factors [28]. In support of this, a phase I trial of the Repare ATR inhibitor RP-3500 monotherapy observed multiple clinical responses in ovarian cancer patients with PARP-inhibitor resistant cancers that harbored actionable *BRCA1* and *RAD51C* mutations [87, 117]. Other responses described in this study included patients with homologous recombination deficiency (HRD), with molecular alterations in *ATM*, *BRCA2* and *RAD51B/C* [87]. ATR inhibition in HRD-cancers is largely under clinical investigation via multiple trials that are actively recruiting patients with deleterious mutations in HRR genes.

ATR deficiency has also been shown to confer a strong synthetic lethal response with many other DDR genes as well as with inducers of DNA replication stress [29]. For example, ATR inhibition is synthetic lethal in cells with genetic defects in genes such as *APOBEC3A* and *B* as well as with overexpression of *cyclin E1 (CCNE1)* and with *c-MYC* amplifications [28, 131–133]. In addition to those mentioned above, molecular defects in DDR genes such as *ERCC1*, *XRCC1*, *CHK1*, and *FANCD2*, and even accumulation of R-loops, all have been shown to produce a synthetic lethal effect in response to ATR inhibition [8, 28, 29]. With so many potential synthetic lethal partners possible, results from ongoing preclinical and clinical studies will be instrumental in identifying biomarkers and factors associated with therapeutic response as ATR inhibitors appear poised to enter the clinic in the coming years.

14.9 Concluding Remarks

This chapter provides a rationale for targeting ATR and summarizes the current landscape of ATR inhibitors in clinical evaluation. As a key component of the DDR, ATR is a promising druggable target that is being widely evaluated in phase I, II and III clinical trials as monotherapy and in combinations with other agents, including DNA repair inhibitors, chemo- and radiotherapy, and immunotherapy. Regardless of the approach taken, ongoing clinical studies must address optimization of the therapeutic window for this drug class. A predominantly reported toxicity across ATR inhibitors trials is myelosuppression, which is a mechanism-based toxicity that ultimately limits the therapeutic window in both monotherapy and combination approaches [134]. This carries key implications particularly for combination strategies due to potentiating of overlapping toxicities that may deepen myelosuppression and reduce drug tolerability. Proposed rational combination strategies should limit overlapping toxicity, which may be achieved by coordinating intermittent dosing schedules to facilitate tissue recovery. Another prevalent challenge is refining the target patient population most likely to benefit from ATR inhibition. Molecular technology advances and companion diagnostics have opened the door to precision oncology and the opportunity to offer personalized treatment strategies to patients [135]. Today, many clinical studies are designed on the basis of mutational status, which has led to the approval of several tumor-agnostic drugs [136]. Interestingly, many ongoing ATR inhibitor trials are recruiting patients based on molecular alteration rather than relying solely on tumor-type. A spectrum of molecular alterations have already been identified as potential predictive biomarkers that may sensitize to ATR inhibition; however, to be clinically efficacious, the biomarkers must be sensitive and easy to measure to allow for successful integration into the clinic. In closing, although several ATR inhibitors in development are poised to address a clinically unmet need, no ATR inhibitor has received FDA-approval for cancer indications thus far. We eagerly await the results from ongoing clinical studies as FDA-approval of ATR inhibitors lies close in sight.

Acknowledgements Timothy A. Yap is supported by MD Anderson Cancer Center Support grant (NIH/NCI P30 CA016672), The National Cancer Institute (NIH/NCI R01-CA255074), the US Department of Defense Ovarian Cancer Research Program (OC200482), and the V Foundation Clinical Scholar Program (VC2020-001). Helen M.R. Robinson, Graeme C.M. Smith are employed at Artios Pharma.

References

1. Ngoi NYL, Peng G, Yap TA (2021) A Tale of Two Checkpoints: ATR Inhibition and PD-(L)1 Blockade. Annu Rev Med 73(1):1–20
2. Helleday T (2018) Targeting the DNA damage response for anti-cancer therapy. Canc Drug Disc Dev 1–9
3. Alhmoud JF, Woolley JF, Moustafa A-EA, Malki MI (2020) DNA damage/repair management in cancers. Cancers 12(4):1050
4. Mazouzi A, Velimezi G, Loizou JI (2014) DNA replication stress: causes, resolution and disease. Exp Cell Res 329(1):85–93
5. Luo J, Solimini NL, Elledge SJ (2009) Principles of cancer therapy: oncogene and non-oncogene addiction. Cell 138(4):807
6. Bartkova J, Hořejší Z, Koed K, Krämer A, Tort F, Zieger K et al (2005) DNA damage response as a candidate anti-cancer barrier in early human tumorigenesis. Nature 434(7035):864–870
7. Gorgoulis VG, Vassiliou L-VF, Karakaidos P, Zacharatos P, Kotsinas A, Liloglou T et al (2005) Activation of the DNA damage checkpoint and genomic instability in human precancerous lesions. Nature 434(7035):907–913

8. Sundar R, Brown J, Russo AI, Yap TA (2017) Targeting ATR in cancer medicine. Curr Prob Cancer 41(4):302–315

9. Branzei D, Foiani M (2010) Maintaining genome stability at the replication fork. Nat Rev Mol Cell Bio 11(3):208–219

10. Ngoi NYL, Pham MM, Tan DSP, Yap TA (2021) Targeting the replication stress response through synthetic lethal strategies in cancer medicine. Trends Cancer 7(10):930–957

11. Berti M, Vindigni A (2016) Replication stress: getting back on track. Nat Struct Mol Biol 23(2):103–109

12. Bradbury A, Hall S, Curtin N, Drew Y (2020) Targeting ATR as Cancer Therapy: A new era for synthetic lethality and synergistic combinations? Pharmacol Therapeut. 207:107450

13. Baillie KE, Stirling PC (2020) Beyond kinases: targeting replication stress proteins in cancer therapy. Trends Cancer 7(5):430–446

14. Lecona E, Fernandez-Capetillo O (2018) Targeting ATR in cancer. Nat Rev Cancer 18(9):586–595

15. Wang X, Wang L, Huang Y, Deng Z, Li C, Zhang J et al (2022) A plant-specific module for homologous recombination repair. Proc Natl Acad Sci 119(16):e2202970119

16. Rundle S, Bradbury A, Drew Y, Curtin NJ (2017) Targeting the ATR-CHK1 axis in cancer therapy. Cancers 9(5):41

17. Bass TE, Cortez D (2019) Quantitative phosphoproteomics reveals mitotic function of the ATR activator ETAA1. J Cell Biol 218(4):1235–1249

18. Zou L, Elledge SJ (2003) Sensing DNA damage through ATRIP Recognition of RPA-ssDNA complexes. Science 300(5625):1542–1548

19. Butler LR, Gilad O, Brown EJ (2018) Targeting the DNA damage response for anti-cancer therapy. Canc Drug Disc Dev 11–33

20. Couch FB, Bansbach CE, Driscoll R, Luzwick JW, Glick GG, Bétous R et al (2013) ATR phosphorylates SMARCAL1 to prevent replication fork collapse. Gene Dev 27(14):1610–1623

21. Matos DA, Zhang J-M, Ouyang J, Nguyen HD, Genois M-M, Zou L (2020) ATR protects the genome against R loops through a MUS81-triggered feedback loop. Mol Cell 77(3):514-527.e4

22. Sørensen CS, Hansen LT, Dziegielewski J, Syljuåsen RG, Lundin C, Bartek J et al (2005) The cell-cycle checkpoint kinase Chk1 is required for mammalian homologous recombination repair. Nat Cell Biol 7(2):195–201

23. Wang LC, Gautier J (2010) The Fanconi anemia pathway and ICL repair: implications for cancer therapy. Crit Rev Biochem Mol 45(5):424–439

24. Sirbu BM, Cortez D (2013) DNA damage response: three levels of DNA repair regulation. Csh Perspect Biol 5(8):a012724

25. Auclair Y, Rouget R, Drobetsky EA (2009) ATR kinase as master regulator of nucleotide excision repair during S phase of the cell cycle. Cell Cycle 8(12):1865–1871

26. Lee T-H, Park J-M, Leem S-H, Kang T-H (2014) Coordinated regulation of XPA stability by ATR and HERC2 during nucleotide excision repair. Oncogene 33(1):19–25

27. Fokas E, Prevo R, Hammond EM, Brunner TB, McKenna WG, Muschel RJ (2014) Targeting ATR in DNA damage response and cancer therapeutics. Cancer Treat Rev 40(1):109–117

28. Kim D, Liu Y, Oberly S, Freire R, Smolka MB (2018) ATR-mediated proteome remodeling is a major determinant of homologous recombination capacity in cancer cells. Nucleic Acids Res 46(16):8311–8325

29. Kantidze OL, Velichko AK, Luzhin AV, Petrova NV, Razin SV (2018) Synthetically lethal interactions of atm, ATR, and DNA-PKcs. Trends Cancer 4(11):755–768

30. Qiu Z, Oleinick NL, Zhang J (2018) ATR/CHK1 inhibitors and cancer therapy. Radiother Oncol 126(3):450–464

31. Weber AM, Ryan AJ (2015) ATM and ATR as therapeutic targets in cancer. Pharmacol Therapeut. 149:124–138

32. Hurley PJ, Wilsker D, Bunz F (2007) Human cancer cells require ATR for cell cycle progression following exposure to ionizing radiation. Oncogene 26(18):2535–2542

33. Mei L, Zhang J, He K, Zhang J (2019) Ataxia telangiectasia and Rad3-related inhibitors and cancer therapy: where we stand. J Hematol Oncol 12(1):43

34. Nishida H, Tatewaki N, Nakajima Y, Magara T, Ko KM, Hamamori Y et al (2009) Inhibition of ATR protein kinase activity by schisandrin B in DNA damage response. Nucleic Acids Res 37:5678–5689. Available from <Go to ISI>://WOS:000271569100009

35. Toledo LI, Murga M, Zur R, Soria R, Rodriguez A, Martinez S et al (2011) A cell-based screen identifies ATR inhibitors with synthetic lethal properties for cancer-associated mutations. Nat Struct Mol Biol 18(6):721–U124. Available from <Go to ISI>://WOS:000291308000014

36. Charrier JD, Durrant SJ, Golec JMC, Kay DP, Knegtel RMA, MacCormick S et al (2011) Discovery of potent and selective inhibitors of ataxia telangiectasia mutated and Rad3 related (ATR) protein kinase as potential anticancer agents. J Med Chem 54:2320–2330. Available from <Go to ISI>://WOS:000289215700028

37. Reaper PM, Griffiths MR, Long JM, Charrier JD, MacCormick S, Charlton PA et al (2011) Selective killing of ATM- or p53-deficient cancer cells through inhibition of ATR. Nat Chem Biol 7:428–430. Available from <Go to ISI>://WOS:000292252100008

38. Huntoon CJ, Flatten KS, Hendrickson AEW, Huehls AM, Sutor SL, Kaufmann SH et al (2013) ATR inhibition broadly sensitizes ovarian cancer cells to chemotherapy independent of BRCA status. Cancer Res 73:3683–3691. Available from <Go to ISI>://WOS:000320380300020

39. Kastan MB, Zhan QM, Eldeiry WS, Carrier F, Jacks T, Walsh WV et al (1992) A mammalian-cell cycle checkpoint pathway utilizing P53 and Gadd45 Is defective in ataxia-telangiectasia. Cell 71:587–597. Available from <Go to ISI>://WOS:A1992JY67600007

40. Wengner AM, Siemeister G, Lucking U, Lefranc J, Wortmann L, Lienau P et al (2020) The novel ATR inhibitor BAY 1895344 is efficacious as monotherapy and combined with DNA damage-inducing or repair-compromising therapies in preclinical cancer models. Mol Cancer Ther 19(1):26–38. Available from <Go to ISI>://WOS:000505667900003

41. Knegtel R, Charrier JD, Durrant S, Davis C, O'Donnell M, Storck P et al (2019) Rational design of 5-(4-(Isopropylsulfonyl)phenyl)-3-(3-(4-((methylamino)methyl)phenyl)isoxazol-5-yl)pyrazin-2-amine (VX-970,M6620): optimization of intra- and intermolecular polar interactions of a new ataxia telangiectasia mutated and Rad3-related (ATR) kinase inhibitor. J Med Chem 62:5547–5561. Available from <Go to ISI>://WOS:000471834500020

42. Hall AB, Newsome D, Wang Y, Boucher DM, Eustace B, Gu Y et al (2014) Potentiation of tumor responses to DNA damaging therapy by the selective ATR inhibitor VX-970. Oncotarget 5(14):5674–5685

43. Nagel R, Avelar AT, Aben N, Proost N, Ven M van de, van der Vliet J et al (2019) Inhibition of the replication stress response is a synthetic vulnerability in SCLC that acts synergistically in combination with cisplatin. Mol Cancer Ther 18:762–770. Available from <Go to ISI>://WOS:000462996800004

44. Kurmasheva RT, Kurmashev D, Reynolds CP, Kang M, Wu J, Houghton PJ et al (2018) Initial testing (stage 1) of M6620 (formerly VX-970), a novel ATR inhibitor, alone and combined with cisplatin and melphalan, by the Pediatric Preclinical Testing Program. Pediatr Blood Cancer 65(2):e26825

45. Leszczynska KB, Dobrynin G, Leslie RE, Ient J, Boumelha AJ, Senra JM et al (2016) Preclinical testing of an Atr inhibitor demonstrates improved response to standard therapies for esophageal cancer. Radiother Oncol 121(2):232–238

46. Combes E, Andrade AF, Tosi D, Michaud HA, Coquel F, Garambois V et al (2019) Inhibition of Ataxia-telangiectasia mutated and RAD3-related (ATR) overcomes oxaliplatin resistance and promotes antitumor immunity in colorectal cancer. Cancer Res 79:2933–2946. Available from <Go to ISI>://WOS:000470291600015

47. Tu XY, Kahila MM, Zhou Q, Yu J, Kalari KR, Wang LW et al (2018) ATR inhibition is a promising radiosensitizing strategy for triple-negative breast cancer. Mol Cancer Ther 17:2462–2472. Available from <Go to ISI>://WOS:000448888000017

48. Middleton MR, Dean E, Evans TRJ, Shapiro GI, Pollard J, Hendriks BS et al (2021) Phase 1 study of the ATR inhibitor berzosertib (formerly M6620, VX-970) combined with gemcitabine +/− cisplatin in patients with advanced solid tumours. Brit J Cancer 125(4):510–59. Available from <Go to ISI>://WOS:000655068600003

49. Yazinski SA, Comaills V, Buisson R, Genois MM, Nguyen HD, Ho CK et al (2017) ATR inhibition disrupts rewired homologous recombination and fork protection pathways in PARP inhibitor-resistant BRCA-deficient cancer cells. Gene Dev 31(3):318–332. Available from <Go to ISI>://WOS:00039579610001

50. Yap TA, O'Carrigan B, Penney MS, Lim JS, Brown JS, Luken MJD et al (2020) Phase I trial of first-in-class ATR inhibitor M6620 (VX-970) as monotherapy or in combination with carboplatin in patients with advanced solid tumors. J Clin Oncol 38(27):3195–+. Available from <Go to ISI>://WOS:000574579100010

51. Konstantinopoulos PA, Cheng SC, Hendrickson AEW, Penson RT, Schumer ST, Doyle LA et al (2020) Berzosertib plus gemcitabine versus gemcitabine alone in platinum-resistant high-grade serous ovarian cancer: a multicentre, open-label, randomised, phase 2 trial. Lancet Oncology 21:957–9568. Available from <Go to ISI>://WOS:000545328900033

52. Konstantinopoulos PA, da Costa AABA, Gulhan D, Lee EK, Cheng S-C, Hendrickson AEW et al (2021) A replication stress biomarker is associated with response to gemcitabine versus combined gemcitabine and ATR inhibitor therapy in ovarian cancer. Nat Commun 12(1):5574

53. Shapiro GI, Wesolowski R, Devoe C, Lord S, Pollard J, Hendriks BS et al (2021) Phase 1 study of the ATR inhibitor berzosertib in combination with cisplatin in patients with advanced solid tumours. Brit J Cancer 125:520–57. Available from <Go to ISI>://WOS:000655068600001

54. Thomas A, Redon CE, Sciuto L, Padiernos E, Ji JP, Lee MJ et al (2018) Phase I study of ATR Inhibitor M6620 in combination with topotecan in patients with advanced solid tumors. J Clin Oncol 2018;36:1594–+. Available from <Go to ISI>://WOS:000434262900008

55. Thomas A, Takahashi N, Rajapakse VN, Zhang XH, Sun YL, Ceribelli M et al (2021) Therapeutic targeting of ATR yields durable regressions in small cell lung cancers with high replication stress. Cancer Cell 39:566–+. Available from <Go to ISI>://WOS:000640027300015

56. Merck_KGaA (2022). Merck KGaA, Darmstadt, Germany, advances development programs in oncology focusing on novel mechanisms and pathways. Cited 27 Dec 2022. Available from https://www.emdgroup.com/en/news/development-projects-in-oncology-03-06-2022.html

57. Foote KM, Nissink JWM, McGuire T, Turner P, Guichard S, Yates JWT et al (2018) Discovery and Characterization<Go to ISI>://WOS:000451496300005 of AZD6738, a potent inhibitor of ataxia telangiectasia mutated and Rad3 related (ATR) kinase with application as an anticancer agent. J Med Chem 61:9889–9907. Available from

58. Jones CD, Blades K, Foote KM, Guichard SM, Jewsbury PJ, McGuire T et al (2013) Abstract 2348: Discovery of AZD6738, a potent and selective inhibitor with the potential to test the clinical efficacy of ATR kinase inhibition in cancer patients. Cancer Res 73(8_Supplement):2348–2348

59. Kwok M, Davies N, Agathanggelou A, Smith E, Oldreive C, Petermann E et al (2016) ATR inhibition induces synthetic lethality and overcomes chemoresistance in TP53- or ATM-defective chronic lymphocytic leukemia cells. Blood 127(5):582–595

60. Wilson Z, Odedra R, Wallez Y, Wijnhoven PWG, Hughes AM, Gerrard J et al (2022) ATR inhibitor AZD6738 (ceralasertib) exerts antitumor activity as a monotherapy and in combination with chemotherapy and the PARP inhibitor olaparib. Cancer Res 82:1140–1152. Available from <Go to ISI>://WOS:000772155800001

61. Sundar R, Brown J, Russo AI, Yap TA (2017) Targeting ATR in cancer medicine. Curr Prob Cancer 41(4):302–315. Available from https://www.ncbi.nlm.nih.gov/pubmed/28662958

62. Dillon M, Guevara J, Mohammed K, Smith SA, Dean E, McLellan L et al (2019) A phase I study of ATR inhibitor, AZD6738, as monotherapy in advanced solid tumours (PATRIOT part A, B). Ann Oncol 30:165–+. Available from <Go to ISI>://WOS:000491295501267

63. Guichard SM, Brown E, Odedra R, Hughes A, Heathcote D, Barnes J et al (2013) The preclinical in vitro and in vivo activity of AZD6738: A potent and selective inhibitor of ATR kinase. Cancer Res 73. Available from <Go to ISI>://WOS:000331220602050

64. Vendetti FP, Lau A, Schamus S, Conrads TP, O'Connor MJ, Bakkenist CJ (2015) The orally active and bioavailable ATR kinase inhibitor AZD6738 potentiates the anti-tumor effects of cisplatin to resolve ATM-deficient non-small cell lung cancer in vivo. Oncotarget 6(42):44289–44305

65. Kim H, Min A, Im S, Jang H, Lee KH, Lau A et al (2017) Anti-tumor activity of the ATR inhibitor AZD6738 in HER2 positive breast cancer cells. Int J Cancer 140(1):109–119

66. Yap TA, Krebs MG, Postel-Vinay S, El-Khouiery A, Soria JC, Lopez J et al (2021) Ceralasertib (AZD6738), an oral ATR kinase inhibitor, in combination with carboplatin in patients with advanced solid tumors: a phase I study. Clin Cancer Res 27:5213–5224. Available from: https://www.ncbi.nlm.nih.gov/pubmed/34301752

67. Kim ST, Smith SA, Mortimer P, Loembe AB, Cho H, Kim KM et al (2021) Phase I study of ceralasertib (AZD6738), a novel DNA damage repair agent, in combination with weekly paclitaxel in refractory cancer. Clin Cancer Res 27:4700–4709. Available from: https://www.ncbi.nlm.nih.gov/pubmed/33975862

68. Paula BH de, Basu B, Mander A, Khan J, Bundi P, Goodwin R et al (2021) ATRiUM: a first-in-human dose escalation phase I trial of ceralasertib (AZD6738) and gemcitabine as combination therapy. Cancer Res 81. Available from <Go to ISI>://WOS:000680263501296

69. Dunlop CR, Wallez Y, Johnson TI, Fernandez SBD, Durant ST, Cadogan EB et al (2020) Complete loss of ATM function augments replication catastrophe induced by ATR inhibition and gemcitabine in pancreatic cancer models. Brit J Cancer. 123:1424–1436. Available from Available from: <Go to ISI>://WOS:000554842400004

70. Bukhari AB, Lewis CW, Pearce JJ, Luong D, Chan GK, Gamper AM (2019) Inhibiting Wee1 and ATR kinases produces tumor-selective synthetic lethality and suppresses metastasis. J Clin Investig 129:1329–1344. Available from <Go to ISI>://WOS:000460125800037

71. Jin J, Fang HH, Yang F, Ji WF, Guan N, Sun ZJ et al (2018) Combined Inhibition of ATR and WEE1 as a novel therapeutic strategy in triple-negative breast cancer. Neoplasia 20:478–488. Available from <Go to ISI>://WOS:000430688400007

72. Krebs MG, Lopez J, El-Khoueiry A, Bang YJ, Postel-Vinay S, Abida W et al (2018) Phase I study of AZD6738, an inhibitor of ataxia telangiectasia Rad3-related (ATR), in combination with olaparib or durvalumab in patients (pts) with advanced solid cancers. Cancer Res 78(13_Supplement):CT026–CT026. Available from <Go to ISI>://WOS:000468818900025

73. Aggarwal R, Umetsu S, Dhawan M, Grabowsky J, Carnevale J, Howell M et al (2021) Interim results from a phase II study of the ATR inhibitor ceralasertib in ARID1A-deficient and ARID1A-intact advanced solid tumor malignancies. Ann Oncol 32:S583–S583. Available from <Go to ISI>://WOS:000700527700488

74. Shah PD, Wethington SL, Pagan C, Latif N, Tanyi J, Martin LP et al (2021) Combination ATR and PARP Inhibitor (CAPRI): a phase 2 study of ceralasertib plus olaparib in patients with recurrent, platinum-resistant epithelial ovarian cancer. Gynecol Oncol. 163(2):246–253. Available from <Go to ISI>://WOS:000714728500005

75. Besse B, Awad M, Forde P, Thomas M, Park K, Goss G et al (2021) HUDSON: an open-label, multi-drug, biomarker-directed, phase II platform study in patients with NSCLC, who progressed on anti-PD(L)1 therapy. J Thorac Oncol 16:S118–S119. Available from <Go to ISI>://WOS:000631349600099

76. Kwon M, Kim G, Kim R, Kim KT, Kim ST, Smith S et al (2022) Phase II study of ceralasertib (AZD6738) in combination with durvalumab in patients with advanced gastric cancer. J Immunother Cancer 10. Available from <Go to ISI>://WOS:000821480200001

77. Hernandez M, Besse B, Awad M, Forde P, Thomas M, Park K et al (2021) Immunomodulatory effects of ceralasertib in combination with durvalumab in NSCLC with progression on anti-PD(L)1 treatment (HUDSON). J Thorac Oncol 16:S350–S350. Available from <Go to ISI>://WOS:000631349600531

78. Lucking U, Wortmann L, Wengner AM, Lefranc J, Lienau P, Briem H et al (2020) Damage incorporated: discovery of the potent, highly selective, orally available ATR inhibitor BAY 1895344 with favorable pharmacokinetic properties and promising efficacy in monotherapy and in combination treatments in preclinical tumor models. J Med Chem 63:7293–7325. Available from <Go to ISI>://WOS:000550753700043

79. Szydzik J, Lind DE, Arefin B, Kurhe Y, Umapathy G, Siaw JT et al (2021) ATR inhibition enables complete tumour regression in ALK-driven NB mouse models. Nat Commun 12. Available from <Go to ISI>://WOS:000722322900021

80. Yap TA, Tan DSP, Terbuch A, Caldwell R, Guo C, Goh BC et al (2021) First-in-human trial of the oral ataxia telangiectasia and RAD3-related (ATR) inhibitor BAY 1895344 in patients with advanced solid tumors. Cancer Discov 11(1):80–91. Available from <Go to ISI>://WOS:000607017700021

81. Austin WR, Armijo AL, Campbell DO, Singh AS, Hsieh T, Nathanson D et al (2012) Nucleoside salvage pathway kinases regulate hematopoiesis by linking nucleotide metabolism with replication stress. J Exp Med 209:2215–2228. Available from <Go to ISI>://WOS:000311295600008

82. Jo U, Murai Y, Takebe N, Thomas A, Pommier Y (2021) Precision Oncology with drugs targeting the replication stress, ATR, and schlafen 11. Cancers 13(18):4601

83. Jo U, Senatorov IS, Zimmermann A, Saha LK, Murai Y, Kim SH et al (2021) Novel and highly potent ATR inhibitor M4344 kills cancer cells with replication stress, and enhances the chemotherapeutic activity of widely used DNA damaging agents. Mol Cancer Ther 20(8):1431–1441

84. Zenke FT, Zimmermann A, Dahmen H, Elenbaas B, Pollard J, Reaper P et al (2019) Abstract 369: Antitumor activity of M4344, a potent and selective ATR inhibitor, in monotherapy and combination therapy. Cancer Res 79(13_Supplement):369

85. Jo U, Senatorov IS, Zimmermann A, Saha LK, Murai Y, Kim SH et al (2021) Novel and highly potent ATR inhibitor M4344 kills cancer cells with replication stress, and enhances the chemotherapeutic activity of widely used DNA damaging agents. Mol Cancer Ther 20:1431–1441. Available from <Go to ISI>://WOS:000680862700011

86. Roulston A, Zimmermann M, Papp R, Skeldon A, Pellerin C, Dumas-Bérube É et al (2021) RP-3500: A novel, potent, and selective atr inhibitor that is effective in preclinical models as a monotherapy and in combination with PARP inhibitors. Mol Cancer Ther 21(2):245–256

87. Yap T, Lee E, Spigel D, Fontana E, Højgaard M, Lheureux S et al (2021) Abstract CC04-01: first-in-human biomarker-driven phase I TRESR trial of ataxia telangiectasia and Rad3-related inhibitor (ATRi) RP-3500 in patients (pts) with advanced solid tumors harboring synthetic lethal (SL) genomic alterations. Mol Cancer Ther 20(12_Supplement):CC04-01–CC04-01

88. Zhang Y, Hreiki J, Wilkinson G, Ploeger B. Alternative dosing schedules for therapeutic window optimization for the ataxia telangiectasia and Rad3-related pathway (Atr) inhibitor elimusertib in patients with advanced solid tumors: M&S-based exploration using phase 1 data. Clin Pharmacol Ther 111:S41–S41. Available from <Go to ISI>://WOS:000752207700140

89. Yap TA, Tolcher AW, Plummer ER, Becker A, Fleuranceau-Morel P, Goddemeier T et al (2021) A first-in-human phase I study of ATR inhibitor M1774 in patients with solid tumors. J Clin Oncol 39:TPS3153–TPS3153. Available from: https://ascopubs.org/doi/abs/10.1200/JCO.2021.39.15_suppl.TPS3153

90. Patel M, Moore KN, Piscitello D, Majithiya J, Luzarraga MR, Millward H et al (2022) Abstract LB520: a pharmacodynamic platform using liquid biopsy to support dose selection for the ATR inhibitor ART0380 (IACS-030380). Cancer Res 82:LB520–LB520. Available from: https://doi.org/10.1158/1538-7445.AM2022-LB520

91. McCabe N, Lord CJ, Tutt AN, Martin N, Smith GCM, Ashworth A (2005) BRCA2-deficient CAPAN-1 cells are extremely sensitive to the inhibition of poly (ADP-ribose) polymerase: an issue of potency. Cancer Biol Ther 4(9):934–936

92. McCabe N, Turner NC, Lord CJ, Kluzek K, Białkowska A, Swift S et al (2006) Deficiency in the repair of DNA damage by homologous recombination and sensitivity to poly(ADP-ribose) polymerase inhibition. Cancer Res 66(16):8109–8115

93. Farmer H, McCabe N, Lord CJ, Tutt ANJ, Johnson DA, Richardson TB et al (2005) Targeting the DNA repair defect in BRCA mutant cells as a therapeutic strategy. Nature 434(7035):917–921

94. Sachdev E, Tabatabai R, Roy V, Rimel BJ, Mita MM (2019) PARP Inhibition in cancer: an update on clinical development. Target Oncol 14(6):657–679

95. Topatana W, Juengpanich S, Li S, Cao J, Hu J, Lee J et al (2020) Advances in synthetic lethality for cancer therapy: cellular mechanism and clinical translation. J Hematol Oncol 13(1):118

96. Brown TJ, Reiss KA (2021) PARP inhibitors in pancreatic cancer. Cancer J 27(6):465–475

97. Tripathi A, Balakrishna P, Agarwal N (2020) PARP inhibitors in castration-resistant prostate cancer. Cancer Treat Res Commun. 24:100199

98. Li X, Heyer W-D (2008) Homologous recombination in DNA repair and DNA damage tolerance. Cell Res 18(1):99–113

99. Haynes B, Murai J, Lee J-M (2018) Restored replication fork stabilization, a mechanism of PARP inhibitor resistance, can be overcome by cell cycle checkpoint inhibition. Cancer Treat Rev 71:1–7

100. Turner NC, Lord CJ, Iorns E, Brough R, Swift S, Elliott R et al (2008) A synthetic lethal siRNA screen identifying genes mediating sensitivity to a PARP inhibitor. Embo J 27(9):1368–1377

101. Sanjiv K, Hagenkort A, Calderón-Montaño JM, Koolmeister T, Reaper PM, Mortusewicz O et al (2016) Cancer-specific synthetic lethality between ATR and CHK1 kinase activities. Cell Rep 17(12):3407–3416

102. Toledo LI, Altmeyer M, Rask M-B, Lukas C, Larsen DH, Povlsen LK et al (2014) ATR prohibits replication catastrophe by preventing global exhaustion of RPA. Cell 156(1–2):374

103. Kim H, George E, Ragland RL, Rafail S, Zhang R, Krepler C et al (2017) Targeting the ATR/CHK1 axis with PARP inhibition results in tumor regression in BRCA-mutant ovarian cancer models. Clin Cancer Res 23(12):3097–3108

104. Krebs MG, Lopez J, El-Khoueiry A, Bang Y-J, Postel-Vinay S, Abida W et al (2018) Abstract CT026: Phase I study of AZD6738, an inhibitor of ataxia telangiectasia Rad3-related (ATR), in combination with olaparib or durvalumab in patients (pts) with advanced solid cancers. Cancer Res 78(13_Supplement):CT026–CT026

105. Wethington SL, Shah PD, Martin LP, Tanyi JL, Latif NA, Morgan MA et al (2021) Combination of PARP and ATR inhibitors (olaparib and ceralasertib) shows clinical activity in acquired PARP inhibitor-resistant recurrent ovarian cancer. J Clin Oncol 39(15_suppl):5516–5516

106. Shah PD, Wethington SL, Pagan C, Latif N, Tanyi J, Martin LP et al (2021) Combination ATR and PARP Inhibitor (CAPRI): a phase 2 study of ceralasertib plus olaparib in patients with recurrent, platinum-resistant epithelial ovarian cancer. Gynecol Oncol 163(2):246–253

107. Schoonen PM, Kok YP, Wierenga E, Bakker B, Foijer F, Spierings DCJ et al (2019) Premature mitotic entry induced by ATR inhibition potentiates olaparib inhibition-mediated genomic instability, inflammatory signaling, and cytotoxicity in BRCA2-deficient cancer cells. Mol Oncol. 13:2422–2440. Available from <Go to ISI>://WOS:000491106400001

108. Parkes EE, Walker SM, Taggart LE, McCabe N, Knight LA, Wilkinson R et al (2017) Activation of STING-dependent innate immune signaling by S-phase-specific DNA damage in breast cancer. J Natl Cancer Inst 109. Available from https://www.ncbi.nlm.nih.gov/pubmed/27707838

109. Pilie P, Tang Z, Park S, Wu C, Dong ZY, Yap T et al (2019) Inhibitors of Ataxia-Telangiectasia Related (ATR) protein lead to innate immune pathway activation and enhanced response to immune therapy in prostate cancer. Journal for Immunotherapy of Cancer. 7. Available from <Go to ISI>://WOS:000496473200135

110. Sheng HL, Huang Y, Xiao YZ, Zhu ZR, Shen MY, Zhou PT et al (2020) ATR inhibitor AZD6738 enhances the antitumor activity of radiotherapy and immune checkpoint inhibitors by potentiating the tumor immune microenvironment in hepatocellular carcinoma. J Immunother Cancer 8. Available from <Go to ISI>://WOS:000553971800001

111. Dillon MT, Bergerhoff KF, Pedersen M, Whittock H, Crespo-Rodriguez E, Patin EC et al (2019) ATR inhibition potentiates the radiation-induced inflammatory tumor microenvironment. Clin Cancer Res 25:3392–3403. Available from <Go to ISI>://WOS:000470293000021

112. Gasser S, Orsulic S, Brown EJ, Raulet DH (2005) The DNA damage pathway regulates innate immune system ligands of the NKG2D receptor. Nature 436:1186–1190. Available from: https://www.ncbi.nlm.nih.gov/pubmed/15995699

113. Sato H, Niimi A, Yasuhara T, Permata TBM, Hagiwara Y, Isono M et al (2017) DNA double-strand break repair pathway regulates PD-L1 expression in cancer cells. Nat Commun 8:1751. Available from https://www.ncbi.nlm.nih.gov/pubmed/29170499

114. Chen CF, Ruiz-Vega R, Vasudeva P, Espitia F, Krasieva TB, de Feraudy S et al (2017) ATR mutations promote the growth of melanoma tumors by modulating the immune microenvironment. Cell Rep 18:2331–2342. Available from: https://www.ncbi.nlm.nih.gov/pubmed/28273450

115. Lee J, Kim ST, Smith S, Mortimer PG, Loembe B, Hong J et al (2020) Results from a phase I, open-label study of ceralasertib (AZD6738), a novel DNA damage repair agent, in combination with weekly paclitaxel in refractory cancer (NCT02630199). J Clin Oncol 38. Available from <Go to ISI>://WOS:000560368301399

116. Louie AD, Huntington K, Carlsen L, Zhou L, El-Deiry WS (2021) Integrating molecular biomarker inputs into development and use of clinical cancer therapeutics. Front Pharmacol 12:747194

117. Ngoi NYL, Westin SN, Yap TA (2022) Targeting the DNA damage response beyond poly(ADP-ribose) polymerase inhibitors: novel agents and rational combinations. Curr Opin Oncol 34(5):559–569

118. Pilie PG, Gheeya JS, Kyewalabye K, Goswamy RV, Wani KM, Le H, et al. Identifying functional loss of ATM gene in patients with advanced cancer. J Clin Oncol 38(15_suppl):3629–3629

119. Rafiei S, Fitzpatrick K, Liu D, Cai M-Y, Elmarakeby HA, Park J et al (2020) ATM loss confers greater sensitivity to ATR inhibition than PARP inhibition in prostate cancer. Cancer Res 80(11):2094–2100

120. Yap TA, Tan DSP, Terbuch A, Caldwell R, Guo C, Goh BC et al (2021) First-in-human trial of the oral ataxia telangiectasia and RAD3-related (ATR) inhibitor BAY 1895344 in patients with advanced solid tumors. Cancer Discov 11(1):80–91

121. Kwok M, Davies N, Agathanggelou A (2016) ATR inhibition induces synthetic lethality and overcomes chemoresistance in TP53- or ATM-defective chronic lymphocytic leukemia cells (vol 127, p 582, 2016). Blood 127:2647–2647. Available from <Go to ISI>://WOS:000378334400022

122. Middleton FK, Pollard JR, Curtin NJ (2018) The impact of p53 dysfunction in ATR inhibitor cytotoxicity and chemo- and radiosensitisation. Cancers 10(8):275

123. Dillon MT, Barker HE, Pedersen M, Hafsi H, Bhide SA, Newbold KL et al (2017) Radiosensitization by the ATR inhibitor AZD6738 through generation of acentric micronuclei. Mol Cancer Ther 16(1):25–34

124. Das S, Whisenant J, Doyle A, Allegra CJ, Berlin J (2019) A phase II study of M6620 and irinotecan in TP53 mutant gastric and gastroesophageal junction (GEJ) adenocarcinoma patients (pts) [NCT03641313]. J Clin Oncol 37(4_suppl):TPS175–TPS175

125. Williamson CT, Miller R, Pemberton HN, Jones SE, Campbell J, Konde A et al (2016) ATR inhibitors as a synthetic lethal therapy for tumours deficient in ARID1A. Nat Commun 7(1):13837

126. Tsai S, Fournier L-A, Chang EY, Wells JP, Minaker SW, Zhu YD et al (2021) ARID1A regulates R-loop associated DNA replication stress. Plos Genet 17(4):e1009238

127. Aggarwal R, Umetsu S, Dhawan M, Grabowsky J, Carnevale J, Howell M et al (2021) 512O Interim results from a phase II study of the ATR inhibitor ceralasertib in ARID1A-deficient and ARID1A-intact advanced solid tumor malignancies. Ann Oncol 32:S583
128. Yap TA, O'Carrigan B, Penney MS, Lim JS, Brown JS, Luken MJ de M et al (2020) Phase I trial of first-in-class ATR inhibitor M6620 (VX-970) as monotherapy or in combination with carboplatin in patients with advanced solid tumors. J Clin Oncol 38(27):3195–3204
129. Krajewska M, Fehrmann RSN, Schoonen PM, Labib S, de Vries EGE, Franke L et al (2015) ATR inhibition preferentially targets homologous recombination-deficient tumor cells. Oncogene 34(26):3474–3481
130. Toh M, Ngeow J (2021) Homologous recombination deficiency: cancer predispositions and treatment implications. Oncol 26(9):e1526–e1537
131. Buisson R, Lawrence MS, Benes CH, Zou L (2017) APOBEC3A and APOBEC3B activities render cancer cells susceptible to ATR inhibition. Cancer Res 77(17):4567–4578
132. Savva C, Souza KD, Ali R, Rakha EA, Green AR, Madhusudan S (2019) Clinicopathological significance of ataxia telangiectasia-mutated (ATM) kinase and ataxia telangiectasia-mutated and Rad3-related (ATR) kinase in MYC overexpressed breast cancers. Breast Cancer Res Tr 175(1):105–115
133. Kok YP, Llobet SG, Schoonen PM, Everts M, Bhattacharya A, Fehrmann RSN et al (2020) Overexpression of Cyclin E1 or Cdc25A leads to replication stress, mitotic aberrancies, and increased sensitivity to replication checkpoint inhibitors. Oncogenesis 9(10):88
134. Ngoi N, Lin HY, Dumbrava EE, Fu S, Karp DD, Naing A et al (2022) Baseline predictors of hematological toxicity in patients with advanced cancer treated with ATR inhibitors in phase I/II clinical trials. J Clin Oncol 40(16_suppl):3111–3111
135. Fernandez-Rozadilla C, Simões AR, Lleonart ME, Carnero A, Carracedo Á (2021) Tumor profiling at the service of cancer therapy. Frontiers Oncol 10:595613
136. Fountzilas E, Tsimberidou AM, Vo HH, Kurzrock R (2022) Clinical trial design in the era of precision medicine. Genome Med 14(1):101

Targeting Polymerase Theta (POLθ) for Cancer Therapy

15

Jeffrey Patterson-Fortin and Alan D. D'Andrea

15.1 Double Strand Break Repair by POLθ-Mediated Microhomology-Mediated End-Joining

Maintenance of genome integrity is of upmost importance for cellular survival [1]. Genome integrity is achieved by DNA repair pathways, collectively known as the DNA damage response (DDR) [2]. Double-stranded breaks (DSBs) are the most cytotoxic form of DNA damage and, if unrepaired, these lesions lead to deleterious outcomes such as permanent changes to DNA sequence or cellular death [3–8]. Consequently, there are at least three pathways which repair DSBs. The majority of DSBs are rapidly repaired by the non-homologous end-joining (NHEJ) pathway, in which DSB DNA ends are directly re-ligated with minimal processing. NHEJ is an error prone and template independent DSB repair pathway that can occur throughout the entire cell cycle. The first step of NHEJ is recognition of the DSB by the Ku70-Ku80 heterodimer [9, 10]. The Ku70-Ku80 heterodimer acts as a scaffold, required for recruiting other NHEJ proteins and for joining DNA ends [9–14]. DNA-dependent protein kinase catalytic subunit (DNA-PKcs) is next recruited, and it binds with high affinity to Ku70-Ku80 heterodimer-DNA ends

J. Patterson-Fortin
Department of Medical Oncology, Dana-Farber Cancer Institute, Boston, MA 02215, USA
e-mail: Jeffrey_patterson-fortin@dfci.harvard.edu

J. Patterson-Fortin · A. D. D'Andrea
Department of Radiation Oncology, Dana-Farber Cancer Institute, Boston, MA 02215, USA

A. D. D'Andrea (✉)
Harvard Medical School, Center for DNA Damage and Repair, Susan F. Smith Center for Women's Cancers (SFSCWC), The Fuller-American Cancer Society, Dana-Farber Cancer Institute, HIM 243, 450 Brookline Ave., Boston, MA 02215, USA
e-mail: Alan_Dandrea@dfci.harvard.edu

[10]. If the DNA end breaks are compatible (ie, either blunt ends or breaks with complementary overhangs), then repair will likely be error-free through ligation by XRCC4-DNA ligase IV proteins. If, however the DNA break ends are not compatible, requiring additional processing (ie, either resection by nucleases or addition of nucleotides by polymerases), then repair will be error prone [15]. During S and G2 phases of the cell cycle, DSB repair can occur by homologous recombination (HR) which is sequence-guided by the available sister chromatid. The first step of HR is the generation of 3' overhanging single-stranded (ssDNA) by end resection. The nuclease activity of the MRN complex, comprised of MRE11, RAD50, and NBS1, stimulated by CtIP, performs end-resection at the site of the DSB [16–21]. Next, the resultant 3' ssDNA ends are first bound by replication protein A (RPA) followed by replacement with the RAD51 recombinase via the action of BRCA2, thus forming a RAD51-ssDNA nucleoprotein filament. This RAD51-ssDNA nucleoprotein filament then searches for a homologous DNA sequence, and performs strand invasion of the sister chromatid, thus forming a synapse with the homologous region on the other strand (D-loop). The homologous sequence ultimately acts as a template to yield an error-free repair product [22–24].

Microhomology-mediated end-joining (MMEJ, alternative named alternative end-joining or polymerase theta-mediated end-joining) is a third pathway that can repair DSBs. Through MMEJ, the DNA polymerase theta (POLθ) enzyme, encoded by *POLQ*, acts as a translesion DNA polymerase essential for the MMEJ repair process [42, 50]. Similar to HR, the MMEJ repair pathway is initiated by end-resection by the MRN complex stimulated by CtIP near the DSB exposing short regions of complementary sequences ranging from 2 to 20 nucleotides (microhomologies) [25–27]. These microhomologies are then used to align the DNA ends with end bridging occurring secondary to the activities of PARP-1 [28, 29]. Next, the resultant 5' flaps, created following alignment of the microhomology regions, are processed by nucleases such as FEN1 [30, 31]. POLθ then binds 3' single-stranded DNA generated by end-resection and uses annealed microhomology sequences as primers for DNA synthesis [32–36]. Ligation of the DNA ends then occurs by the activity of XRCC1-LIG3 [37, 38] (Simsek et al. 2011). Similar to NHEJ, MMEJ is error prone. The POLθ activity of MMEJ creates a specific mutational signature of (1) microhomology deletions, and (2) templated insertions providing a genomic biomarker of MMEJ [39–41].

POLθ is structurally and functionally distinct from other polymerases, consisting of three domains with distinct activities that are all required for POLθ activity (Fig. 15.1). The N-terminal domain contains a superfamily 2 (SF2) Hel308-typeS helicase domain that has helicase activity, ATPase activity, and RAD51-binding motifs. This domain may have both MMEJ independent and dependent activities [42]. In terms of MMEJ-independent activity, the helicase domain can unwind short double-stranded DNA with a 3'–5' polarity in an ATP-dependent manner though of unknown significance [43]. In terms of MMEJ-dependent activities, the helicase domain, with its ATPase activity, can facilitate removal of RAD51 and RPA from ssDNA to inhibit HR. This stripping activity of POLθ is essential in HR deficient cells, presumably due to the build-up of toxic levels of RAD51

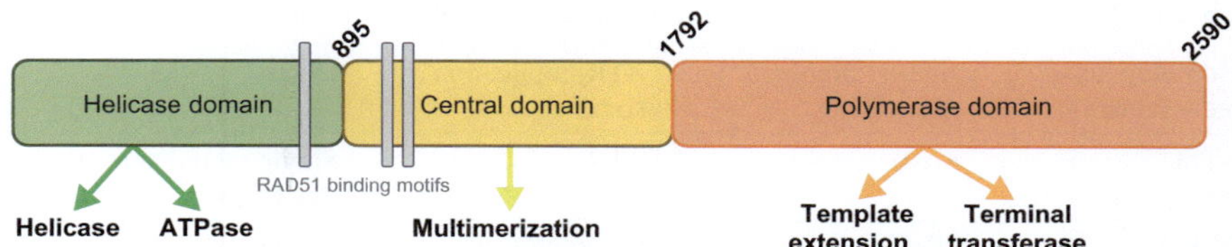

Fig. 15.1 Domains of POLθ. POLθ is a 2590 residue enzyme with three distinct domains: (1) a helicase domain, (2) a central domain, and (3) a polymerase domain. The N-terminal helicase domain has helicase activity, ATPase activity, and one RAD51-binding motif. The helicase domain facilitates removal of RAD51 and RPA to suppress HR, and prevents snap-back replication, allowing the polymerase domain to perform MMEJ on long ssDNA substrates. The unstructured central domain contains 2 RAD51 binding motifs involved in suppressing HR and regulates POLθ multimerization. The C-terminal polymerase domain synthesizes DNA during MMEJ repair, either by template extension or by terminal transferase activity. See text for more detail. Figure created using Biorender

in the absence of POLθ [42, 44] (Mateos-Gomez et al., 2017). In addition, the helicase domain, independent of its ATPase activity, allows the POLθ C-terminal polymerase to perform MMEJ on long ssDNA substrates with 3′ terminal microhomology [45]. The central domain of POLθ is a long unstructured region that links the N-terminal helicase domain and the C-terminal polymerase domain (Fig. 15.1). Similar to the N-terminal domain, the central domain contains RAD51-binding motifs and functions as an anti-recombinase, by inhibiting HR and promoting MMEJ [42]. This domain also regulates POLθ multimerization and MMEJ substrate choice, preventing MMEJ on short ssDNA and promoting MMEJ on long ssDNA [45]. The C-terminal domain of POLθ contains an A-family polymerase domain that performs gap filling by template extension or terminal transferase activity [34–36, 62]. In addition to its role in MMEJ, POLθ can function in other repair pathways, including base excision repair and translesion synthesis. It also has recently being shown to possess reverse transcriptase activity [46]. In summary, MMEJ is an error prone DSB repair pathway mediated by the unique multidomain and multifunctional POLθ enzyme.

15.2 Synthetic Lethality of POLθ in Cancers

POLθ is expressed at low levels in normal tissue but is overexpressed in a variety of malignancies, including lung, gastric, colorectal, breast, and ovarian cancers, and this portends a poorer prognosis [42, 47–49]. Although POLθ expression is tightly regulated, the mechanism of this regulation and corresponding overexpression in cancers remain unresolved. Nonetheless, its overexpression in HR-deficient cancers, which are known to be selectively dependent on POLθ-mediated MMEJ for viability, makes POLθ a promising synthetic lethal anti-cancer target. It is an especially good target since POLθ is dispensable for growth and survival of normal cells [42, 50]. In the clinic, the concept of synthetic lethality has been translated

Table 15.1 Known synthetic lethal interactors with POLθ depletion or inhibition

Homologous recombination	Non-homologous end-joining	ATR, replication stress	Others
ATM	Ku70	ATR	Single-strand annealing (RAD52)
BRCA1	PRKDC	Camptothecin	Shelterin (POT1)
BRCA2	53BP1	Etoposide	Translesion synthesis (POLH)
FANCD2	REV7	Hydroxyurea	
GEN1	SHLD2		
PALB2			
RAD51C			
SLX4			

Grouping of validated synthetic lethal interactors with POLθ depletion or inhibition. See text for further details

therapeutically by targeting PARP1 in HR-deficient cancers harboring mutations in BRCA1 or BRCA2. Patients with germline mutations in either of these two genes can develop HR deficient ovarian, breast, pancreatic, or prostate cancer [51, 52]. Indeed, there exists a number of synthetic lethal relationships that can be exploited with POLθ inhibitors (Table 15.1).

The *POLQ* gene was originally cloned and mapped by Sharief and colleagues [53]. Later Shima and colleagues performed a mutagenesis screen for chromosome instability mutants and used a screen of increased peripheral blood micronuclei as a quantitative indicator of chromosomal damage. This group identified a recessive mutation, termed *chaos1*, that increased both spontaneous and mitomycin C-induced micronuclei. Interestingly, the *chaos1* mouse was shown to have biallelic mutations in the *POLQ* gene, suggesting a role for POLθ in DSB repair [54]. Later, Shima and colleagues demonstrated the first example of a POLθ synthetic lethal interaction [55]. To investigate POLθ's role in DSB repair, they bred *POLQ*-deficient mice with ATM (ataxia telangiectasia mutated)-deficient mice. Double knockout embryos or new born mice either failed to survive or exhibited severe growth retardation and enhanced chromosome instability [55]. This synthetic lethal interaction between POLθ and ATM was confirmed when *POLQ*-depleted ovarian cancer cells were exposed to an ATM inhibitor (Ku55933) [42]. Subsequent studies revealed that POLθ inhibition or depletion is synthetic lethal with other DSB repair processes such as NHEJ (Ku70, PRKDC), HR (BRCA1, BRCA2, PALB2, RAD51, GEN1, SLX4), Faconi Anemia interstrand crosslink repair (FANCD2, FANCF) and single-strand annealing (RAD52). Similarly, because POLθ inhibition results in increased DNA resection at DSBs, it is not unexpected that POLθ inhibition or depletion would be synthetic lethal with antagonists of DNA end-resection (53BP1, REV7, SHLD2) [41, 56, 57]. ssDNA activates the ATR (Ataxia telangiectasia and Rad3 related) checkpoint which responds to ssDNA breaks in a multistep pathway that involves DNA-damage sensing, signal transduction, and execution to protect replication forks from collapsing and to promote replication fork restart [58, 59]. Accordingly, POLθ depletion is synthetic lethal with pharmacological ATR inhibition or ATR depletion [60]. Similarly, because the ATR pathway responds to replication stress, agents that induce replication stress and fork collapse, such as camptothecin (a topoisomerase I inhibitor) etoposide (a topoisomerase II inhibitor), or hydroxyurea, are synthetic lethal with POLθ depletion [60]. Finally, Zatreanu and colleagues employed a siRNA chemosensitization screen to identify determinants of POLθ inhibition. They identified the telomere protective protein complex (Shelterin) POT1 component and the translesion synthesis associated gene, *POLH* in the screen [57]. In summary, POLθ and MMEJ has several validated synthetic lethal interactions with other DDR processes. Indeed, approximately half of the 300 murine DDR genes analyzed in a CRISPR KO screen in *POLQ*-deficient mouse embryonic fibroblasts demonstrated synthetic lethality [41]. Thus, targeting POLθ in cancers with known synthetic lethal mutations or deficiencies has substantial clinical potential.

15.3 Development of POLθ Inhibitors

As discussed in the first section, POLθ is comprised of two known enzymatically active domains: the ATPase containing N-terminal helicase domain and the polymerase containing C-terminal domain. The crystal structures of both domains have been solved, providing insight to both drug targets [61, 62]. CRISPR-mediated mutagenesis of either domain was synthetic lethal in *BRCA1*-deficient mouse embryonic stem cells, indicating that pharmacological inhibition of either domain could recapitulate this synthetic lethal relationship (Mateo-Gomez 2017). Indeed, two independent groups recently published small molecular inhibitors that target either the helicase or polymerase domains respectively, and a number of independent biotechnology companies are actively developing POLθ inhibitors [56, 57].

The first research group performed a high-throughput small-molecule screen of 23,513 bioactive compounds for inhibitors of POLθ ATPase activity and identified an antibiotic, novobiocin, as a top hit [56]. They repurposed novobiocin as a POLθ inhibitor, demonstrating that the drug selectively kills HR-deficient tumor cells, both in vitro and in vivo, in genetically engineered mouse models (GEMMs) and xenograft and patient-derived xenograft (PDX) models. Specifically, they showed that novobiocin-mediated POLθ inhibition is synthetic lethal in *BRCA1*, *BRCA2*, *FANCF*, and *RAD51C*-deficiency backgrounds (Table 15.1). Importantly, novobiocin-mediated POLθ inhibition was additive with PARP inhibition in killing HR-deficient tumors. PARP inhibitors or POLθ inhibitors (NVB) can inhibit the recruitment of POLθ protein to sites of DNA damage. Moreover, these agents also have distinct functions in killing HR deficient tumor cells. (Sect. 15.1). In addition, novobiocin-mediated POLθ inhibition was able to overcome PARP inhibitor resistance secondary to two different mechanisms: in vitro, in BRCA1-deficient breast cancers with resistance to PARP inhibitor secondary to downregulation of the Shieldin complex; and in vivo, *in* a PDX model of PARP inhibitor resistant BRCA1 deficient ovarian cancer with biallelic loss of *TP53BP1* [56]. Thus, pharmacological targeting of the ATPase containing helicase domain of POLθ is an effective therapeutic strategy in treating HR-deficient cancers and in overcoming PARP inhibitor resistance.

The second research group in contrast, performed a high-throughput DNA primer extension small-molecule screen to discover inhibitors of the POLθ polymerase activity. This group initially identifyied ART558, an allosteric inhibitor of the POLθ polymerase domain, and later developing ART812, a more potent in vivo POLθ polymerase inhibitor [57]. Consistently, they showed that ART558-mediated POLθ inhibition was synthetic lethal in HR-deficient tumor cells, additive with PARP inhibitors, and able to overcome PARP inhibitor resistance. Specifically, they showed that ART558-mediated POLθ polymerase activity was synthetic lethal in *BRCA1*-deficient breast cancer cells in vitro. ART558 also killed genetically engineered *BRCA2*-deficient colorectal cancer cells and *BRCA2*-deficient pancreatic cancer cells. Similar to novobiocin's ability to re-sensitize PARP inhibitor resistance secondary to Shieldin or *TP53BP1* loss, ART558 was able to kill these cancers as well, through inhibition of the POLθ polymerase activity. The authors then recapitulated their work in an in vivo xenograft model in rats bearing *BRCA1*-deficient breast cancer cells, demonstrating significant tumor inhibition with ART812 [57]. Thus, pharmacological targeting of the polymerase domain of POLθ has the same functional outcome as pharmacological targeting of the ATPase domain. These two contemporaneous studies have demonstrated a number of advances while also raising new questions.

First, the successful pharmacological inhibition of the POLθ ATPase containing helicase domain or the POLθ polymerase domain demonstrated proof-of-concept that POLθ inhibition reiterates the phenotypes obtained from genomic perturbation of POLθ. Second, the studies have confirmed a role for POLθ in genomic maintenance, as its inhibition by a small molecule inhibitor leads to an increase in a marker of DNA damage-namely, γH2AX. Third, the work has independently demonstrated that POLθ likely limits further DNA end-resection. Accordingly, inhibition of POLθ leads to the accumulation of ssDNA and ultimately to cell death via apoptosis. Fourth, the work has provided proof that POLθ inhibition is additive with PARP inhibition, and indeed, can re-sensitize PARP inhibitor resistant cancers.

However, additional questions remain. First, which domain of POLθ should be targeted? As discussed in Sect. 15.1, the ATPase containing helicase domain may have both MMEJ independent and MMEJ-dependent functions. Similarly, the polymerase domain also has MMEJ independent and dependent functions. Perhaps simultaneous inhibition of both enzymatic domains would improve the killing of HR deficient tumor cells. Second, the polymerase domain of POLθ was recently shown to possess reverse transcriptase activity similar to HIV's reverse transcriptase activity [46]. Given the efficacy of targeting the POLθ polymerase domain, it is possible that HIV reverse transcriptase inhibitors could be repurposed to inhibit

POLθ or to be used in combination with the known POLθ inhibitors. Third, newer POLθ inhibitors, such as agents which promote the degradation of POLθ, could be generated. In summary, small molecule inhibition of either POLθ enzymatic domain is synthetic lethal in HR-deficient tumors, recapitulating the previously reported synthetic lethal studies in which POLθ was depleted by CRISPR knockout [42, 50, 56, 57]. Fourth, although POLθ inhibition has been shown to be additive with PARP inhibition in the re-sensitization of PARP inhibitor resistant cancers, little is known regarding the appropriate scheduling regimen of a POLθ and PARP inhibitor combination. It is hoped that the continued development and refinement of POLθ inhibitors will translate into clinically effective treatments for patients and continued molecular understanding about POLθ.

15.4 Clinical Use of POLθ Inhibitors

In Sect. 15.2, the known synthetic lethal relationships with POLθ depletion or inhibition were detailed, suggesting that patients with cancers with these specific genetic alterations could benefit from treatment with a POLθ inhibitor based on robust pre-clinical data (Table 15.1). Whether this pre-clinical data can translate to clinically effective treatments remains to be seen, but the first clinical trial for a POLθ inhibitor, ART4215, (Artios Pharma, NCT04991480) which specifically inhibits the POLθ polymerase domain has begun. Also, a clinical trial of novobiocin which targets the POLθ helicase domain is anticipated in 2022. In Sect. 15.3, the development of two different POLθ inhibitors was detailed and notable for their efficacy in HR-deficient cancers. Both of these POLθ inhibitor trials will enroll patients with breast cancers that harbor defects in HR, such as patients with *BRCA1* or *BRCA2* germline mutations. For these patients, POLθ inhibition is expected to have monotherapy activity (Fig. 15.2). In some cases, patients will receive POLθ inhibitors as monotherapy or in combination with a PARP inhibitor. Combination with PARP inhibitors is especially important since these agents are not curative and acquired resistance can rapidly emerge [63–65]. First, given the pre-clinical data, it is expected that the combination POLθ and PARP inhibition would augment PARP inhibitor activity by deepening responses or by prolonging clinical benefit. Indeed, the treatment with PARPi plus POLθi upfront could possibly delay or prevent the development of PARPi resistance. Second, POLθ expression is upregulated in HR-deficient cancers, and these cancers often exhibit a MMEJ specific mutational signature of microhomology deletions and templated insertions consistent with a microhomology-rich insertion and deletion 6 (ID6) signature [66]. Indeed, it has been proposed that upregulation of this mutational signature indicates a direct upregulation of MMEJ and could serve as a predictive biomarker of a cancer's dependence on POLθ [67]. Similarly, analysis of whole exome sequences has also revealed a specific nucleotide variant (SNV) substitution signature, COSMIC signature 3, as a marker of HR deficiency, correlated with functional loss of *BRCA1, BRCA2, PALB2,* and *RAD51C* [68, 69]. Thus, COSMIC signature 3 could also serve as a predictive biomarker of HR deficiency

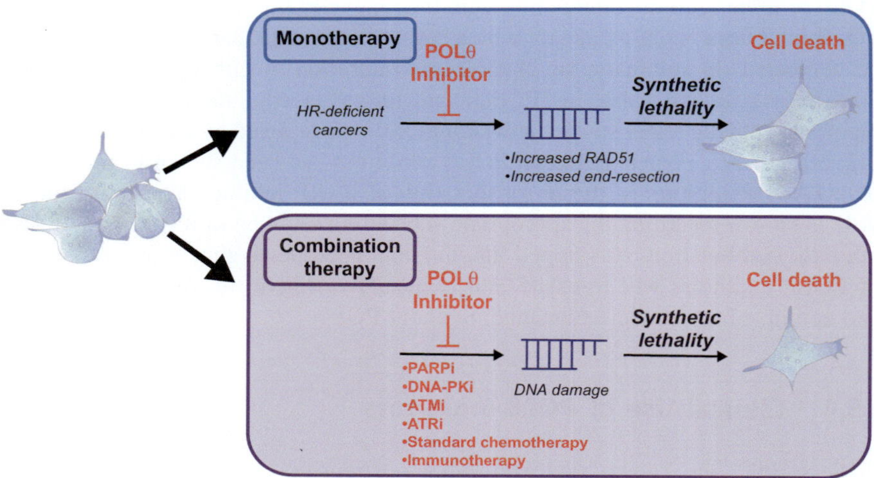

Fig. 15.2 Clinical Use of POLθ Inhibitors. Schematic representation of treatment rationale for POLθ inhibitors on the basis of synthetic lethality. In a HR-deficient cancer cell, monotherapy POLθ inhibition will increase both RAD51 deposition and DNA end-resection to toxic levels, leading to cell death. Alternatively, POLθ inhibition could be combined with standard chemotherapy, targeted DNA repair inhibitors, or immunotherapy in both HR-deficient and HR-proficient tumors. Figure created using Biorender

and synthetic lethal interaction with POLθ depletion or inhibition, though further prospective studies to establish this relationship are required. Nonetheless, error-prone MMEJ could drive genomic plasticity and contribute to the acquisition of PARP inhibitor resistance which could be prevented by POLθ inhibition de novo in combination with PARP inhibition [39–41]. Third, if PARP inhibitor resistance has developed by rewiring of DNA end-resection via loss of *TP53BP1*, *REV7* (*MAD2L2*), or other components of the Shieldin complex, for example *SHLD2*, these tumors remain dependent on POLθ and thus sensitive to POLθ inhibition [56, 57, 70, 71]. Thus, using POLθ inhibitors in combination with PARP inhibitors or in cancers with acquired PARP inhibitor resistance could be beneficial. Nonetheless, these first-in-human studies are critical for determining whether POLθ inhibition will turn out to be a useful treatment of primary HR-deficient cancers or tumors with acquired PARPi resistance.

Though the pre-clinical data has demonstrated the synthetic lethal relationship between POLθ depletion or inhibition with HR-deficiency, there are also other synthetic lethality relationships with POLθ inhibition, as highlighted in Table 15.1. First, the MMEJ pathway was first identified as an alternative DSB repair pathway in NHEJ-deficient yeast and hamster cells as these cells retained some degree of end-joining activity, and hence initially termed as alternative end-joining [72, 73]. Thus, these observations raise the possibility that NHEJ and MMEJ may be synthetic lethal. Indeed, biallelic mutation of *Ku70* (NHEJ) and *POLQ* resulted in a synthetic-sick phenotype in mouse embryonic fibroblasts (Wyatt 2016). More recently, pharmacologic inhibition of DNA-PK and genetic depletion of *POLQ* restored radiomimetic sensitivity of *TP53*-deficient cancers [74]. Whether the combination of a NHEJ inhibitor, such as peposertib (EMD Serono), with a POLθ inhibitor, such as novobiocin, with or without an additional DNA damaging agent (i.e., radiation) would be effective for a p53 mutant tumor is unknown. Since both peposertib and novobiocin are well-tolerated, orally- available medications, such a combination trial is feasible [56, 75]. Second, as described above, the original synthetic lethal POLθ interactor was ATM [55]. A number of ATM inhibitors are currently undergoing clinical trial for cancer therapy in combination with other drugs (i.e., NCT02588105) or radiation (i.e., NCT03423628). Combination small molecule ATM inhibition and POLθ inhibition would be predicted to be synthetic lethal. Third, inhibition of POLθ leads to increased DNA end-resection, the accumulation of ssDNA, and the activation of ATR. In addition, POLθ repairs DSBs upon replication fork collapse and is required for an adequate response to replication stress [60]. Thus, combining POLθ inhibition in combination with ATR inhibitors or with topoisomerase inhibitors that induce replication stress is another likely viable treatment strategy. Fourth, POLθ inhibitors could be combined with standard cytotoxic chemotherapy. For example, in metastatic castration-resistant prostate cancer, *POLQ* overexpression predicts a poor response to chemotherapy (docetaxel). In vitro, *POLQ* knockdown enhances docetaxel sensitivity, suggesting that POLθ inhibition may synergize with cytotoxic chemotherapy [76]. Finally, therapeutically effective DNA-damaging anti-tumor agents require the activation of host cytotoxic immune responses [77, 78]. Indeed, PARP inhibitors have been shown to activate the cGAS/STING innate immune response in HR-deficient cells leading to intratumoral CD8+ T-cell infiltration and anti-tumor immune responses in HR-deficient cancers, critical for their efficacy [77, 78]. Thus, given that POLθ inhibition leads to the formation of micronuclei, a known trigger of immunogenic responses, these findings suggest that POLθ inhibitors could be used in combination with STING agonists or with immune checkpoint blockade [79]. In summary, POLθ inhibitors are currently entering clinical trial to first demonstrate safety, second to demonstrate efficacy against HR-deficient cancers, and third to demonstrate synergy with PARP inhibitors, based on robust pre-clinical data [56, 57]. But given the known POLθ synthetic lethal interactions (Table 15.1), it is likely that POLθ inhibition can be used as a targeted therapy in cancers beyond HR-deficient cancers, and in combination with synergistic agents to minimize toxicity while maximizing efficacy (Fig. 15.2).

15.5 Predictive Biomarkers for POLθ Inhibitor Responsiveness

POLθ inhibitors are a new class of anti-cancer drugs that are advancing in clinical trials. It still remains unclear which clinical setting is most appropriate for these agents. Also, it will be especially important to determine which biomarkers will be most predictive of a POLθ inhibitor clinical response. Table 15.1 outlines known pre-clinical synthetic lethal interactors with POLθ inhibition and predicts that cancers with one or more of these alterations will be responsive to POLθ inhibition. Immunohistochemistry for expression of these known synthetic lethal interactors could be performed. Absence of expression of these biomarkers in a tumor could better predict drug responsiveness. In addition, because replication stress correlates with *POLQ* expression. Assessment of biomarkers of replication stress, such as pRPA and pKAP1, by immunohistochemistry could provide an "up" assay, for predicting POLθ inhibitor response [80]. Alternatively, pathogenic genomic alterations identified by next-generation sequencing is also a useful biomarker tool. This could include targeted sequencing for genomic alterations in DDR genes such as *BRCA1* or *BRCA2*, or to identify common genomic signatures such as COSMIC signature 3 which may capture more patients, or to identify common transcriptional signature such as upregulation of POLθ expression which correlates with response to novobiocin-mediated POLθ inhibition. The development of a biomarker for POLθ inhibition is important as meta-analysis of clinical trial participants has demonstrated that the use of biomarker-guided therapy increases objective response rates and improves overall survival [81–83]. Furthermore, the development of biomarkers of POLθ inhibitor responsiveness may allow for the identification of resistance mechanisms and inform how to appropriately adjust cancer treatment. Finally, in terms of pharmacodynamic markers of POLθ inhibition, two gain of signal assays are predicted to correlate with POLθ inhibition. Mechanistically, because POLθ inhibition increases ssDNA, assessment of RPA or RAD51, proteins that bind ssDNA, by immunohistochemistry could correlate with POLθ inhibitor efficacy [56, 57]. Maximizing the potential POLθ inhibitors will require the development of biomarkers to guide their clinical utilization and to monitor their clinical efficacy.

15.6 Summary

In summary, MMEJ is an error-prone DSB repair pathway mediated by POLθ. POLθ is often upregulated in cancers and its depletion or inhibition is synthetic lethal with loss of other DNA repair pathway genes, suggesting a dependence on POLθ and hence a promising precision medicine cancer target. Indeed, POLθ inhibitors are now entering the cancer clinic, based on their robust pre-clinical data. The agents are likely to have monotherapy activity when used in the genetically appropriate cancers (i.e., HR-deficient cancers) (Fig. 15.2). Alternatively, they combine well with other therapeutic agents, based on their underlying POLθ synthetic lethal relationships. Continued development of POLθ inhibitors will not only advance our understanding of POLθ's activities and mechanisms of action but will also appropriately define which patients who will benefit from targeting POLθ for cancer therapy.

References

1. Ceccaldi R, Rondinelli B, D'Andrea AD (2016) Repair pathway choices and consequences at the double-strand break. Trends Cell Biol 26(1):52–64
2. Nilles N, Fahrenkrog B (2017) Taking a bad turn: compromised DNA damage response in leukemia. Cells 6(2)
3. Sung P, Klein H (2006) Mechanism of homologous recombination: mediators and helicases take on regulatory functions. Nat Rev Mol Cell Biol 7(10):739–750
4. Heyer W-D, Ehmsen KT, Liu J (2010) Regulation of homologous recombination in eukaryotes. Annu Rev Genet 44:113–139
5. Chapman JR, Taylor MRG, Boulton SJ (2012) Playing the end game: DNA double-strand break repair pathway choice. Mol Cell 47(4):497–510
6. Bunting SF, Nussenzweig A (2013) End-joining, translocations and cancer. Nat Rev Cancer 13(7):443–454
7. Helleday T, Eshtad S, Nik-Zainal S (2014) Mechanisms underlying mutational signatures in human cancers. Nat Rev Genet 15(9):585–598
8. Carvalho CMB, Lupski JR (2016) Mechanisms underlying structural variant formation in genomic disorders. Nat Rev Genet 17(4):224–238
9. Mari P-O, Florea BI, Persengiev SP, Verkaik NS, Brüggenwirth HT, Modesti M et al (2006) Dynamic assembly of end-joining complexes requires interaction between Ku70/80 and XRCC4. Proc Natl Acad Sci U S A 103(49):18597–18602
10. Uematsu N, Weterings E, Yano K, Morotomi-Yano K, Jakob B, Taucher-Scholz G et al (2007) Autophosphorylation of DNA-PKCS regulates its dynamics at DNA double-strand breaks. J Cell Biol 177(2):219–229
11. McElhinny AS, Warner CM (2000) Cross-linking of Qa-2 protein, the Ped gene product, increases the cleavage rate of C57BL/6 preimplantation mouse embryos. Mol Hum Reprod 6(6):517–522
12. Costantini S, Woodbine L, Andreoli L, Jeggo PA, Vindigni A (2007) Interaction of the Ku heterodimer with the DNA ligase IV/Xrcc4 complex and its regulation by DNA-PK. DNA Repair (Amst). 6(6):712–722
13. Meek K, Dang V, Lees-Miller SP (2008) DNA-PK: the means to justify the ends? Adv Immunol 99:33–58
14. Yano K, Morotomi-Yano K, Akiyama H (2009) Cernunnos/XLF: a new player in DNA double-strand break repair. Int J Biochem Cell Biol 41(6):1237–1240
15. Bétermier M, Bertrand P, Lopez BS (2014) Is non-homologous end-joining really an inherently error-prone process? PLoS Genet 10(1):e1004086
16. Sartori AA, Lukas C, Coates J, Mistrik M, Fu S, Bartek J et al (2007) Human CtIP promotes DNA end resection. Nature 450(7169):509–514
17. Stracker TH, Petrini JHJ (2011) The MRE11 complex: starting from the ends. Nat Rev Mol Cell Biol 12(2):90–103
18. Symington LS, Gautier J (2011) Double-strand break end resection and repair pathway choice. Annu Rev Genet 45:247–271
19. Anand R, Ranjha L, Cannavo E, Cejka P (2016) Phosphorylated CtIP functions as a Co-factor of the MRE11-RAD50-NBS1 endonuclease in DNA end resection. Mol Cell 64(5):940–950
20. Daley JM, Jimenez-Sainz J, Wang W, Miller AS, Xue X, Nguyen KA et al (2017) Enhancement of BLM-DNA2-mediated long-range DNA end resection by CtIP. Cell Rep 21(2):324–332
21. Wilkinson OJ, Martín-González A, Kang H, Northall SJ, Wigley DB, Moreno-Herrero F et al (2019) CtIP forms a tetrameric dumbbell-shaped particle which bridges complex DNA end structures for double-strand break repair. Elife 8
22. Jasin M, Rothstein R (2013) Repair of strand breaks by homologous recombination. Cold Spring Harb Perspect Biol 5(11):a012740

23. Hustedt N, Durocher D (2016) The control of DNA repair by the cell cycle. Nat Cell Biol 19(1):1–9
24. Densham RM, Morris JR (2019) Moving mountains—The BRCA1 promotion of DNA resection. Front Mol Biosci 6:79
25. Garcia V, Phelps SEL, Gray S, Neale MJ (2011) Bidirectional resection of DNA double-strand breaks by Mre11 and Exo1. Nature 479(7372):241–244
26. Cannavo E, Cejka P (2014) Sae2 promotes dsDNA endonuclease activity within Mre11-Rad50-Xrs2 to resect DNA breaks. Nature 514(7520):122–125
27. Daley JM, Niu H, Miller AS, Sung P (2015) Biochemical mechanism of DSB end resection and its regulation. DNA Repair (Amst). 32:66–74
28. Mansour WY, Rhein T, Dahm-Daphi J (2010) The alternative end-joining pathway for repair of DNA double-strand breaks requires PARP1 but is not dependent upon microhomologies. Nucleic Acids Res 38(18):6065–6077
29. Robert I, Dantzer F, Reina-San-Martin B (2009) Parp1 facilitates alternative NHEJ, whereas Parp2 suppresses IgH/c-myc translocations during immunoglobulin class switch recombination. J Exp Med 206(5):1047–1056
30. Zou G-M, Maitra A (2008) Small-molecule inhibitor of the AP endonuclease 1/REF-1 E3330 inhibits pancreatic cancer cell growth and migration. Mol Cancer Ther 7(7):2012–2021
31. Sharma S, Javadekar SM, Pandey M, Srivastava M, Kumari R, Raghavan SC (2015) Homology and enzymatic requirements of microhomology-dependent alternative end joining. Cell Death Dis 6:e1697
32. Hogg M, Sauer-Eriksson AE, Johansson E (2012) Promiscuous DNA synthesis by human DNA polymerase θ. Nucleic Acids Res 40(6):2611–2622
33. McVey M, Lee SE (2008) MMEJ repair of double-strand breaks (director's cut): deleted sequences and alternative endings. Trends Genet 24(11):529–538
34. Kent T, Chandramouly G, McDevitt SM, Ozdemir AY, Pomerantz RT (2015) Mechanism of microhomology-mediated end-joining promoted by human DNA polymerase θ. Nat Struct Mol Biol 22(3):230–237
35. Wyatt DW, Feng W, Conlin MP, Yousefzadeh MJ, Roberts SA, Mieczkowski P et al (2016) Essential roles for polymerase θ-mediated end joining in the repair of chromosome breaks. Mol Cell 63(4):662–673
36. Yousefzadeh MJ, Wyatt DW, Takata K-I, Mu Y, Hensley SC, Tomida J et al (2014) Mechanism of suppression of chromosomal instability by DNA polymerase POLQ. PLoS Genet 10(10):e1004654
37. Audebert M, Salles B, Calsou P (2004) Involvement of poly(ADP-ribose) polymerase-1 and XRCC1/DNA ligase III in an alternative route for DNA double-strand breaks rejoining. J Biol Chem 279(53):55117–55126
38. Wang H, Rosidi B, Perrault R, Wang M, Zhang L, Windhofer F et al (2005) DNA ligase III as a candidate component of backup pathways of nonhomologous end joining. Cancer Res 65(10):4020–4030
39. Chan SH, Yu AM, McVey M (2010) Dual roles for DNA polymerase theta in alternative end-joining repair of double-strand breaks in Drosophila. PLoS Genet 6(7):e1001005
40. Carvajal-Garcia J, Cho J-E, Carvajal-Garcia P, Feng W, Wood RD, Sekelsky J et al (2020) Mechanistic basis for microhomology identification and genome scarring by polymerase theta. Proc Natl Acad Sci U S A 117(15):8476–8485
41. Feng W, Simpson DA, Carvajal-Garcia J, Price BA, Kumar RJ, Mose LE et al (2019) Genetic determinants of cellular addiction to DNA polymerase theta. Nat Commun 10(1):4286
42. Ceccaldi R, Liu JC, Amunugama R, Hajdu I, Primack B, Petalcorin MIR et al (2015) Homologous-recombination-deficient tumours are dependent on Polθ-mediated repair. Nature 518(7538):258–262
43. Ozdemir AY, Rusanov T, Kent T, Siddique LA, Pomerantz RT (2018) Polymerase θ-helicase efficiently unwinds DNA and RNA-DNA hybrids. J Biol Chem 293(14):5259–5269
44. Seki M, Marini F, Wood RD (2003) POLQ (Pol theta), a DNA polymerase and DNA-dependent ATPase in human cells. Nucleic Acids Res 31(21):6117–6126

45. Black SJ, Ozdemir AY, Kashkina E, Kent T, Rusanov T, Ristic D et al (2019) Molecular basis of microhomology-mediated end-joining by purified full-length Polθ. Nat Commun 10(1):4423
46. Chandramouly G, Zhao J, McDevitt S, Rusanov T, Hoang T, Borisonnik N, et al (2021) Polθ reverse transcribes RNA and promotes RNA-templated DNA repair. Sci Adv 7(24)
47. Kawamura K, Bahar R, Seimiya M, Chiyo M, Wada A, Okada S et al (2004) DNA polymerase theta is preferentially expressed in lymphoid tissues and upregulated in human cancers. Int J cancer 109(1):9–16
48. Lemée F, Bergoglio V, Fernandez-Vidal A, Machado-Silva A, Pillaire M-J, Bieth A et al (2010) DNA polymerase theta up-regulation is associated with poor survival in breast cancer, perturbs DNA replication, and promotes genetic instability. Proc Natl Acad Sci U S A 107(30):13390–13395
49. Higgins GS, Harris AL, Prevo R, Helleday T, McKenna WG, Buffa FM (2010) Overexpression of POLQ confers a poor prognosis in early breast cancer patients. Oncotarget 1(3):175–184
50. Mateos-Gomez PA, Gong F, Nair N, Miller KM, Lazzerini-Denchi E, Sfeir A (2015) Mammalian polymerase θ promotes alternative NHEJ and suppresses recombination. Nature 518(7538):254–257
51. Mateo J, Carreira S, de Bono JS (2019) PARP inhibitors for advanced prostate cancer: validating predictive biomarkers. Eur Urol 76(4):459–460
52. Curtin NJ, Szabo C (2020) Poly(ADP-ribose) polymerase inhibition: past, present and future. Nat Rev Drug Discov 19(10):711–736
53. Sharief FS, Vojta PJ, Ropp PA, Copeland WC (1999) Cloning and chromosomal mapping of the human DNA polymerase theta (POLQ), the eighth human DNA polymerase. Genomics 59(1):90–96
54. Shima N, Hartford SA, Duffy T, Wilson LA, Schimenti KJ, Schimenti JC (2003) Phenotype-based identification of mouse chromosome instability mutants. Genetics 163(3):1031–1040
55. Shima N, Munroe RJ, Schimenti JC (2004) The mouse genomic instability mutation chaos1 is an allele of Polq that exhibits genetic interaction with Atm. Mol Cell Biol 24(23):10381–10389
56. Zhou J, Gelot C, Pantelidou C, Li A, Yücel H, Davis RE et al (2021) A first-in-class polymerase theta inhibitor selectively targets homologous-recombination-deficient tumors. Nat cancer. 2(6):598–610
57. Zatreanu D, Robinson HMR, Alkhatib O, Boursier M, Finch H, Geo L et al (2021) Polθ inhibitors elicit BRCA-gene synthetic lethality and target PARP inhibitor resistance. Nat Commun 12(1):3636
58. Zou L (2007) Single- and double-stranded DNA: building a trigger of ATR-mediated DNA damage response. Genes Dev 21(8):879–885
59. Zeman MK, Cimprich KA (2014) Causes and consequences of replication stress. Nat Cell Biol 16(1):2–9
60. Wang Z, Song Y, Li S, Kurian S, Xiang R, Chiba T et al (2019) DNA polymerase θ (POLQ) is important for repair of DNA double-strand breaks caused by fork collapse. J Biol Chem 294(11):3909–3919
61. Newman JA, Cooper CDO, Aitkenhead H, Gileadi O (2015) Structure of the helicase domain of DNA polymerase theta reveals a possible role in the microhomology-mediated end-joining pathway. Structure 23(12):2319–2330
62. Zahn KE, Averill AM, Aller P, Wood RD, Doublié S (2015) Human DNA polymerase θ grasps the primer terminus to mediate DNA repair. Nat Struct Mol Biol 22(4):304–311
63. Ledermann J, Harter P, Gourley C, Friedlander M, Vergote I, Rustin G et al (2012) Olaparib maintenance therapy in platinum-sensitive relapsed ovarian cancer. N Engl J Med 366(15):1382–1392
64. Mirza MR, Monk BJ, Herrstedt J, Oza AM, Mahner S, Redondo A et al (2016) Niraparib Maintenance therapy in platinum-sensitive, recurrent ovarian cancer. N Engl J Med 375(22):2154–2164

65. Golan T, Hammel P, Reni M, Van Cutsem E, Macarulla T, Hall MJ et al (2019) Maintenance olaparib for germline BRCA-mutated metastatic pancreatic cancer. N Engl J Med 381(4):317–327

66. Alexandrov LB, Kim J, Haradhvala NJ, Huang MN, Tian Ng AW, Wu Y et al (2020) The repertoire of mutational signatures in human cancer. Nature 578(7793):94–101

67. Ramsden DA, Carvajal-Garcia J, Gupta GP (2022) Mechanism, cellular functions and cancer roles of polymerase-theta-mediated DNA end joining. Nat Rev Mol Cell Biol 23(2):125–140

68. Polak P, Kim J, Braunstein LZ, Karlic R, Haradhavala NJ, Tiao G et al (2017) A mutational signature reveals alterations underlying deficient homologous recombination repair in breast cancer. Nat Genet 49(10):1476–1486

69. Alexandrov LB, Nik-Zainal S, Wedge DC, Aparicio SAJR, Behjati S, Biankin AV et al (2013) Signatures of mutational processes in human cancer. Nature 500(7463):415–421

70. Lord CJ, Ashworth A (2013) Mechanisms of resistance to therapies targeting BRCA-mutant cancers. Nat Med 19(11):1381–1388

71. D'Andrea AD (2018) Mechanisms of PARP inhibitor sensitivity and resistance. DNA Repair (Amst). 71:172–176

72. Boulton SJ, Jackson SP (1996) Saccharomyces cerevisiae Ku70 potentiates illegitimate DNA double-strand break repair and serves as a barrier to error-prone DNA repair pathways. EMBO J 15(18):5093–5103

73. Kabotyanski EB, Gomelsky L, Han JO, Stamato TD, Roth DB (1998) Double-strand break repair in Ku86- and XRCC4-deficient cells. Nucleic Acids Res 26(23):5333–5342

74. Kumar RJ, Chao HX, Simpson DA, Feng W, Cho M-G, Roberts VR, et al. Dual inhibition of DNA-PK and DNA polymerase theta overcomes radiation resistance induced by p53 deficiency. NAR Cancer. 2020;2(4):zcaa038.

75. van Bussel MTJ, Awada A, de Jonge MJA, Mau-Sørensen M, Nielsen D, Schöffski P et al (2021) A first-in-man phase 1 study of the DNA-dependent protein kinase inhibitor peposertib (formerly M3814) in patients with advanced solid tumours. Br J Cancer 124(4):728–735

76. Kuei C-H, Lin H-Y, Lin M-H, Lee H-H, Lin C-H, Lee W-J et al (2020) DNA polymerase theta repression enhances the docetaxel responsiveness in metastatic castration-resistant prostate cancer. Biochim Biophys acta Mol basis Dis 1866(12):165954

77. Pantelidou C, Sonzogni O, De Oliveria TM, Mehta AK, Kothari A, Wang D et al (2019) PARP inhibitor efficacy depends on CD8+ T-cell recruitment via intratumoral STING pathway activation in BRCA-deficient models of triple-negative breast cancer. Cancer Discov 9(6):722–737

78. Ding L, Kim H-J, Wang Q, Kearns M, Jiang T, Ohlson CE et al (2018) PARP inhibition elicits STING-dependent antitumor immunity in brca1-deficient ovarian cancer. Cell Rep 25(11):2972-2980.e5

79. Pantelidou C, Jadhav H, Kothari A, Liu R, Guerriero JL, Shapiro GI (2021) STING agonism enhances anti-tumor immune responses and therapeutic efficacy of PARP inhibition in BRCA-associated breast cancer. bioRxiv. 2021.01.26.428337

80. Cheng B, Ren X, Kerppola TK (2014) KAP1 represses differentiation-inducible genes in embryonic stem cells through cooperative binding with PRC1 and derepresses pluripotency-associated genes. Mol Cell Biol 34(11):2075–2091

81. Jardim DL, Fontes Jardim DL, Schwaederle M, Wei C, Lee JJ, Hong DS, et al. Impact of a biomarker-based strategy on oncology drug development: a meta-analysis of clinical trials leading to FDA approval. J Natl Cancer Inst. 2015;107(11).

82. Schwaederle M, Zhao M, Lee JJ, Lazar V, Leyland-Jones B, Schilsky RL et al (2016) Association of biomarker-based treatment strategies with response rates and progression-free survival in refractory malignant neoplasms: a meta-analysis. JAMA Oncol 2(11):1452–1459

83. Schwaederle M, Zhao M, Lee JJ, Eggermont AM, Schilsky RL, Mendelsohn J et al (2015) Impact of precision medicine in diverse cancers: a meta-analysis of Phase II clinical trials. J Clin Oncol 33(32):3817–3825

Targeting DNA-PK

16

Jan Philipp Novotny, Adrian Mariño-Enríquez,
and Jonathan A. Fletcher

16.1 Introduction

DNA-PK is a heterotrimeric complex formed in the presence of DNA that is composed of the catalytic subunit of DNA-PK (DNA-PKcs) and the Ku70/80 heterodimer [1, 2]. Ku70/80 is also known as the DNA binding subunit of DNA-PK. DNA-PKcs is one of the largest and most abundant proteins in eukaryotes, spanning 4128 amino acids and weighing $\approx$ 469 kDa [3]. This protein was discovered in 1985 as a DNA-activated protein kinase in a HeLa extract contaminated with double-stranded DNA [1, 4, 5]. The key observation was that this new DNA-activated protein kinase phosphorylated the alpha isoform of heat shock protein 90 on a SQ/ST motif, which is a known phosphatidylinositol 3-kinase-related kinase (PIKK) substrate motif [6, 7]. Indeed, DNA-PKcs is the largest member of the PIKK family, which otherwise includes ataxia-telangiectasia mutated (ATM), ataxia- and Rad3-related (ATR), and the mammalian target of rapamycin (mTOR) [8].

All PIKKs share a common domain structure, with a kinase domain located in the C-terminal region, flanked by FAT (FRAP, ATM, TRRAP) and PIKK regulatory domains (PRD). At the N-terminus, PIKKs feature alpha helical HEAT (Huntingtin, Elongation factor 3, A subunit of protein phosphatase 2A and TOR1)

J. P. Novotny (✉) · A. Mariño-Enríquez · J. A. Fletcher
Department of Pathology, Brigham and Women's Hospital, Boston, USA
e-mail: JanPhilipp.Novotny@med.uni-heidelberg.de

A. Mariño-Enríquez
e-mail: admarion@bwh.harvard.edu

J. A. Fletcher
e-mail: Jfletcher@bwh.harvard.edu

© The Author(s), under exclusive license to Springer Nature Switzerland AG 2023
T. A. Yap and G. I. Shapiro (eds.), *Targeting the DNA Damage Response for Cancer Therapy*, Cancer Treatment and Research 186,
https://doi.org/10.1007/978-3-031-30065-3_16

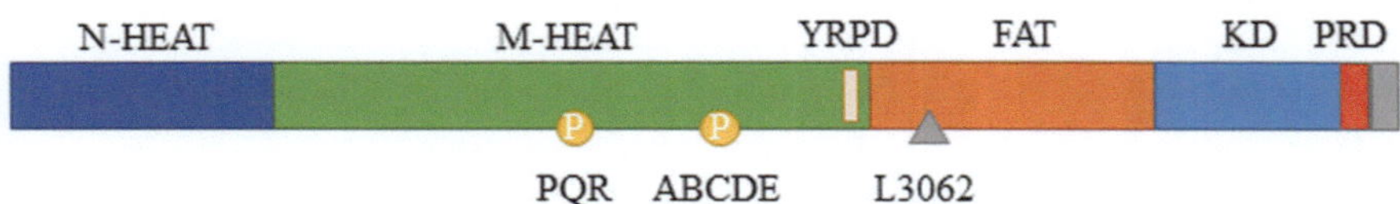

Fig. 16.1 Graphical depiction of the DNA-PKcs domain architecture

repeats (Fig. 16.1) [3]. Though the PIKK kinase domain contains motifs similar to those in phosphatidylinositol 3-kinases (PI3Ks, e.g. PIK3CA), PIKKs are serine/threonine kinases which do not phosphorylate lipids.

The gene encoding DNA-PKcs (also known as XRCC7) is *PRKDC*, located on chromosome 8q11 [9]. Phylogenetic studies demonstrate ancient origins of DNA-PKcs with remarkable amino acid sequence conservation among Eukaryota, particularly within the YPRD motif which is located between a phosphorylation cluster (ABCDE) and the FAT domain [3]. The ABCDE cluster contains 6 redundant autophosphorylation sites and together with autophosphorylation sites in another cluster (termed PQR) these enable DNA-PK regulation of V(D)J recombination and DNA damage repair (DDR) by non-homologous end-joining [10–12]. DNA-PKcs is further regulated through phosphorylation by other PIKK family members, including ATM, within the ABCDE cluster and at T3205.

DNA-PK has been implicated in varied biological processes but is best known for its key function in non-homologous end-joining. In this function, DNA-PKcs orchestrates the repair of DNA double strand breaks (DSBs) [13]. In addition to its well-known roles in DNA damage repair, it is increasingly apparent that DNA-PKcs serves roles in regulation of mitosis [14], transcription [15], RNA processing [16], and innate immune response [17]. Although initial preclinical and clinical studies of DNA-PK inhibition have targeted the DDR roles, it is likely that future clinical studies, while continuing to refine the DDR-inhibition strategies, will also be mindful of opportunities to leverage inhibition of other DNA-PK functions.

16.1.1 Insights from SCID Mice and Other DNA-PK Loss-of-Function Phenotypes

Severe combined immunodeficiency (SCID) in humans is characterized by compromised B- and T-cell development and function [18]. The mouse counterpart to human SCID was identified in 1983 by M. Bosma based on the absence of serum immunoglobulins [19]. Subsequent studies demonstrated that the agammaglobulinemia resulted from defective V(D)J recombination, which in turn was caused by DNA-PK definciency due to inactivating mutation in *PRKDC* [20]. V(D)J recombination is critical for T- and B-cell development and function and requires antigen receptor gene assembly from Variable, Diverse and Joining gene segments. This process is NHEJ-dependent and is initiated by creation of DNA DSBs by recombination activated 1 and 2 (RAG1 and RAG2), which are lymphocyte specific endonucleases [21]. Because this process generates DSBs with hairpin overhangs, these DNA ends need to be end-processed by the endonuclease Artemis before the V(D)J segments can be ligated. Artemis activation is regulated by DNA-PKcs [22, 23]. Because the *PRKDC* mutation in SCID mice results in loss of DNA-PKcs expression, these mice are characterized by accumulation of hairpin intermediates during V(D)J recombination and absence of functional antigen receptors [24, 25].

Studies in mice have characterized three distinct categories of DNA-PKcs alterations, which are summarized below: (1) *complete loss of DNA-PKcs expression*, which can result from spontaneously occurring *PRKDC* mutations in animals [26, 27]; (2) induced loss-of-function mutations in the *DNA-PKcs kinase domain*; and (3) knock-in mutations *preventing (auto)phosphorylation* at the ABCDE and PQR clusters.

(1) DNA-PKcs null mice demonstrate complete loss of T- and B-cells in line with a SCID phenotype but do not show any other impairment [28, 29].
(2) The D3992A substitution, which results in kinase dead (KD) DNA-PKcs is embryonically lethal in mice and results in neuronal apoptosis, similar to that observed in Xrcc4 and LigIV knock-out mice [30, 31]. However, embryonic lethality can be rescued by Ku loss [30]. Furthermore, cells derived from DNA-PKcs KD mice demonstrate greater sensitivity to ionizing radiation than those from DNA-PKcs null mice [30].
(3) Alanine substitutions precluding phosphorylation within the DNA-PKcs ABCDE phosphorylation cluster contribute to bone marrow failure and early death in mice [32]. In contrast, mice with alanine substitutions in the PQR phosphorylation cluster develop normally but have moderate sensitivity to ionizing radiation [32].

Interestingly and in contrast to observations in mice and horses, various components of the DNA-PK heterotrimeric complex are essential in human cells. Indeed, all patients with DNA-PKcs mutations reported in the literature have detectable, albeit reduced DNA-PKcs expression, while naturally occurring DNA-PKcs mutations in other animals can result in null phenotypes. The first patient with mutated *PRKDC* was described by van der Burg and contained a monoallelic L3062R missense mutation within the FAT domain, which did not affect DNA-PK kinase activity but impaired Artemis endonuclease activation [33]. Clinically, this patient demonstrated a SCID phenotype with absence of B and T cells and normal NK cell counts. A patient with *PRKDC* compound heterozygous mutations had a A3574V substitution (FAT domain) on one allele and an abnormally spliced transcript with loss of exon 16 from the other allele, likely resulting in loss of function [34]. This patient had dysmorphic features and growth failure, microcephaly, seizures, and substantial neurological impairment in addition to the $B^-T^-NK^+$ phenotype. Two unrelated patients with homozygous DNA-PKcs p.L3062R mutation exhibited defective DSB repair and V(D)J associated with progressive decline in B- and T-cells along with signs of autoimmunity [35, 36]. Interestingly, two siblings with DNA-PKcs p.L3061R mutation both had immune deficiency but differed in the presence of an autoimmune disorder [36]. While it is unclear whether these patients suffered from mono- or biallelic *PRKDC* mutations, the cases exemplify the variability of symptoms resulting from similar DNA-PKcs mutations.

Several conclusions can be drawn from those observations: (a) the essentiality of DNA-PKcs in humans suggests additional functions compared to non-hominids; (b) the downstream effects of DNA-PKcs mutations depend on which functions they impede; (c) DNA-PKcs appears to have a role in preventing autoimmunity in humans; and (d) the differences observed in animal models must be taken into account when extrapolating DNA-PKcs findings from animals to humans.

16.1.2 DNA-PK Roles in DNA Damage Repair

DNA damage provoked by endogenous or exogeneous mechanisms represents a constant threat to genomic integrity that must be dealt with effectively by intrinsic repair functions. Therefore, DNA damage repair is a key process for genome maintenance and replication fidelity [37]. Upon DNA damage, the DDR system is engaged, recruiting repair factors and activating cell cycle control checkpoints to permit DNA damage repair. DSBs represent the most toxic form of DNA damage, leading to cell death or chromosomal aberrations [38]. In eukaryotes, DSBs can be repaired by several complementary DDR mechanisms. Of those, homologous recombination (HR) and non-homologous end-joining (NHEJ) are the most well studied. The cell's choice of DDR pathways is context dependent and, in case of HR, restricted to S and G2 phase of the cell cycle because this pathway requires the presence of a sister chromatid to serve as template [39]. In contrast, NHEJ is active throughout the cell cycle but error-prone [40]. NHEJ is also the dominant repair pathway in the G2 phase for ionizing radiation damage distant from the replication fork [41].

DNA-PK is a key factor in NHEJ, consisting of a heterotrimeric complex composed of DNA-PKcs and the Ku70/Ku80 heterodimers, which are also known as the DNA binding subunit. Ku heterodimerization forms a DNA-binding ring which fits around the major and minor DNA grooves and translocates inward upon DNA binding. Because the heterodimer does not make any direct base contacts, it is thought that the Ku-DNA interaction proceeds in a sequence independent manner [42, 43]. Inward translocation of the Ku heterodimer recruits DNA-PKcs to interact with the DNA DSB and form the DNA-PK holoenzyme (Fig. 16.2). Assembly of the complex between adjacent DNA breaks forms a synaptic complex to keep the broken ends in proximity, protecting them from unscheduled processing [44–46]. Depending on the damage encountered, non-ligatable DNA needs to be processed prior to ligation via the XLF-XRCC4-LIGIV complex. This is carried out primarily by the $5'$–$3'$ nuclease Artemis along with other factors such as the $3'$-DNA phosphatase/$5'$-DNA kinase polynucleotide kinase phosphatase (PNKP) [47–49].

The mechanisms by which DNA-PK orchestrates DNA-end processing are incompletely understood, but recent evidence sheds light on how features of the DNA ends influence DNA-PK autophosphorylation and thereby downstream

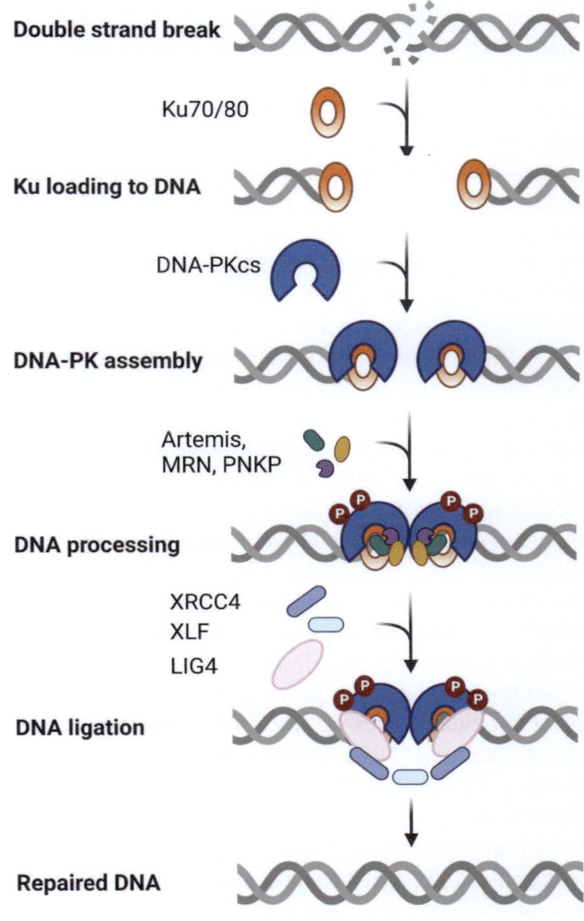

Fig. 16.2 Schematic illustration of NHEJ mediated DNA double strand break repair. Ku70/80 and DNA-PKcs form the DNA-PK holoenzyme and recruit downstream effectors that proceed with DNA end-processing and ligation. Created with BioRender.com

events. Two main phosphorylation clusters have been identified in DNA-PKcs. The ABCDE cluster spanning residues 2609–2647 contains 6 functionally redundant phosphorylation sites that are required for Artemis activation. Phosphorylation within the ABCDE cluster induces a conformational change that releases Artemis from its autoinhibited state and thereby allows for end-processing [50, 51]. Conversely, blocking phosphorylation within the ABCDE region delays DNA-PKcs release from DSBs and impedes end-processing [51]. Hairpin DNA-ends that are generated during V(D)J recombination, a process dependent on NHEJ, promote DNA-PKcs autophosphorylation at the ABCDE cluster. This leads to phosphorylation of the Artemis C-terminal region which is thought to facilitate its de-inhibition [52]. Once end-processing is complete, phosphorylation at the DNA-PKcs PQR cluster limits further processing [12, 53]. In the case of blunt DNA ends or ends with 3' overhang, the ABCDE cluster protects open DNA and cannot be phosphorylated, which promotes DNA end protection and favors phosphorylation of downstream factors, such as Ku70/80 [54]. This is in line with the observation that hairpinned DNA ends do not activate DNA-PK to phosphorylate TP53 and that TelN restricted DNA, which generates covalently closed DNA ends, leads to autophosphorylation within the ABCDE cluster but fails to activate DNA-PK downstream substrates [51].

Substantial evidence indicates that DNA-PKcs has extensive post-translational modifications, of which phosphorylation is the best studied. In addition to autophosphorylation, the ABCDE cluster can also be phosphorylated by the PIKK family members ATM and ATR, both of which serve key functions in DDR [55, 56]. In fact, it has been shown that ATM can compensate for DNA-PKcs dysfunction, exemplifying the crosstalk among DDR kinases [57]. Other DNA-PKcs post-translational modifications include ubiquitination, PARylation, NEDylation, and acetylation. However, as is the case with phosphorylating events, the biologic impact of these modifications is only very incompletely understood. DNA-PKcs is ubiquitinated and tagged for proteosomal degradation by Ring Finger Protein 144A (RNF144A), which was the first ubiquitinase known to target DNA-PKcs. RNF114A expression is induced by cell exposure to DNA damaging agents, and RNF114A depletion results in DNA-PKcs accumulation and decreased chemosensitivity [58]. Likewise, knock-down of the chaperone protein VCP (valosine containing protein), which binds ubiquitinated DNA-PKcs, results in DNA-PKcs accumulation, elevated DNA-PK activity, and increased DNA damage repair efficiency [59].

ADP-ribosylation by poly (ADP-ribose) polymerases (PARPs) regulates numerous biological processes and PARP inhibitors were the first approved anti-cancer drugs targeting DNA damage response in BRCA1/2 mutated breast cancer. Notably, PARP and DNA-PK can be co-recruited to sites of DNA damage, and PARP proteins can interact with DNA-PK to maintain genomic integrity after DNA DSB induction [60, 61]. PARylation by PARP proteins stimulates DNA-PK activity *in vitro* and PARP1 knock-down reduces DNA-PKcs expression and activity in nasopharyngeal carcinoma *in vitro* [62, 63]. Conversely, DNA-PK modulates PARP function by phosphorylating PARP in a DNA dependent manner—although the biological impact is poorly understood [64]. Further studies are needed to determine whether cancers with homologous recombination repair deficiency (which are responsive clinically to PARP-inhibition) are hyper-dependent on DNA-PK as a compensatory mechanism for DSB repair. However, the known biologic interactions between PARP and DNA-PK, and the evidence that NHEJ is a compensatory repair mechanism in cells with HRD, provide rationale for exploring therapeutic combination approaches or sequential approaches drawing upon inhibition of PARP and DNA-PK. As discussed later in this chapter, there is also evidence that DNA-PK co-inhibition in cancer cells with homologous recombination repair deficiency can actually impair response to PARP inhibitors. Given the many cross-connections between PARP proteins and DNA-PK, it is likely the clinical benefit, if any, of co-inhibiting these repair kinases will vary greatly in different cancers.

DNA-PK activity is also regulated by crosstalk with nuclear receptors and indeed nuclear receptor signaling can induce DNA double strand breaks and stimulate recruitment of DNA-PK and other DDR factors [65, 66]. In particular, androgen and estrogen receptor signaling regulate transcriptional activity of the *PRKDC* promoter [67–70]. In addition, DNA-PK can act as a transcriptional co-regulator and phosphorylate various nuclear receptors [71]. These observations raise intriguing questions as to whether DNA-PK signaling roles differ in malignancies with substantial dependence on nuclear receptors.

Many epithelioid caners express epidermal growth factor receptor (EGFR), and high EGFR expression levels have been associated with poor outcomes. Radiation induces EGFR expression and co-treating cells with an EGFR antibody resulted in sensitization to ionizing radiation (IR). These insights had profound clinical impact on how EGFR positive cancers are treated with radiation therapy [72]. Subsequent studies demonstrated that EGFR interacts with DNA-PK and that IR causes EGFR translocation to the nucleus, which then enhances DDR by interaction with DNA-PKcs [73]. Treatment with a monoclonal EGFR antibody inhibits this re-distribution, thereby prevent interaction with DNA-PKcs and explaining why the antibody sensitizes cancer cells to radiation [74–76]. Thus, co-treatment with an anti-EGFR antibody such as cetuximab is now a standard approach to increase sensitivity to radiation therapy in patients.

16.1.3 DNA-PK Roles in Immunity and Autoimmune Disorders

Innate immunity is activated in response to various pathogens, and host detection of cytosolic DNA is a key step in mounting an anti-viral response. Nucleic acids and other pathogen-associated molecular patterns (PAMPs) are sensed by pattern recognition receptors (PRRs), triggering an immune response [77]. Indeed, genomic instability is a major contributor of cytosolic DNA, which itself is potent activator of a type I interferon response [78, 79]. The cGAS-STING pathway is one mechanism that has emerged as a key surveillance system orchestrating anti-pathogen and anti-tumor immunity [80]. Upon binding to cytosolic DNA, cGAS catalyzes the production of cGAMP, which subsequently activates the stimulator of interferon genes (STING). STING then translocates from the ER to the Golgi, inducing serial phosphorylation events and ultimately activating TBK1 and interferon regulatory factor 3 (IRF3) which results in production of type I interferons. DNA-PK inhibits cGAS by phosphorylation events, accounting for the autoimmune disorders that often accompany DNA-PKcs defects [80]. In addition, DNA-PK can activate IRF3 dependent interferon-1 response independently of cGAS and STING, although the evidence for these roles has been conflicting, depending on the cell types (nonneoplastic vs. neoplastic) and species in which the studies were performed [17, 81]. This is in line with the report of a second, STING-independent DNA sensing pathway in human cells that appears to be undetectable in murine cells [82]. As one example of an apparently cGAS-STING independent role, DNA-PK mediates IRF3 on threonine 135, causing IRF3 nuclear retention and delayed proteolysis in the setting of viral infection [81]. The importance of DNA-PK signaling to activate innate immune responses is further highlighted by studies interrogating infections with the vaccinia virus (VAVC) [83, 84]. These studies demonstrated that the VACV encoded protein C16 binds to the Ku70/80 heterodimer, which blocks DNA-PK-dependent DNA sensing and thereby attenuates innate immune activation.

DNA-PK roles in immunity, like the key DNA-PK roles in DNA damage repair, are an area of active study. It is likely that the intersection of these biologic themes will engender opportunities to enhance both cytotoxicity and immune response by targeting DNA-PKcs in combination therapies for various cancers. Another promising avenue is the role of DNA-PK modulating T-cell tolerance by interaction with the transcription factor autoimmune regulator (AIRE) [85]. DNA-PK phosphorylates AIRE on T68 and S156, thereby regulating AIRE transactivating functions. Consequently, DNA-PK inhibition or loss decreases expression of AIRE target genes.

16.1.4 DNA-PK Inhibition as Therapeutic Strategy

Genomic instability is a hallmark of many cancers and in some cases is attributable to inactivation of DDR proteins that normally serve as guardians of genomic integrity. Well known examples include the mutations and deletions that inactivate homologous recombination repair pathway proteins and which denote vulnerability to PARP inhibitor therapies. Nonetheless, even in cancers with evident genomic instability, other repair pathways have essential roles in preventing the instability (and resultant genotoxicity) from getting entirely out of hand. As discussed above, there is evidence that homologous recombination deficient cancer cells can become hyper-dependent on DNA-PK as an alternate pathway to maintain at least partial capabilities for DSB repair.

For this reason, DNA-PK is an attractive target for anti-cancer therapies. And beyond the possibility of compensatory DNA-PK hyper-dependence in cancers with deficiencies in other DDR pathways, DNA-PK is generally known to limit genotoxic instability induced by DNA damaging chemotherapies. High DNA-PKcs expression levels are accordingly associated with resistance to cytotoxic therapies and thereby associated with worse prognosis [86, 87]. Conversely, DNA-PKcs null mice demonstrate increased sensitivity to DNA damaging therapy, and multiple studies demonstrate that DNA-PKcs inhibition is synthetically lethal in combination with DNA damaging agents (DDAs) [88–90].

Various evidence suggests that mechanisms of cell death resulting from DNA-PK inhibition (DNA-PKi) are influenced by the functional status of cell cycle control. For example, when treating acute myeloid leukemia cells wtih the selective DNA-PKcs inhibitor peposertib, Haines et al. demonstrated that DNA-PKi combined with DNA damaging chemotherapy potentiated compensatory ATM signaling. This led to increased TP53 expression and induction of TP53-dependent apoptosis [87]. In contrast, malignancies with dysfunctional TP53 fail to engage cell cycle checkpoints in response to combinations of DDA with DNA-PKi and enter mitosis prior to completion of DNA damage repair [91]. Such failure of scheduled DSB repair fosters incremental genomic damage, culminating in mitotic catastrophe and apoptotic cell death. TP53 functional status can thus impact cell fate after DNA-PKi, specifically determining the mechanisms of cell death. Interestingly, DNA-PKi monotherapy, although clinically well-tolerated, has very limited efficacy against most solid malignancies. This indicates that NHEJ inhibition alone is insufficient to drive genomic instability to genotoxic levels *in vivo* [92]. Current clinical evaluations therefore focus on DNA-PKi as a sensitizer towards conventionally dosed DDAs, such as ionizing radiation or topoisomerase II inhibitors, which induce DNA double strand breaks.

Several clinical trials using new-generation DNA-PKcs inhibitors targeting the ATP binding pocket are underway or have been reported upon. In contrast to prior compounds, new-generation small-molecule inhibitors have greater selectivity for DNA-PKcs over PI3K and other PIKK family members [90]. The first in human phase I trial testing the oral DNA-PK inhibitor peposertib (formerly known as M3814), enrolled 31 patients with advanced solid tumors and did not reach the maximum tolerated dose (MTD). Several clinical trials explored peposertib in combination with chemotherapy, e.g. pegylated liposomal doxorubicin (NCT04092270), or radiation therapy (NCT02516813) [93]. The phase I/IIa first in human trial of AZD7648 completed recruitment and will assess AZD7648 as monotherapy and in combination with either pegylated liposomal doxorubicin or olaparib (NCT03907969) [94].

The aforementioned clinical trials of DNA-PKi combined with DNA damaging therapies at conventional dose levels demonstrated a narrow therapeutic index and substantial toxicity [93]. These challenges highlight the need for better tolerated DNA-PKi combination therapies and also for biomarkers that identify cancers particularly dependent on DNA-PK/NHEJ, in which even low doses of DNA-PKi might be active. Notably, the genetic background of various immunodeficient mouse models must be carefully considered when performing DNA-PKi preclinical evaluations. As discussed above, standard SCID mice, which are DNA-PKcs null (DNA-PKcs$^{-/-}$) are not informative for DNA-PKi toxicities to nonneoplastic cells although toxicities with DNA damaging agents are heightened in these mice due to the intrinsic DNA damage repair deficiency.

DNA damage repair is a multi-step process with extensive crosstalk among DDR factors, which can elicit compensatory repair pathway activation upon inhibiting specific DDR effectors. Synthetic lethality of PARPi in homologous recombination (HR) deficient cancer is well described and it is possible that HR-deficiency sensitizes some cancers to NHEJ pathway inhibition. Surprisingly, other evidence suggests that DNA-PKi can abrogate the impact of PARPi in HR deficient cancer [95]. In addition to TP53 status, genomic and functional assays interrogating HR-deficiency might therefore prove to be useful in predicting DNA-PKi efficacy.

Effective DNA-PKi combination therapies will likely be defined by further studies of the relationships between DNA-PK and other DSB repair mechanisms—particularly compensatory mechanisms. For example, many deficient cancers are dependent on CDK2 for G2/M cell cycle arrest, and therefore inhibiting CDK2 by targeting the ATR-CHK1-WEE1 pathway can consolidate response to DNA-PKi [96]. Additionally, DNA-PKi synthetic lethality has been observed in ATM defective cancer and likewise ATM signaling can rescue cells from DNA-PKi, providing rationale for co-targeting ATM and DNA-PK.

Altogether, DNA-PK inhibition is emerging as a promising but challenging therapeutic approach in cancer. While primarily targeted for its role in NHEJ DNA damage repair, DNA-PK also regulates other important biologic pathways. These additional roles provide new opportunities to advance cancer treatment but also increase the likelihood of substantial toxicity in the clinic, which underscores the need for compelling and novel rationales that can guide effective clinical translation.

References

1. Lees-Miller SP, Chen Y-R, Anderson CW (1990) Human cells contain a DNA-activated protein kinase that phosphorylates simian virus 40 T antigen, mouse p53, and the human Ku autoantigen. Mol Cell Biol. https://doi.org/10.1128/mcb.10.12.6472
2. Gottlieb TM, Jackson SP (1993) The DNA-dependent protein kinase: requirement for DNA ends and association with Ku antigen. Cell. https://doi.org/10.1016/0092-8674(93)90057-w
3. Lees-Miller JP et al (2020) Uncovering DNA-PKcs ancient phylogeny, unique sequence motifs and insights for human disease. Prog Biophys Mol Biol 163:87–108
4. Walker AI, Hunt T, Jackson RJ, Anderson CW (1985) Double-stranded DNA induces the phosphorylation of several proteins including the 90,000 mol. wt. heat-shock protein in animal cell extracts. EMBO J (1985). https://doi.org/10.1002/j.1460-2075.1985.tb02328.x
5. Carter T, Vancurová I, Sun I, Lou W, DeLeon S (1990) A DNA-activated protein kinase from HeLa cell nuclei. Mol Cell Biol. https://doi.org/10.1128/mcb.10.12.6460
6. O'Neill T et al (2000) Utilization of oriented peptide libraries to identify substrate motifs selected by ATM*. J Biol Chem 275:22719–22727
7. Lees-Miller SP, Sakaguchi K, Ullrich SJ, Appella E, Anderson CW (1992) Human DNA-activated protein kinase phosphorylates serines 15 and 37 in the amino-terminal transactivation domain of human p53. Mol Cell Biol 12:5041–5049
8. Manning G, Whyte DB, Martinez R, Hunter T, Sudarsanam S (2002) The protein kinase complement of the human genome. Science 298:1912–1934
9. Ladenburger EM, Fackelmayer FO, Hameister H, Knippers R (1997) MCM4 and PRKDC, human genes encoding proteins MCM4 and DNA-PKcs, are close neighbours located on chromosome 8q12→q13. Cytogenet Genome Res 77:268–270
10. Douglas P et al (2002) Identification of in vitro and in vivo phosphorylation sites in the catalytic subunit of the DNA-dependent protein kinase. Biochemical Journal. https://doi.org/10.1042/bj20020973
11. Chan DW et al (2002) Autophosphorylation of the DNA-dependent protein kinase catalytic subunit is required for rejoining of DNA double-strand breaks. Genes Dev. https://doi.org/10.1101/gad.1015202
12. Cui X et al (2005) Autophosphorylation of DNA-dependent protein kinase regulates DNA end processing and may also alter double-strand break repair pathway choice. Mol Cell Biol. https://doi.org/10.1128/mcb.25.24.10842-10852.2005
13. Davis AJ, Chen BPC, Chen DJ (2014) DNA-PK: a dynamic enzyme in a versatile DSB repair pathway. DNA Repair 17:21–29
14. Jette N, Lees-Miller SP (2015) The DNA-dependent protein kinase: a multifunctional protein kinase with roles in DNA double strand break repair and mitosis. Prog Biophys Mol Biol. https://doi.org/10.1016/j.pbiomolbio.2014.12.003

15. Goodwin JF et al (2015) DNA-PKcs-mediated transcriptional regulation drives prostate cancer progression and metastasis. Cancer Cell 28:97–113

16. Shao Z et al (2020) DNA-PKcs has KU-dependent function in rRNA processing and haematopoiesis. Nature 579:291–296

17. Ferguson BJ, Mansur DS, Peters NE, Ren H, Smith GL (2012) DNA-PK is a DNA sensor for IRF-3-dependent innate immunity. Elife 1:e00047

18. Notarangelo LD (2010) Primary immunodeficiencies. J Allergy Clin Immun 125:S182–S194

19. Bosma GC, Custer RP, Custer RP, Bosma MJ (1983) A severe combined immunodeficiency mutation in the mouse. Nature. https://doi.org/10.1038/301527a0

20. Jhappan C, Morse HC, Fleischmann RD, Gottesman MM, Merlino G (1997) DNA-PKcs: a T-cell tumour suppressor encoded at the mouse SCID locus. Nat Genet 17:483–486

21. Kienker LJ, Shin EK, Meek K (2000) Both V(D)J recombination and radioresistance require DNA-PK kinase activity, though minimal levels suffice for V(D)J recombination. Nucleic Acids Res 28:2752–2761

22. Ma Y, Pannicke U, Schwarz K, Schwarz K, Lieber MR (2002) Hairpin opening and overhang processing by an Artemis/DNA-dependent protein kinase complex in nonhomologous end joining and V(D)J recombination. Cell. https://doi.org/10.1016/s0092-8674(02)00671-2

23. Franco S et al (2008) DNA-PKcs and Artemis function in the end-joining phase of immunoglobulin heavy chain class switch recombination. J Exp Medicine 205:557–564

24. Zhu C, Roth DB (1995) Characterization of coding ends in thymocytes of SCID mice: implications for the mechanism of V(D)J recombination. Immunity 2:101–112

25. Priestley A et al (1998) Molecular and biochemical characterisation of DNA-dependent protein kinase-defective rodent mutant irs-20. Nucleic Acids Res 26:1965–1973

26. Wiler R et al (1995) Equine severe combined immunodeficiency: a defect in V(D)J recombination and DNA-dependent protein kinase activity. Proc National Acad Sci 92:11485–11489

27. Meek K et al (2009) SCID dogs: similar transplant potential but distinct intra-uterine growth defects and premature replicative senescence compared with SCID mice. J Immunol 183:2529–2536

28. Kurimasa A et al (1999) Catalytic subunit of DNA-dependent protein kinase: impact on lymphocyte development and tumorigenesis. Proc National Acad Sci 96:1403–1408

29. Gao Y et al (1998) A targeted DNA-PKcs-null mutation reveals DNA-PK-independent functions for KU in V(D)J recombination. Immunity 9:367–376

30. Jiang W et al (2015) Differential phosphorylation of DNA-PKcs regulates the interplay between end-processing and end-ligation during nonhomologous end-joining. Mol Cell 58:172–185

31. Biosci ZC, Menolfi D, Zha S (2020) ATM, ATR and DNA-PKcs kinases-the lessons from the mouse models: inhibition ≠ deletion. (2020). https://doi.org/10.1186/s13578-020-0376-x

32. Zhang S et al (2011) Congenital bone marrow failure in DNA-PKcs mutant mice associated with deficiencies in DNA repair. J Cell Biol 193:295–305

33. van der Burg M et al (2009) A DNA-PKcs mutation in a radiosensitive T-B– SCID patient inhibits Artemis activation and nonhomologous end-joining. J Clin Invest 119:91–98

34. Woodbine L et al (2013) PRKDC mutations in a SCID patient with profound neurological abnormalities. J Clin Invest 123:2969–2980

35. Mathieu A-L et al (2015) PRKDC mutations associated with immunodeficiency, granuloma, and autoimmune regulator–dependent autoimmunity. J Allergy Clin Immun 135:1578-1588.e5

36. Esenboga S et al (2018) Two siblings with PRKDC defect who presented with cutaneous granulomas and review of the literature. Clin Immunol 197:1–5

37. Jalal S, Earley JN, Turchi JJ (2011) DNA repair: from genome maintenance to biomarker and therapeutic target. Clin Cancer Res 17:6973–6984

38. Jeggo PA, Löbrich M (2007) DNA double-strand breaks: their cellular and clinical impact? Oncogene 26:7717–7719

39. Saleh-Gohari N, Helleday T (2004) Conservative homologous recombination preferentially repairs DNA double-strand breaks in the S phase of the cell cycle in human cells. Nucleic Acids Res 32:3683–3688

40. Rodgers K, McVey M (2016) Error-prone repair of DNA double-strand breaks. J Cell Physiol 231:15

41. Zhao B, Rothenberg E, Ramsden DA, Lieber MR (2020) The molecular basis and disease relevance of non-homologous DNA end joining. Nat Rev Mol Cell Biol 21:765–781

42. Blier PR, Griffith AJ, Craft J, Hardin JA (1993) Binding of Ku protein to DNA. Measurement of affinity for ends and demonstration of binding to nicks. J Biol Chem 268:7594–601

43. Abbasi S, Parmar G, Kelly RD, Balasuriya N, Schild-Poulter C (2021) The Ku complex: recent advances and emerging roles outside of non-homologous end-joining. Cell Mol Life Sci. https://doi.org/10.1007/s00018-021-03801-1

44. DeFazio LG, Stansel RM, Griffith JD, Chu G (2002) Synapsis of DNA ends by DNA-dependent protein kinase. EMBO J. https://doi.org/10.1093/emboj/cdf299

45. Budman J, Kim SA, Chu G (2007) Processing of DNA for nonhomologous end-joining is controlled by kinase activity and XRCC4/ligase IV*. J Biol Chem 282:11950–11959

46. Wu Q et al (2019) Understanding the structure and role of DNA-PK in NHEJ: how X-ray diffraction and cryo-EM contribute in complementary ways. Prog Biophysics Mol Biology 147:26–32

47. Chang HHY, Pannunzio NR, Adachi N, Lieber MR (2017) Non-homologous DNA end joining and alternative pathways to double-strand break repair. Nat Rev Mol Cell Bio 18:495–506

48. Darroudi F et al (2007) Role of Artemis in DSB repair and guarding chromosomal stability following exposure to ionizing radiation at different stages of cell cycle. Mutat Res Fundam Mol Mech Mutagen 615:111–124

49. Karimi-Busheri F, Rasouli-Nia A, Allalunis-Turner J, Weinfeld M (2007) Human polynucleotide kinase participates in repair of DNA double-strand breaks by nonhomologous end joining but not homologous recombination. Cancer Res 67:6619–6625

50. Goodarzi AA et al (2006) DNA-PK autophosphorylation facilitates Artemis endonuclease activity. EMBO J. https://doi.org/10.1038/sj.emboj.7601255

51. Meek K (2020) Activation of DNA-PK by hairpinned DNA ends reveals a stepwise mechanism of kinase activation. Nucleic Acids Res. https://doi.org/10.1093/nar/gkaa614

52. Niewolik D et al (2006) DNA-PKcs dependence of Artemis endonucleolytic activity, differences between hairpins and 5′ or 3′ overhangs*. J Biol Chem 281:33900–33909

53. Neal JA, Meek K (2011) Choosing the right path: does DNA-PK help make the decision? Mutat Res. https://doi.org/10.1016/j.mrfmmm.2011.02.010

54. Liu L et al (2022) Autophosphorylation transforms DNA-PK from protecting to processing DNA ends. Mol Cell 82:177-189.e4

55. Chen BPC et al (2007) Ataxia telangiectasia mutated (ATM) is essential for DNA-PKcs phosphorylations at the Thr-2609 cluster upon DNA double strand break. J Biol Chem. https://doi.org/10.1074/jbc.m611605200

56. Meek K, Dang V, Lees-Miller SP (2008) Chapter 2 DNA-PK the means to justify the ends? Adv Immunol 99:33–58

57. Zhou Y, Paull TT (2013) DNA-dependent protein kinase regulates DNA end resection in concert with Mre11-Rad50-Nbs1 (MRN) and ataxia telangiectasia-mutated (ATM)*. J Biol Chem 288:37112–37125

58. Ho S-R, Mahanic CS, Lee Y-J, Lin W-C (2014) RNF144A, an E3 ubiquitin ligase for DNA-PKcs, promotes apoptosis during DNA damage. Proc National Acad Sci 111:E2646–E2655

59. Jiang N et al (2013) Valosin-containing protein regulates the proteasome-mediated degradation of DNA-PKcs in glioma cells. Cell Death Dis 4:e647–e647

60. Morrison C et al (1997) Genetic interaction between PARP and DNA-PK in V(D)J recombination and tumorigenesis. Nat Genet 17:479–482

61. Spagnolo L, Barbeau J, Curtin NJ, Morris EP, Pearl LH (2012) Visualization of a DNA-PK/PARP1 complex. Nucleic Acids Res 40:4168–4177

62. Han Y et al (2019) DNA-PKcs PARylation regulates DNA-PK kinase activity in the DNA damage response. Mol Med Rep 20:3609–3616

63. Zhang L et al (2022) Positive feedback regulation of Poly(ADP-ribose) polymerase 1 and the DNA-PK catalytic subunit affects the sensitivity of nasopharyngeal carcinoma to etoposide. ACS Omega 7:2571–2582

64. Ariumi Y et al (1999) Suppression of the poly(ADP-ribose) polymerase activity by DNA-dependent protein kinase in vitro. Oncogene 18:4616–4625

65. Goodwin JF et al (2013) A hormone–DNA repair circuit governs the response to genotoxic insult. Cancer Discov 3:1254–1271

66. Haffner MC, Marzo AMD, Meeker AK, Nelson WG, Yegnasubramanian S (2011) Transcription-induced DNA double strand breaks: both oncogenic force and potential therapeutic target? Clin Cancer Res 17:3858–3864

67. Baek M-H et al (2017) Androgen receptor as a prognostic biomarker and therapeutic target in uterine leiomyosarcoma. J Gynecol Oncol 29:e30

68. Yin Y et al (2017) Androgen receptor variants mediate DNA repair after prostate cancer irradiation. Cancer Res 77:4745–4754

69. Giguère V (2020) DNA-PK, nuclear mTOR, and the androgen pathway in prostate cancer. Trends Cancer 6:337–347

70. Ingram DR et al (2014) Estrogen receptor alpha and androgen receptor are commonly expressed in well-differentiated liposarcoma. BMC Clin Pathol 14:42

71. Malewicz M et al (2011) Essential role for DNA-PK-mediated phosphorylation of NR4A nuclear orphan receptors in DNA double-strand break repair. Gene Dev 25:2031–2040

72. Bonner JA et al (2006) Radiotherapy plus cetuximab for squamous-cell carcinoma of the head and neck. New Engl J Med 354:567–578

73. Liccardi G, Hartley JA, Hochhauser D (2011) EGFR nuclear translocation modulates DNA repair following Cisplatin and ionizing radiation treatment. Cancer Res 71:1103–1114

74. Dittmann K, Mayer C, Rodemann H-P (2005) Inhibition of radiation-induced EGFR nuclear import by C225 (Cetuximab) suppresses DNA-PK activity. Radiother Oncol 76:157–161

75. Bandyopadhyay D, Mandal M, Adam L, Mendelsohn J, Kumar R (1998) Physical interaction between epidermal growth factor receptor and DNA-dependent protein kinase in mammalian cells*. J Biol Chem 273:1568–1573

76. Huang SM, Harari PM (2000) Modulation of radiation response after epidermal growth factor receptor blockade in squamous cell carcinomas: inhibition of damage repair, cell cycle kinetics, and tumor angiogenesis. Clin Cancer Res Official J Am Assoc Cancer Res 6:2166–2174

77. Li D, Wu M (2021) Pattern recognition receptors in health and diseases. Signal Transduct Target Ther 6:291

78. Tijhuis AE, Johnson SC, McClelland SE (2019) The emerging links between chromosomal instability (CIN), metastasis, inflammation and tumour immunity. Mol Cytogenet 12:17

79. Bakhoum SF et al (2018) Chromosomal instability drives metastasis through a cytosolic DNA response. Nature 553:7689, 553:467–472 (2018)

80. Lu C et al (2021) DNA sensing in mismatch repair-deficient tumor cells is essential for anti-tumor immunity. Cancer Cell 39:96-108.e6

81. Karpova AY, Trost M, Murray JM, Cantley LC, Howley PM (2002) Interferon regulatory factor-3 is an in vivo target of DNA-PK. Proc National Acad Sci 99:2818–2823

82. Burleigh K et al (2020) Human DNA-PK activates a STING-independent DNA sensing pathway. Sci Immunol. https://doi.org/10.1126/sciimmunol.aba4219

83. Scutts SR et al (2018) DNA-PK is targeted by multiple vaccinia virus proteins to inhibit DNA sensing. Cell Rep 25:1953-1965.e4

84. Peters NE et al (2013) A mechanism for the inhibition of DNA-PK-mediated DNA sensing by a virus. Plos Pathog 9:e1003649

85. Liiv I et al (2008) DNA-PK contributes to the phosphorylation of AIRE: importance in transcriptional activity. Biochim Biophys Acta Bba—Mol Cell Res 1783:74–83

86. Zhang Y et al (2019) PRKDC is a prognostic marker for poor survival in gastric cancer patients and regulates DNA damage response. Pathol—Res Pract 215:152509

87. Zhang Y et al (2019) High expression of PRKDC promotes breast cancer cell growth via p38 MAPK signaling and is associated with poor survival. Mol Genetics Genom Med 7:e908

88. Zenke FT et al (2020) Pharmacologic inhibitor of DNA-PK, M3814, potentiates radiotherapy and regresses human tumors in mouse models. Mol Cancer Ther 19:1091–1101
89. Gordhandas SB et al (2022) Pre-clinical activity of the oral DNA-PK inhibitor, peposertib (M3814), combined with radiation in xenograft models of cervical cancer. Sci REP-UK 12:974
90. Fok JHL et al (2019) AZD7648 is a potent and selective DNA-PK inhibitor that enhances radiation, chemotherapy and olaparib activity. Nat Commun 10:5065
91. Sun Q et al (2019) Therapeutic implications of p53 status on cancer cell fate following exposure to ionizing radiation and the DNA-PK inhibitor M3814. Mol Cancer Res 17:2457–2468
92. van Bussel MTJ et al (2021) A first-in-man phase 1 study of the DNA-dependent protein kinase inhibitor peposertib (formerly M3814) in patients with advanced solid tumours. Brit J Cancer 124:728–735
93. Mau-Sorensen M et al (2018) 1845P Safety, clinical activity and pharmacological biomarker evaluation of the DNA-dependent protein kinase (DNA-PK) inhibitor M3814: results from two phase I trials. Ann Oncol 29, viii654
94. Yap TA et al (2020) Abstract CT248: AZD7648: a phase I/IIa first-in-human trial of a novel, potent and selective DNA-PK inhibitor in patients with advanced malignancies. Cancer Res 80:CT248–CT248
95. Patel AG, Sarkaria JN, Kaufmann SH (2011) Nonhomologous end joining drives poly(ADP-ribose) polymerase (PARP) inhibitor lethality in homologous recombination-deficient cells. Proc National Acad Sci 108:3406–3411
96. Hafsi H et al (2018) Combined ATR and DNA-PK inhibition radiosensitizes tumor cells independently of their p53 status. Front Oncol 8:245

WRN Is a Promising Synthetic Lethal Target for Cancers with Microsatellite Instability (MSI)

Edmond M. Chan, Kyla J. Foster, and Adam J. Bass

17.1   Introduction

Synthetic lethality is a phenomenon in which two or more genetic or epigenetic alterations, which are each tolerable in isolation, are lethal if they exist in combination. Discovering and exploiting synthetic lethal interactions has been a major aim in developing novel oncologic therapies. Indeed, the success of PARP inhibitors in cancers with DNA homologous recombination (HR) deficiency highlights the potential of this therapeutic approach and implies such opportunities can arise in malignancies with other DNA repair deficiencies [1–4].

The promise of finding synthetic lethal targets that could guide drug development spurred several herculean efforts to systematically map genetic cancer vulnerabilities using functional genomic tools. These efforts (the Broad Institute's Dependency Map project, the Wellcome Sanger Institute's Dependency

E. M. Chan (✉)
Department of Medicine, Division of Hematology and Oncology, Columbia University, New York, USA
e-mail: emc2291@cumc.columbia.edu

Herbert Irving Comprehensive Cancer Center, Columbia University, New York, USA

Broad Institute of MIT and Harvard, Cambridge, USA

New York Genome Center, New York, USA

K. J. Foster
University of California, San Francisco, USA
e-mail: kyla.foster@ucsf.edu

A. J. Bass
Novartis Institutes for BioMedical Research, Cambridge, USA
e-mail: ab5147@cumc.columbia.edu

© The Author(s), under exclusive license to Springer Nature Switzerland AG 2023
T. A. Yap and G. I. Shapiro (eds.), *Targeting the DNA Damage Response for Cancer Therapy*, Cancer Treatment and Research 186,
https://doi.org/10.1007/978-3-031-30065-3_17

Map project, and Novartis Institutes for BioMedical Research's Project DRIVE) screened hundreds of cell lines to determine the fitness effects of single gene depletion at genome scale [5–7]. With extensive characterization of over a thousand cell lines by the Cancer Cell Line Encyclopedia (CCLE), genetic vulnerabilities were correlated with specific cancer cell line characteristics, such as deficiency in a DNA repair pathway [8]. By separating MSI from MSS cell lines, several groups of researchers independently identified *Werner syndrome RecQ helicase (WRN)* as selectively critical for the survival of MSI and MMR deficient cancer cell line models [6, 9–11]. In this chapter, we explore and discuss the preclinical work nominating WRN as a promising synthetic lethal target for cancers with MSI.

17.2 Microsatellite Instability and DNA Mismatch Repair

MSI is a state of genetic hypermutability that arises from DNA mismatch repair (MMR) deficiency. MMR is a highly conserved pathway that recognizes base pair mismatches and insertion/deletion (indel) mutations following errors in DNA replication and recombination [12]. When MMR is defective, mutations fail to be corrected, allowing mutations to accumulate with successive cell doublings [13]. This type of hypermutability is especially pronounced at microsatellites, repetitive DNA sequences of 1–6 nucleotide subunits subject to a higher rate of replication errors due to slippage of the DNA replication machinery [14].

The MMR machinery is composed of at least seven proteins, which associate to form heterodimers that recognize and initiate repair of mismatches and insertion/deletion events. MMR initiates with assembling of a hMutS heterodimer onto DNA. There are two hMutS heterodimers, hMutSα and hMutSβ, that recognize mispairing. hMutSα is formed by the hMSH2/hMSH6 heterodimer and preferentially recognizes smaller mismatches such as base–base and mispairing of 1 or 2 nucleotides. hMutSβ, the hMSH2/hMSH3 heterodimer, recognizes insertion/deletion loops following larger mismatch events [15]. Upon recognition of mispairing by the MutS complex, the hMLH1/hPMS2 heterodimer known as hMutLα is recruited to DNA. hMutLα is an endonuclease, generating a single strand break for entry of exonuclease EXO1 and initiating subsequent repair steps [16]. The roles of the other two hMutL complexes, hMutLβ (hMLH1/hPMS1) and hMutLγ (h-MLH1/h-MLH3), are less well understood and play a less significant, role in cancer [17].

In human cancers, MSI arises from two broad mechanisms. Lynch syndrome, formerly known as Hereditary Non-Polyposis Colorectal Cancer (HNPCC), is an autosomal dominant condition arising from germline mutations in an MMR gene. There are at least four definitive Lynch Syndrome genes: *MSH2, MLH1, MSH6,* and *PMS2* [18], with reports of two additional Lynch Syndrome genes (*MLH3* [19] and *EXO1* [20]). Lynch Syndrome is characterized by the development of tumors earlier in life, often in a patient's third decade of life. Multiple tumors may be present and often include colorectal, endometrial, gastric, ovarian, urinary tract, small intestinal cancers, amongst others [21].

More commonly, MSI arises in sporadic tumors rather than from patients with Lynch Syndrome. In most sporadic MSI colorectal cancers, hMLH1 and hPMS2 proteins are lost due to epigenetic silencing of *MLH1*, typically due to hypermethylation, as part of the hypermethylator phenotype known as CpG island methylator phenotype (CIMP) [22]. It has been observed that methylation increases in age, possibly in a response to chronic inflammation and injury [23, 24]. Hence, it is unsurprising that patients with sporadic MSI colorectal cancers tend to be older than those with Lynch Syndrome. Unlike Lynch Syndrome tumors, MSI colon cancers tend to arise from the right side of the colon and frequently harbor *BRAF* V600E mutations. This is an important distinction since it is rare for a Lynch Syndrome colon cancer to possess a *BRAF* V600E mutation [25].

At present, several methods to detect MSI and/or MMR deficiency are employed in the clinic. The prior gold standard was established by the 1997 National Cancer Institute-sponsored MSI workshop. Known as the Bethesda panel, this assay is performed by fluorescence multiplex polymerase chain reaction (PCR) and capillary electrophoresis of five microsatellite loci [three dinucleotide (NR27, NR21, NR24) and two mononucleotide repeats (BAT25, BAT26)] from tumor tissue compared to normal tissue. If tumors demonstrate two or more of the five markers with instability, tumors are identified as MSI-high. If only one of the five markers demonstrates instability, the tumors are considered MSI-low. MSS tumors are distinguished from MSI-H and MSI-L tumors by the absence of instability at the defined markers [26]. Currently, clinical research tends to classify MSS and MSI-L as the same. It is worth noting that this method detects the mutational burden or 'genomic scarring' of prior MMR deficiency, regardless of the current state of MMR proficiency.

MSI can also be inferred by immunohistochemical (IHC) analyses of MMR loss. IHC detects the presence of the MMR proteins hMLH1, hPMS2, hMSH2, and hMSH6. If the result demonstrates loss of any one of these proteins, it suggests MMR deficiency. Since IHC detection of MMR protein is cheaper and more readily performed, IHC is more frequently performed and used to infer MSI status [27]. In clinical practice, MMR deficiency is treated as MSI-H [28]. However, it is worth noting that results from MMR IHC and MSI status may not be concordant. For example, an MSI-H tumor may arise in the setting of functionally deleterious mutation of a MMR gene, but the protein may still be detected with IHC. Conversely, MMR deficiency induced by *MSH6* mutations may not meet the criteria of MSI-H diagnosis.

With the increasing use of next generation sequencing (NGS) to identify cancer mutations [29–32], methods to detect MSI are evolving. The predilection of both insertion/deletion mutations as well as other characteristic features of the mutational pattern (or mutation signature) has aided the ability to infer MSI status from somatic sequencing data. Indeed, the use of NGS was shown to reliably infer MSI status and gained FDA approval for detection of MSI. MSISensor, an algorithm based on the Memorial Sloan Kettering Integrated Mutation Profiling of Actionable Cancer Targets (IMPACT), detects the percentage of unstable microsatellites in tumor and paired normal tissue [33] to determine MSI status. The FoundationOne CDx (F1CDx) assay was also FDA approved for the detection of MSI [29].

17.3   Clinical Characteristics of Microsatellite Instability

MSI-H is found in approximately 3% of all cancers [34]. By primary tumor location, 15% of colorectal [13], 20–30% of endometrial, 12–20% of ovarian, and 10–30% of gastric cancers are characterized by MSI-H. MSI also appears rarely in breast, urothelial, prostate, pancreatic, hepatobiliary, and follicular thyroid cancers [35–41].

The MSI-H phenotype is associated with distinct prognostic, predictive, and therapeutic implications. With MSI-H colorectal cancer, tumors are more likely to be poorly differentiated and associated with prominent inflammatory infiltrate [42, 43]. MSI-H colorectal cancer is more frequently seen in women and when metastatic, is more likely involves the lymph nodes and peritoneum as opposed to the liver [44]. MSI-H is also a positive prognostic sign in early-stage colorectal cancer, where outcomes, including recurrence rates, were better for patients with MMR deficient tumors as compared to MMR proficient cancers [45, 46]. Notably, even *BRAF* V600E mutations do not confer a negative prognosis in early stage MSI-H colorectal cancer as compared to *BRAF*-mutated MSS cancers [47].

The diagnosis of MSI-H also informs treatment decisions. Data from several studies have demonstrated the lack of efficacy of single agent 5-Fluorouracil (5-FU) as adjuvant therapy in stage II MSI-H colorectal cancer [45, 46, 48]. However, it is worth mentioning that patients with stage III MSI colorectal cancer benefited from adjuvant fluoropyrimidine-based therapy, especially with oxaliplatin/5-FU/leucovorin therapy [49].

More recently, seminal work has demonstrated the impressive benefit of immune checkpoint blockade (ICB) in MSI-H cancers. The PD-1 (Programmed Death-1) inhibitors pembrolizumab and nivolumab are now FDA approved for use in MSI-H/MMR deficient cancers [50, 51]. It is noteworthy that the FDA-approval for pembrolizumab in patients was the first approval to be biomarker-based, regardless of the primary tumor. More recently, the cytotoxic T-lymphocyte-associated antigen 4 (CTLA-4) inhibitor ipilimumab was approved in combination with nivolumab for the use of MSI-H/MMR deficient cancers [52]. In the first line setting, pembrolizumab demonstrated significantly improved progression-free survival with fewer adverse effects than chemotherapy for MSI-H/MMR deficient metastatic colorectal cancer [53]. While these discoveries have been paradigm changing, it is worth noting that not all patients with MSI-H cancers respond to ICB, with response rates ranging from 31–55%. Relapses are not infrequent and adverse effects may limit the use of ICB in this context [50–52]. Despite these encouraging advances, the partial response and adverse effects observed in patients warrant the development of additional combinatorial therapies that can augment ICB and be effective against ICB-resistant MSI cancers.

17.4   Synthetic Lethality of WRN Loss and Microsatellite Instability

The discovery of WRN as a synthetic lethal target was driven by large functional screening studies. These efforts sought to identify genetic vulnerabilities of cancer by determining the fitness effects of single gene depletion at genome-scale across hundreds of cell lines (Fig. 17.1a) [5–7]. Researchers then segregated cell lines on the basis of their MSI status [8, 54] and sought to identify genes that are critical for the survival of MSI but not MSS cells (Fig. 17.1a). Taking this approach, four independent groups identified the *Werner Syndrome RecQ helicase* (*WRN*) as the most significant preferential genetic dependency in MSI cancers (Fig. 17.1b) [6, 9–11]. The robustness of this discovery is reflected by its consistency across four independent research groups leveraging three distinct functional genomic screens—two using CRISPR-based perturbations and one utilizing RNAi.

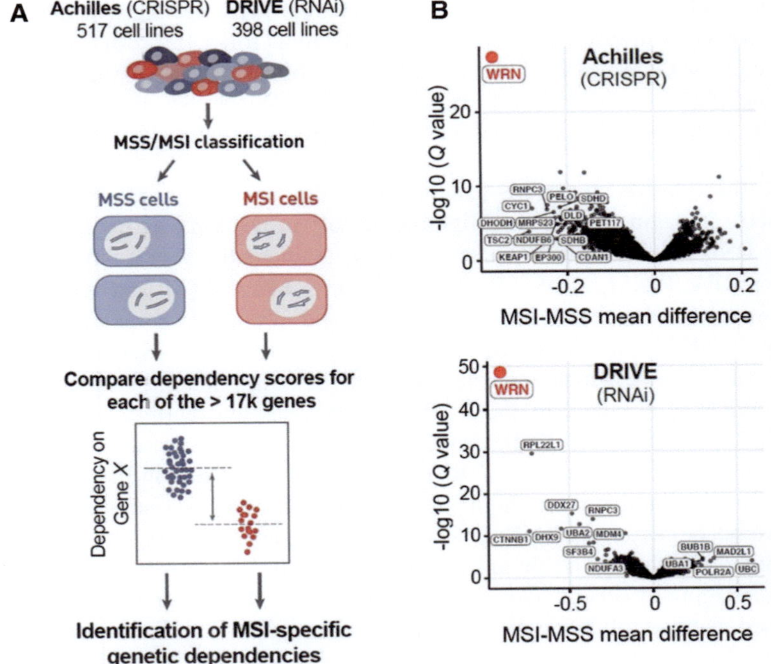

Fig. 17.1 a. Schematic of functional genomic screening analyses to identify preferential MSI genetic dependencies. b. Volcano plots identifying WRN as the top preferential dependency in MSI cells. P values plotted against the mean difference of dependency scores between MSI and MSS cells from Projects Achilles and DRIVE. Figures adapted from [9]

17.5   WRN Background

WRN is one of the five members of the RecQ family of helicases in humans [55]. WRN plays a critical role in DNA repair and maintenance. WRN's function is highlighted by the observation that WRN deficient cells demonstrate telomere shortening, chromosomal instability, and increased sensitivity to DNA-damage agents [56, 57]. Indeed, WRN Syndrome (WS), an autosomal recessive disease characterized by premature aging, increased propensity for cardiovascular disease and cancer, and a shortened life expectancy of 30–50 years old, is attributed to the defects in DNA metabolism stemming from biallelic *WRN* loss.

WRN resolves a variety of DNA structures including duplex DNA, bubble structures, G-quadruplex (especially in telomere G-rich DNA), and four-way DNA structures such as Holliday junctions (HJ), D-loops, and cruciform structures. The resolution of these structures is critical to many cellular functions, including replication fork stalling, double strand break (DSB) repair, base excision repair (BER) and telomere maintenance [58].

While WRN typically resides in the nucleoli, WRN responds to DNA replication stress by translocating to stalled replication forks [59, 60]. At collapsed replication forks, WRN stabilizes the interaction of Rad51 with replication breaks, blocking MRE11-mediated fork degradation [61]. WRN also initiates replication forks by unwinding HJ intermediates associated with regressed replication forks [62, 63].

Cell lines derived from WS patients are highly sensitive to DSBs and numerous DNA damaging agents, highlighting its role in DNA repair [64, 65]. WRN's role in DSB repair is further underscored by its interactions with the DNA repair proteins RPA, Rad51, Rad52, PARP1, p53, DNA-PKcs, ATM, and ATR [66–72]. WRN regulates the choice between classical and alternative nonhomologous end joining (c-NHEJ and alt-NHEJ, respectively). It promotes c-NHEJ via helicase and exonuclease activities and inhibits alt-NHEJ using non-enzymatic functions. When WRN is recruited to the DSBs it suppresses the recruitment of MRE11 and CtIP, protecting the DSBs from end resection [73]. Furthermore, WS cell lines demonstrate a HR defect. WRN plays an important role in the resolution of recombination intermediates. In the absence of WRN, aberrant mitotic recombination promotes genetic instability, mitotic arrest, or gene rearrangements [74, 75]. Separately, WRN plays a role in base excision repair. WS cells are sensitive to the DNA damaging effects of hydrogen peroxide and cells lacking WRN accumulate increased damage following oxidative DNA damage [76–78]. WRN has also been implicated in telomere metabolism, by processing telomeric DNA and activation of DNA damage responses [79]. WRN also is required at telomeres to dissociate D-loop end structures, promoting DNA replication progression or recombination repair [80].

WRN is composed of four main domains and is unique within the RecQ family of helicases by possessing a $3'$–$5'$ exonuclease. WRN's helicase activity is driven by its ATPase domain in tandem with its DNA binding RecQ C-terminal (RQC) domain. WRN also possesses a Helicase-and-Ribonuclease D C-terminal (HRDC) domain, which is less well understood. Studies suggest that the HRDC is critical for protein interactions and may interact with DNA [81, 82].

17.6   Validation of the MSI/WRN Synthetic Lethal Relationship

The convergence upon WRN by multiple screening efforts underscored the likelihood that WRN is synthetic lethal with MSI. Focused validation by multiple groups indeed confirmed the requirement for WRN across multiple MSI models. Genetic depletion of WRN by CRISPR-mediated knockout or RNAi-based knockdown substantially decreased cellular fitness of MSI, but not MSS, cancer cell line models (Fig. 17.2) [6, 9–11]. This viability impairment was found to be secondary to apoptosis or G2/S cell cycle arrest in WRN-depleted MSI cells [9]. Xenograft mouse models of MSI cancers confirmed that this phenotype was not an artifact of traditional 2-D cell culture conditions [9]. The essentiality of *WRN* for MSI cancer cells was further validated with organoid cancer models recently derived from patients with MSI cancers [9, 83, 84]. Organoid modeling demonstrated that *WRN* remains essential even in MSI models resistant to chemotherapeutics or ICB, asserting WRN inhibition as a tractable therapeutic strategy in chemo- or ICB-resistant MSI cancers [84]. The conclusions demonstrated in these studies were rigorously bolstered by experiments demonstrating that the viability effects of endogenous *WRN* knockout are reversed by *WRN* cDNA expression. This critical set of experiments demonstrated that loss of WRN, rather than off-target effects, was responsible for impaired MSI cell viability [9].

Notably, non-cancerous cells were largely excluded from these aforementioned studies. It is inferred that normal cells are acutely resistant to WRN depletion since normal cells are inherently MSS. While further work is required to confidently make this claim, there are multiple lines of evidence to suggest that normal cells tolerate transient loss of WRN. WS, being a condition with latent features,

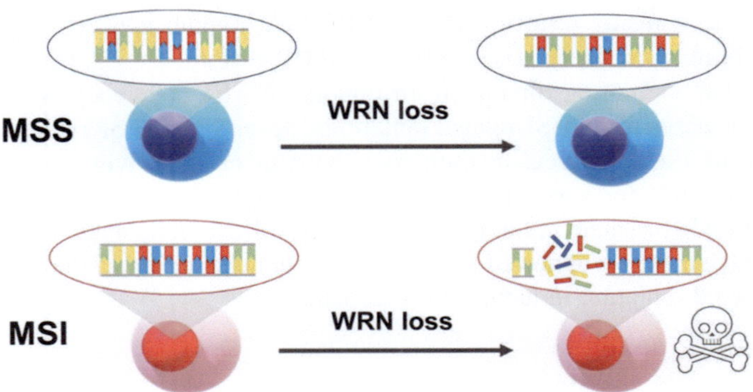

Fig. 17.2 Schematic of the effects following WRN loss in MSI and MSS cell lines

typically manifests following decades of biallelic *WRN* loss [85]. Murine models of biallelic *WRN* loss fail to recapitulate many phenotypes of human WS and demonstrate no overt signs of accelerated senescence. While this discordance may be a consequence of multiple factors, one distinct possibility is that mice with biallelic *WRN* loss do not live long enough to develop WS [86].

To focus drug discovery efforts, researchers queried which, if any, of WRN's enzymatic activities were critical for MSI. While WRN has the distinction of being the only RecQ helicase with exonuclease activity, its exonuclease activity was demonstrated to be dispensable for the acute survival of MSI cancers. In contrast, inactivation of WRN's helicase activity by point mutations of WRN's ATPase, phenocopied *WRN* knockout or knockdown [9–11, 82]. These data confirmed the importance of WRN helicase, but not exonuclease, activity for the survival of MSI cells.

While MMR deficiency and MSI are associated and clinically treated as similar entities, it is important to note their distinctness. MMR deficiency refers to impairment of this particular DNA repair mechanism. On the other hand, MSI is a result of prolonged MMR deficiency and manifests as an elevated mutational burden, especially at microsatellites. The importance of this distinction is highlighted by the mechanistic difference between the WRN/MSI and PARP1 inhibitor/BRCA1/2 relationships. On one hand, ongoing HR impairment is required for PARP1 inhibitor sensitivity with BRCA1/2 mutant cancers. This relationship is underscored by the reversion mutations observed in BRCA1/2 mutant cancers to promote resistance to PARP1 inhibition [87]. Reversion mutations are secondary mutations that convert the initial inactivating mutation of BRCA1/2 into a partially functional protein that restores HR.

In contrast, ongoing MMR deficiency does not appear to be critical for WRN dependency. Acute loss of MMR in an otherwise MSS cell line has no effect on sensitivity to WRN loss, demonstrating that MMR loss is not sufficient for this phenotype [88]. While there is some evidence to suggest that MMR restoration may rescue MSI cells from WRN depletion, these results are modest at best and do not represent true rescue [9]. Taken together, these data suggest that unlike the resistance mechanisms restoring HR in BRCA1/2 mutant cancers, resistance to WRN inhibition will likely arise outside of MMR restoration.

Rather than stemming directly from ongoing MMR deficiency, WRN dependency likely arises from MSI-related mutations. Several pieces of evidence support this statement. Firstly, increasing mutational burden correlates with stronger dependency upon WRN for survival. These data argue that the requirement for WRN stems from MSI-related mutations, rather than MMR deficiency. As discussed later, this statement is supported by mechanistic understanding of the specific type of MSI-related mutation inducing *WRN* dependency.

17.7 Mechanistic Underpinnings of WRN Dependency

The consequences of WRN loss are remarkably detrimental to the DNA integrity of MSI cells. Multiple groups have demonstrated widespread DSBs in MSI cells following *WRN* silencing [6, 9–11, 88]. Consistent with viability effects, the degree of DNA damage in MSI cells following WRN loss far exceeds that of their MSS counterparts (Fig. 17.3). Loss of WRN in dependent MSI cancer cells can be so catastrophic that DNA damage was observed on the chromosomal level, with shattering of chromosomes [9, 10, 88]. While WRN participates in DSB repair, these observations are unexpected because of the degree of DNA damage in MSI cells, far exceeding what is expected when WRN is lost in isolation.

When researchers asked where DSBs were located following WRN loss, they discovered DSBs occur at TA-dinucleotide repeats scattered across the MSI genome. Notably, only a minority (~ 8%) of all TA repeats were affected by WRN loss. For the remainder of the chapter, we will refer to these TA repeats as fragile TA repeats. However, these loci of DSBs were highly conserved across different MSI cell lines, suggesting a common process at these loci. When researchers sequenced these MSI models with long-read sequencing, they uncovered previously uncharacterized expansion mutations at fragile TA repeats, ranging from expansions of dozens to hundreds of base pairs. It is worth noting that these expanded TA repeats could not be detected by conventional 'short-read' next-generation sequencing (e.g. Illumina sequencing), thus explaining why they were previously uncharacterized in prior sequencing studies [88, 89].

Long TA repeats have the propensity to fold into non-B form cruciform-like structures, which can have deleterious consequences when unresolved [90]. When researchers interrogated for cruciform structures, they discovered that cruciform DNA formed specifically in MSI, but not MSS, at these TA repeats. Moreover, they

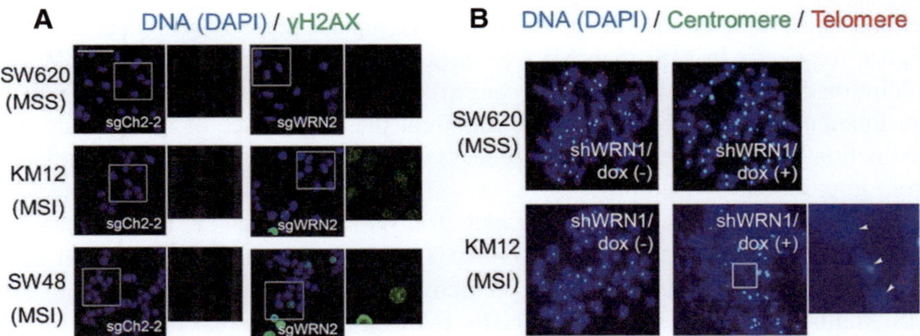

Fig. 17.3 a. Immunofluorescence for the DNA damage marker γH2AX and DAPI staining for DNA in representative MSS and MSI cell lines. sgCh2-2: negative control. sgWRN2: sgRNA to knock out WRN. b. Chromosomal analyses without and with doxycycline induction of shRNA targeting WRN (shWRN1) [dox (−) and dox (+) respectively] in representative MSS and MSI cells. Figures adapted from [9]

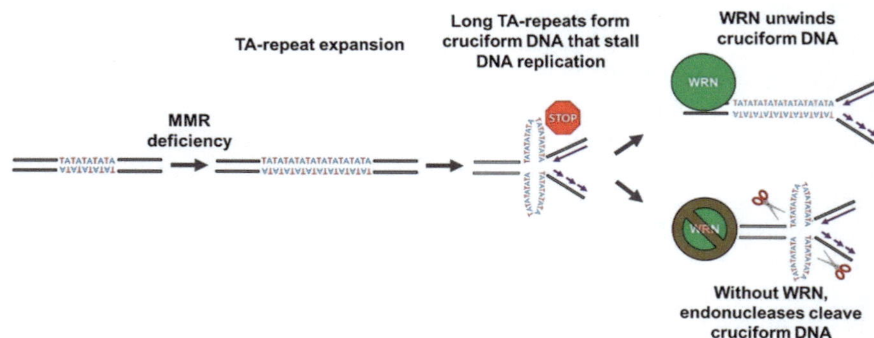

Fig. 17.4 Schematic representation of WRN dependency in MSI cells

demonstrated WRN's ability to unwind these cruciform DNA. In the absence of WRN, cruciform DNA accumulates at these loci and stalls DNA replication forks. When this replication fork remains stalled at mitosis, the replication intermediates are cleaved by endonucleases such as MUS81, thereby inducing catastrophic DSBs (Fig. 17.4). The importance of MUS81 in this process was highlighted by MUS81 depletion. The loss of MUS81 or its scaffold SLX4 substantially attenuates the DSBs at TA repeats following WRN depletion, consistent with endonuclease-mediated cleavage of cruciform structures [88]. While MUS81 or SLX4 loss attenuates DSBs upon WRN loss, it is unclear whether it is sufficient to induce resistance to WRN inhibition.

17.8 Perspectives

With mechanistic understanding of WRN dependency in MSI cancers, it is worth reiterating several points. Since expanded TA repeats were observed at a much higher frequency in MSI than MSS cells, it stands to reason that selective WRN inhibition could effectively kill MSI cancer cells while sparing normal cells, which are inherently MSS. These data also highlight the importance of recognizing the distinction between the DNA repair process and the genomic consequences arising from impairment of such processes.

While MSI is a predictive biomarker for *WRN* dependency, the mechanism underlying this phenomenon suggests that TA repeat length characterization may be more a specific and/or sensitive predictive biomarker compared to relying on MSI status alone. This may be especially relevant to tumors that inactivate MMR as a later event. In such cancers (e.g. glioblastomas rendered resistant to the alkylating agent temozolomide by MMR inactivation), it is unclear if TA repeats are sufficiently expanded to induce *WRN* dependency [91]. In these cases, TA repeat characterization of tumors could be critical to select appropriate patients for WRN-based therapies.

Taken together, these preclinical data have garnered significant interest in the development of WRN inhibitors for the treatment of patients with MSI cancers. Still, key preclinical questions remain unresolved. Is WRN required to unwind cruciform DNA in normal cells and how does inhibition of its helicase function affect healthy cells over a course of months to years?

Small molecule inhibitors may not necessarily phenocopy genetic depletion as is the case with PARP inhibitors. PARP1 inhibitors function in part by trapping PARP1 and PARP2 on DNA, which promotes DNA replication fork collapse and DSBs [92, 93]. This mechanism of action cannot be recapitulated by genetic depletion of PARP1 or 2. Would small molecule inhibitors of WRN helicase activity phenocopy WRN loss? Studies using tool compounds of WRN inhibition appear to trap WRN onto DNA, inducing toxic DNA lesions [94]. Will more specific and clinically tractable WRN helicase inhibitors similarly trap WRN onto the DNA and if so, would normal cells be able to tolerate these lesions?

Beyond TA repeat fragility, there may be additional reasons why MSI cells are sensitive to loss of WRN helicase. The inability of WRN to participate in repair following DSBs at TA repeats may exacerbate DSBs observed in WRN-depleted MSI cells. Furthermore, combined WRN and MMR deficiencies may have additional consequences for the MSI cell. Both WRN and MMR are implicated in resolving HR intermediates [74, 95]. Indeed, studies demonstrate that the yeast WRN homolog *Sgs1* is redundant with MMR for suppressing recombination between divergent DNA sequences [96]. For MSI cells able to tolerate DSBs with WRN inhibition, it is unclear how increased genomic instability stemming from MMR and WRN loss will influence MSI cancers and the development of therapeutic resistance.

No mammalian helicase inhibitor has been developed an approved for clinical use at present. While it is outside the scope of this chapter to discuss the challenges associated with developing WRN inhibitors or degraders, drug discovery efforts need to develop a new class of drug, optimizing potency, specificity, pharmacokinetics, and bioavailability of such compounds to target WRN. These and other questions will need to be addressed to fully exploit WRN's potential as a synthetic lethal target for the treatment of MSI cancers.

References

1. Moore K, Colombo N, Scambia G, Kim B-G, Oaknin A, Friedlander M et al (2018) Maintenance Olaparib in patients with newly diagnosed advanced ovarian cancer. N Engl J Med 379(26):2495–2505
2. Ray-Coquard I, Pautier P, Pignata S, Pérol D, González-Martín A, Berger R et al (2019) Olaparib plus Bevacizumab as first-line maintenance in ovarian cancer. N Engl J Med 381(25):2416–2428
3. Coleman RL, Oza AM, Lorusso D, Aghajanian C, Oaknin A, Dean A et al (2017) Rucaparib maintenance treatment for recurrent ovarian carcinoma after response to platinum therapy (ARIEL3): a randomised, double-blind, placebo-controlled, phase 3 trial. Lancet 390(10106):1949–1961

4. Topatana W, Juengpanich S, Li S, Cao J, Hu J, Lee J et al (2020) Advances in synthetic lethality for cancer therapy: cellular mechanism and clinical translation. J Hematol Oncol 13(1):1–22

5. Meyers RM, Bryan JG, McFarland JM, Weir BA, Sizemore AE, Xu H et al (2017) Computational correction of copy number effect improves specificity of CRISPR-Cas9 essentiality screens in cancer cells. Nat Genet 49(12):1779–1784

6. Behan FM, Iorio F, Picco G, Gonçalves E, Beaver CM, Migliardi G et al (2019) Prioritization of cancer therapeutic targets using CRISPR-Cas9 screens. Nature 568(7753):511–516

7. McDonald ER 3rd, de Weck A, Schlabach MR, Billy E, Mavrakis KJ, Hoffman GR et al (2017) Project DRIVE: a compendium of cancer dependencies and synthetic lethal relationships uncovered by large-scale, deep RNAi screening. Cell 170(3):577–92.e10

8. Ghandi M, Huang FW, Jané-Valbuena J, Kryukov GV, Lo CC, McDonald ER 3rd et al (2019) Next-generation characterization of the cancer cell line Encyclopedia. Nature 569(7757):503–508

9. Chan EM, Shibue T, McFarland JM, Gaeta B, Ghandi M, Dumont N et al (2019) WRN helicase is a synthetic lethal target in microsatellite unstable cancers. Nature 568(7753):551–556

10. Lieb S, Blaha-Ostermann S, Kamper E, Rippka J, Schwarz C, Ehrenhöfer-Wölfer K et al (2019) Werner syndrome helicase is a selective vulnerability of microsatellite instability-high tumor cells. Elife 25(8):e43333

11. Kategaya L, Perumal SK, Hager JH, Belmont LD (2019) Werner syndrome helicase is required for the survival of cancer cells with microsatellite instability. iScience 13:488–497

12. Li G-M (2008) Mechanisms and functions of DNA mismatch repair. Cell Res 18(1):85–98

13. Boland CR, Goel A (2010) Microsatellite instability in colorectal cancer. Gastroenterology 138(6):2073–87.e3

14. Ellegren H (2004) Microsatellites: simple sequences with complex evolution. Nat Rev Genet 5(6):435–445

15. Brown MW, Kim Y, Williams GM, Huck JD, Surtees JA, Finkelstein IJ (2016) Dynamic DNA binding licenses a repair factor to bypass roadblocks in search of DNA lesions. Nat Commun 3(7):10607

16. Kadyrov FA, Dzantiev L, Constantin N, Modrich P (2006) Endonucleolytic function of MutLα in human mismatch repair. Cell 126(2):297–308

17. Hsieh P, Yamane K (2008) DNA mismatch repair: molecular mechanism, cancer, and ageing. Mech Ageing Dev 129(7–8):391–407

18. Peltomäki P. Lynch Syndrome Genes [Internet]. Vol. 4, Familial Cancer. 2005. p. 227–32. Available from: https://doi.org/10.1007/s10689-004-7993-0

19. Lipkin SM, Wang V, Jacoby R, Banerjee-Basu S, Baxevanis AD, Lynch HT et al (2000) MLH3: a DNA mismatch repair gene associated with mammalian microsatellite instability. Nat Genet 24(1):27–35

20. Wu Y, Berends MJ, Post JG, Mensink RG, Verlind E, Van Der Sluis T et al (2001) Germline mutations of EXO1 gene in patients with hereditary nonpolyposis colorectal cancer (HNPCC) and atypical HNPCC forms. Gastroenterology 120(7):1580–1587

21. Lynch HT, Lynch PM, Lanspa SJ, Snyder CL, Lynch JF, Boland CR (2009) Review of the Lynch syndrome: history, molecular genetics, screening, differential diagnosis, and medicolegal ramifications. Clin Genet 76(1):1–18

22. van Rijnsoever M, Grieu F, Elsaleh H, Joseph D, Iacopetta B (2002) Characterisation of colorectal cancers showing hypermethylation at multiple CpG islands. Gut 51(6):797–802

23. Advani SM, Advani P, DeSantis SM, Brown D, VonVille HM, Lam M et al (2018) Clinical, pathological, and molecular characteristics of CpG Island methylator phenotype in colorectal cancer: a systematic review and meta-analysis. Transl Oncol 11(5):1188–1201

24. Issa JP, Ahuja N, Toyota M, Bronner MP, Brentnall TA (2001) Accelerated age-related CpG island methylation in ulcerative colitis. Cancer Res 61(9):3573–3577

25. Lynch HT, Lynch JF, Lynch PM (2007) Toward a consensus in molecular diagnosis of hereditary nonpolyposis colorectal cancer (Lynch syndrome). J Natl Cancer Inst 99(4):261–263

26. Umar A, Boland CR, Terdiman JP, Syngal S, de la Chapelle A, Rüschoff J et al (2004) Revised Bethesda Guidelines for hereditary nonpolyposis colorectal cancer (Lynch syndrome) and microsatellite instability. J Natl Cancer Inst 96(4):261–268

27. Chen W, Frankel WL (2019) A practical guide to biomarkers for the evaluation of colorectal cancer. Mod Pathol 32(Suppl 1):1–15

28. Pawlik TM, Raut CP, Rodriguez-Bigas MA (2004) Colorectal carcinogenesis: MSI-H versus MSI-L. Dis Markers 20(4–5):199–206

29. Colomer R, Mondejar R, Romero-Laorden N, Alfranca A, Sanchez-Madrid F, Quintela-Fandino M (2020) When should we order a next generation sequencing test in a patient with cancer? EClinicalMedicine. 25:100487

30. Nagahashi M, Shimada Y, Ichikawa H, Kameyama H, Takabe K, Okuda S et al (2019) Next generation sequencing-based gene panel tests for the management of solid tumors. Cancer Sci 110(1):6–15

31. Cheng DT, Mitchell TN, Zehir A, Shah RH, Benayed R, Syed A et al (2015) Memorial Sloan Kettering-integrated mutation profiling of actionable cancer targets (MSK-IMPACT): a hybridization capture-based next-generation sequencing clinical assay for solid tumor molecular oncology. J Mol Diagn 17(3):251–264

32. Garcia EP, Minkovsky A, Jia Y, Ducar MD, Shivdasani P, Gong X et al (2017) Validation of OncoPanel: a targeted next-generation sequencing assay for the detection of somatic variants in cancer. Arch Pathol Lab Med 141(6):751–758

33. Middha S, Zhang L, Nafa K, Jayakumaran G, Wong D, Kim HR et al (2017) Reliable pan-cancer microsatellite instability assessment by using targeted next-generation sequencing data. JCO Precis Oncol [Internet]. Available from: https://doi.org/10.1200/PO.17.00084

34. Bonneville R, Krook MA, Kautto EA, Miya J, Wing MR, Chen H-Z et al (2017) Landscape of microsatellite instability across 39 cancer types. JCO Precis Oncol [Internet]. 2017. Available from: https://doi.org/10.1200/PO.17.00073

35. Abida W, Cheng ML, Armenia J, Middha S, Autio KA, Vargas HA et al (2019) Analysis of the prevalence of microsatellite instability in prostate cancer and response to immune checkpoint blockade. JAMA Oncol 5(4):471–478

36. Ozer E, Yuksel E, Kizildag S, Sercan O, Ozen E, Canda T et al (2002) Microsatellite instability in early-onset breast cancer. Pathol Res Pract 198(8):525–530

37. Fraune C, Simon R, Hube-Magg C, Makrypidi-Fraune G, Kähler C, Kluth M et al (2020) MMR deficiency in urothelial carcinoma of the bladder presents with temporal and spatial homogeneity throughout the tumor mass. Urol Oncol 38(5):488–495

38. Kullmann F, Strissel PL, Strick R, Stoehr R, Eckstein M, Bertz S et al (2021) Frequency of microsatellite instability (MSI) in upper tract urothelial carcinoma: comparison of the Bethesda panel and the Idylla MSI assay in a consecutively collected, multi-institutional cohort. J Clin Pathol [Internet]. Available from: https://jcp.bmj.com/content/early/2021/09/27/jclinpath-2021-207855.abstract

39. Wilentz RE, Goggins M, Redston M, Marcus VA, Adsay NV, Sohn TA et al (2000) Genetic, immunohistochemical, and clinical features of medullary carcinoma of the pancreas: A newly described and characterized entity. Am J Pathol 156(5):1641–1651

40. Goeppert B, Roessler S, Renner M, Singer S, Mehrabi A, Vogel MN et al (2019) Mismatch repair deficiency is a rare but putative therapeutically relevant finding in non-liver fluke associated cholangiocarcinoma. Br J Cancer 120(1):109–114

41. Genutis LK, Tomsic J, Bundschuh RA, Brock PL, Williams MD, Roychowdhury S et al (2019) Microsatellite instability occurs in a subset of follicular thyroid cancers. Thyroid 29(4):523–529

42. Saeterdal I, Bjørheim J, Lislerud K, Gjertsen MK, Bukholm IK, Olsen OC et al (2001) Frameshift-mutation-derived peptides as tumor-specific antigens in inherited and spontaneous colorectal cancer. Proc Natl Acad Sci U S A 98(23):13255–13260

43. Xiao H, Yoon YS, Hong S-M, Roh SA, Cho D-H, Yu CS et al (2013) Poorly differentiated colorectal cancers: correlation of microsatellite instability with clinicopathologic features and survival. Am J Clin Pathol 140(3):341–347

44. Kim CG, Ahn JB, Jung M, Beom SH, Kim C, Kim JH et al (2016) Effects of microsatellite instability on recurrence patterns and outcomes in colorectal cancers. Br J Cancer 115(1):25–33

45. Hutchins G, Southward K, Handley K, Magill L, Beaumont C, Stahlschmidt J et al (2011) Value of mismatch repair, KRAS, and BRAF mutations in predicting recurrence and benefits from chemotherapy in colorectal cancer. J Clin Oncol 29(10):1261–1270

46. Sargent DJ, Shi Q, Yothers G, Tejpar S, Bertagnolli MM, Thibodeau SN et al (2014) Prognostic impact of deficient mismatch repair (dMMR) in 7,803 stage II/III colon cancer (CC) patients (pts): a pooled individual pt data analysis of 17 adjuvant trials in the ACCENT database. J Clin Orthod 32(15_suppl):3507–3507

47. Sanz-Garcia E, Argiles G, Elez E, Tabernero J (2017) BRAF mutant colorectal cancer: prognosis, treatment, and new perspectives. Ann Oncol 28(11):2648–2657

48. Sargent DJ, Marsoni S, Monges G, Thibodeau SN, Labianca R, Hamilton SR et al (2010) Defective mismatch repair as a predictive marker for lack of efficacy of fluorouracil-based adjuvant therapy in colon cancer. J Clin Oncol 28(20):3219–3226

49. André T, de Gramont A, Vernerey D, Chibaudel B, Bonnetain F, Tijeras-Raballand A et al (2015) Adjuvant fluorouracil, leucovorin, and oxaliplatin in stage II to III colon cancer: updated 10-year survival and outcomes according to BRAF mutation and mismatch repair status of the MOSAIC study. J Clin Oncol 33(35):4176–4187

50. Le DT, Uram JN, Wang H, Bartlett BR, Kemberling H, Eyring AD et al (2015) PD-1 blockade in tumors with mismatch-repair deficiency. N Engl J Med 372(26):2509–2520

51. Overman MJ, McDermott R, Leach JL, Lonardi S, Lenz H-J, Morse MA et al (2017) Nivolumab in patients with metastatic DNA mismatch repair-deficient or microsatellite instability-high colorectal cancer (CheckMate 142): an open-label, multicentre, phase 2 study. Lancet Oncol 18(9):1182–1191

52. Overman MJ, Lonardi S, Wong KYM, Lenz H-J, Gelsomino F, Aglietta M et al (2018) Durable clinical benefit with nivolumab plus ipilimumab in DNA mismatch repair-deficient/ microsatellite instability-high metastatic colorectal cancer. J Clin Oncol 36(8):773–779

53. André T, Shiu K-K, Kim TW, Jensen BV, Jensen LH, Punt C et al (2020) Pembrolizumab in microsatellite-instability-high advanced colorectal cancer. N Engl J Med 383(23):2207–2218

54. Iorio F, Knijnenburg TA, Vis DJ, Bignell GR, Menden MP, Schubert M et al (2016) A landscape of pharmacogenomic interactions in cancer. Cell 166(3):740–754

55. Luo J (2010) WRN protein and Werner syndrome. N Am J Med Sci 3(4):205–207

56. A role for WRN in telomere-based DNA damage responses [Internet]. PNAS. [cited 2022 Apr 18]. Available from: https://www.pnas.org/doi/https://doi.org/10.1073/pnas.0607332103

57. Agrelo R, Cheng W-H, Setien F, Ropero S, Espada J, Fraga MF et al (2006) Epigenetic inactivation of the premature aging Werner syndrome gene in human cancer. Proc Natl Acad Sci U S A 103(23):8822–8827

58. Kitano K (2014) Structural mechanisms of human RecQ helicases WRN and BLM. Front Genet 29(5):366

59. Marciniak RA, Lombard DB, Johnson FB, Guarente L (1998) Nucleolar localization of the Werner syndrome protein in human cells. Proc Natl Acad Sci U S A 95(12):6887–6892

60. Constantinou A, Tarsounas M, Karow JK, Brosh RM, Bohr VA, Hickson ID et al (2000) Werner's syndrome protein (WRN) migrates Holliday junctions and co-localizes with RPA upon replication arrest. EMBO Rep 1(1):80–84

61. Su F, Mukherjee S, Yang Y, Mori E, Bhattacharya S, Kobayashi J et al (2014) Nonenzymatic role for WRN in preserving nascent DNA strands after replication stress. Cell Rep 9(4):1387–1401

62. Sharma S, Otterlei M, Sommers JA, Driscoll HC, Dianov GL, Kao H-I et al (2004) WRN helicase and FEN-1 form a complex upon replication arrest and together process branchmigrating DNA structures associated with the replication fork [Internet]. Mol Biol Cell 15:734–750. Available from: https://doi.org/10.1091/mbc.e03-08-0567

63. Machwe A, Xiao L, Lloyd RG, Bolt E (2007) … regression in vitro by the Werner syndrome protein (WRN): Holliday junction formation, the effect of leading arm structure and a potential

role for WRN …. Nucleic acids [Internet]. Available from: https://academic.oup.com/nar/art icle-abstract/35/17/5729/2402088

64. Ogburn CE, Oshima J, Poot M, Chen R, Hunt KE, Gollahon KA et al (1997) An apoptosis-inducing genotoxin differentiates heterozygotic carriers for Werner helicase mutations from wild-type and homozygous mutants. Hum Genet 101(2):121–125

65. Poot M, Yom JS, Whang SH, Kato JT, Gollahon KA, Rabinovitch PS (2001) Werner syndrome cells are sensitive to DNA cross-linking drugs. FASEB J 15(7):1224–1226

66. Brosh RM Jr, Orren DK, Nehlin JO, Ravn PH, Kenny MK, Machwe A et al (1999) Functional and physical interaction between WRN helicase and human replication protein A. J Biol Chem 274(26):18341–18350

67. Sakamoto S, Nishikawa K, Heo SJ, Goto M, Furuichi Y, Shimamoto A (2001) Werner helicase relocates into nuclear foci in response to DNA damaging agents and co-localizes with RPA and Rad51. Genes Cells 6(5):421–430

68. Baynton K, Otterlei M, Bjørås M, von Kobbe C, Bohr VA, Seeberg E (2003) WRN interacts physically and functionally with the recombination mediator protein RAD52. J Biol Chem 278(38):36476–36486

69. Lebel M (2003) Genetic cooperation between poly (ADP-ribose) polymerase-1 in preventing chromosome breaks, complex chromosomal rearrangements and cancer in mice. Am J Pathol 162:1559–1569

70. Blander G, Kipnis J, Leal JF, Yu CE, Schellenberg GD, Oren M (1999) Physical and functional interaction between p53 and the Werner's syndrome protein. J Biol Chem 274(41):29463–29469

71. Li B, Comai L (2002) Displacement of DNA-PKcs from DNA ends by the Werner syndrome protein. Nucleic Acids Res 30(17):3653–3661

72. Pichierri P, Rosselli F, Franchitto A (2003) Werner's syndrome protein is phosphorylated in an ATR/ATM-dependent manner following replication arrest and DNA damage induced during the S phase of the cell cycle [Internet]. Oncogene 22:1491–1500. Available from: https://doi. org/10.1038/sj.onc.1206169

73. Shamanna RA, Lu H, de Freitas JK, Tian J, Croteau DL, Bohr VA (2016) WRN regulates pathway choice between classical and alternative non-homologous end joining. Nat Commun 6(7):13785

74. Saintigny Y, Makienko K, Swanson C, Emond MJ, Monnat RJ Jr (2002) Homologous recombination resolution defect in Werner syndrome. Mol Cell Biol 22(20):6971–6978

75. Prince PR, Emond MJ, Monnat RJ Jr (2001) Loss of Werner syndrome protein function promotes aberrant mitotic recombination. Genes Dev 15(8):933–938

76. Von Kobbe C, May A, Grandori C, Bohr VA (2004) Werner syndrome cells escape hydrogen peroxide-induced cell proliferation arrest. FASEB J 18(15):1970–1972

77. Szekely AM, Bleichert F, Nümann A, Van Komen S, Manasanch E, Ben Nasr A et al (2005) Werner protein protects nonproliferating cells from oxidative DNA damage [Internet]. Mol Cell Biol. 25:10492–10506. Available from: https://doi.org/10.1128/mcb.25.23.10492-10506. 2005

78. Rossi ML, Ghosh AK, Bohr VA (2010) Roles of Werner syndrome protein in protection of genome integrity. DNA Repair 9(3):331–344

79. Eller MS, Liao X, Liu S, Hanna K, Bäckvall H, Opresko PL et al (2006) A role for WRN in telomere-based DNA damage responses. Proc Natl Acad Sci U S A 103(41):15073–15078

80. Opresko PL, Otterlei M, Graakjaer J, Bruheim P, Dawut L, Kølvraa S et al (2004) The Werner syndrome helicase and exonuclease cooperate to resolve telomeric D loops in a manner regulated by TRF1 and TRF2. Mol Cell 14(6):763–774

81. Lan L, Nakajima S, Komatsu K, Nussenzweig A, Shimamoto A, Oshima J et al (2005) Accumulation of Werner protein at DNA double-strand breaks in human cells. J Cell Sci 118(Pt 18):4153–4162

82. Newman JA, Gavard AE, Lieb S, Ravichandran MC, Hauer K, Werni P et al (2021) Structure of the helicase core of Werner helicase, a key target in microsatellite instability cancers. Life Sci Alliance [Internet]. 4(1). Available from: https://doi.org/10.26508/lsa.202000795

83. Lazzari L, Corti G, Picco G, Isella C, Montone M, Arcella P et al (2019) Patient-derived xenografts and matched cell lines identify pharmacogenomic vulnerabilities in colorectal cancer. Clin Cancer Res 25(20):6243–6259

84. Picco G, Cattaneo CM, van Vliet EJ, Crisafulli G, Rospo G, Consonni S et al (2021) Werner helicase is a synthetic-lethal vulnerability in mismatch repair-deficient colorectal cancer refractory to targeted therapies, chemotherapy, and immunotherapy. Cancer Discov 11(8):1923–1937

85. Muftuoglu M, Oshima J, von Kobbe C, Cheng W-H, Leistritz DF, Bohr VA (2008) The clinical characteristics of Werner syndrome: molecular and biochemical diagnosis. Hum Genet 124(4):369–377

86. Lombard DB, Beard C, Johnson B, Marciniak RA, Dausman J, Bronson R et al (2000) Mutations in the WRN gene in mice accelerate mortality in a p53-null background. Mol Cell Biol 20(9):3286–3291

87. Tobalina L, Armenia J, Irving E, O'Connor MJ, Forment JV (2021) A meta-analysis of reversion mutations in BRCA genes identifies signatures of DNA end-joining repair mechanisms driving therapy resistance. Ann Oncol 32(1):103–112

88. van Wietmarschen N, Sridharan S, Nathan WJ, Tubbs A, Chan EM, Callen E et al (2020) Repeat expansions confer WRN dependence in microsatellite-unstable cancers. Nature 586(7828):292–298

89. Kim T-M, Laird PW, Park PJ (2013) The landscape of microsatellite instability in colorectal and endometrial cancer genomes. Cell 155(4):858–868

90. Kaushal S, Wollmuth CE, Das K, Hile SE, Regan SB, Barnes RP et al (2019) Sequence and nuclease requirements for breakage and healing of a structure-forming (AT)n sequence within fragile site FRA16D. Cell Rep 27(4):1151–64.e5

91. Indraccolo S, Lombardi G, Fassan M, Pasqualini L, Giunco S, Marcato R et al (2019) Genetic, epigenetic, and immunologic PROFILING of MMR-deficient relapsed glioblastoma. Clin Cancer Res 25(6):1828–1837

92. Murai J, Huang S-YN, Das BB, Renaud A, Zhang Y, Doroshow JH et al (2012) Trapping of PARP1 and PARP2 by clinical PARP inhibitors. Cancer Res 72(21):5588–5599

93. Hopkins TA, Ainsworth WB, Ellis PA, Donawho CK, DiGiammarino EL, Panchal SC et al (2019) PARP1 trapping by PARP inhibitors drives cytotoxicity in both cancer cells and healthy bone marrow. Mol Cancer Res 17(2):409–419

94. Aggarwal M, Banerjee T, Sommers JA, Iannascoli C, Pichierri P, Shoemaker RH et al (2013) Werner syndrome helicase has a critical role in DNA damage responses in the absence of a functional fanconi anemia pathway. Cancer Res 73(17):5497–5507

95. Spies M, Fishel R (2015) Mismatch repair during homologous and homeologous recombination. Cold Spring Harb Perspect Biol 7(3):a022657

96. Myung K, Datta A, Chen C, Kolodner RD (2001) SGS1, the Saccharomyces cerevisiae homologue of BLM and WRN, suppresses genome instability and homeologous recombination. Nat Genet 27(1):113–116